The Prostaglandin System

Endoperoxides, Prostacyclin, and Thromboxanes

NATO ADVANCED STUDY INSTITUTES SERIES

A series of edited volumes comprising multifaceted studies of contemporary scientific issues by some of the best scientific minds in the world, assembled in cooperation with NATO Scientific Affairs Division.

Series A: Life Sciences

Recent Volumes in this Series

This series is published by an international board of publishers in conjunction with NATO Scientific Affairs Division

A Life Sciences	Plenum Publishing Corporation
B Physics	London and New York
C Mathematical and Physical Sciences	D. Reidel Publishing Company Dordrecht, Boston and London
D Behavioral and Social Sciences	Sijthoff & Noordhoff International Publishers
E Applied Sciences	Alphen aan den Rijn, The Netherlands, and Germantown, U.S.A.

The Prostaglandin System

Endoperoxides, Prostacyclin, and Thromboxanes

Edited by

F. Berti
University of Milan
Milan, Italy

and

G. P. Velo
University of Padua
Verona, Italy

PLENUM PRESS • NEW YORK AND LONDON
Published in cooperation with NATO Scientific Affairs Division

Library of Congress Cataloging in Publication Data

Nato Advanced Study Institute on Advances in Endoperoxide, Prostacyclin, and
    Thromboxane Research, Erice, Italy, 1979.
    The prostaglandin system.

    (Nato advanced study institutes series: Series A, Life sciences; v. 36)
    Includes index.
        1. Prostaglandins—Congresses. 2. Prostacyclin—Congresses. 3. Thromboxanes—
    Congresses. 4. Peroxides—Congresses. I. Berti, Ferruccio. II. Velo, G. P. III. Title.
    IV. Series. [DNLM: 1. Prostaglandin endoperoxides—Congresses. 2. Thromboxanes—
    Congresses. 3. Prostaglandins—Congresses. QU 90 N106p 1979]
    QP801.P68N36 1979   612'.0157   80-28197
    ISBN 0-306-40645-4

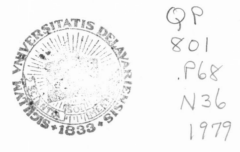
Proceedings of a NATO Advanced Study Institute on Advances in
Endoperoxide, Prostacyclin, and Thromboxane Research
held September 2–13, 1979, in Erice, Sicily

© 1981 Plenum Press, New York
A Division of Plenum Publishing Corporation
233 Spring Street, New York, N.Y. 10013

Printed in the United States of America

PREFACE

    Prostaglandin research is one of the most explosive fields in
the biological science, and there have been a number of international
symposia on this subject. In planning the second Advanced Course
in Erice (Sicily) at the "Ettore Majorana" center it was
realized that large congresses might not represent the best way to
facilitate communication within specialized areas of biologic
and medical research. In fact small meetings where in depth
discussion is confined to a limited number of scientists, are now
generally considered successful vehicles of scientific information.
With this in mind, we made an effort in collecting a number of
experts in both experimental and clinical use of these important
arachidonate metabolites. We have been very fortunate in bringing
together a faculty of international authorities who contributed to
the course with brilliant presentations and lively discussion.
Thus, this book represents an up-to-date overview of the physiology
and pharmacology of different products derived from arachidonic
acid metabolism, associated with outstanding suggestions of their
clinical potential. It is our hope that from this Advanced Course,
and its resulting publication, new ideas concerning the physiopathological role of these compounds will arise together with
new directions for future research.

    We are deeply indebted to NATO for its interest and generous
support which made this Second Course a reality.

F. Berti and G. P. Velo

CONTENTS

TRANSBILAYER LOCALIZATION AND MOVEMENT OF LYSOPHOSPHATIDYLCHOLINE

AND PHOSPHATIDYLCHOLINE IN MODEL - AND BIOMEMBRANES

H. Van den Bosch, A. M. H. P. van den Besselaar,
O. M. de Oliveira Filgueiras, J. H. E. Moonen and
B. de Kruyff

Laboratory of Biochemistry
State University of Utrecht
The Netherlands

INTRODUCTION

It has long been recognized that biological membranes
represent vectorial structures with a topological asymmetry of
their protein constituents, notably transport factors, receptors
and glycoproteins. Only more recently has an asymmetric disposition
of the phospholipids in the transverse plane of the membrane been
appreciated. Classical in this respect are studies on the
phospholipid distribution in the erythrocyte membrane. The use
of specific phospholipases has led to the conclusion that
sphingomyelin, and the majority of phosphatidylcholine are located
in the outer half of the bilayer while phosphatidylserine and
most of the phosphatidylethanolamine are situated in the inner
monolayer (1). The use of impermeable reagents to detect the
amino-phospholipids phosphatidylethanolamine and phosphatidylserine, gave results consistent with this distribution (2).
It is obvious that the asymmetric arrangement of phospholipids in
biomembranes, if a general phenomenon, can have important
implications for the availability of phospholipid classes or
-species for the functioning of membrane proteins in general and
of phospholipid metabolizing enzymes in particular. For example,
can phospholipases A located in a given monolayer only release
fatty acids from phospholipids in that monolayer or are the
phospholipids in that monolayer in dynamic equilibrium with those
in the other monolayer through a rapid transbilayer movement? Is
further metabolism of the reaction products of such a phospholipase
activity, i.e. lysophospholipids and free fatty acids, restricted
to the monolayer in which they are formed or can they move to the
other monolayer as well?

In this contribution I like to discuss some of the recent
results we have obtained on the transbilayer localization and
movement of lysophosphatidylcholine (LPC) and phosphatidylcholine
(PC) in various membranes.

LYSOPHOSPHOLIPASES AS TOOLS IN DETERMINING LYSOPHOSPHOLIPID LOCALIZATION

The use of lysophospholipases as tools to determine the
transbilayer distribution of LPC was born of the observations
that several tissues, f.e. bovine liver, contain both membrane-
bound and soluble lysophospholipases (3). This raised the
question of whether the soluble enzyme could participate in the
deacylation of membrane-bound LPC. Experiments with liver
microsomal membranes in which LPC was generated through the action
of pancreatic phospholipases A_2 demonstrated that the soluble
enzyme was able to act on membrane-embedded LPC substrate (4).
Thus, intracellularly the soluble enzyme can contribute to the
catabolism of phosphoglycerides in those subcellular membranes
that can be reached by the enzyme and thus it can aid in maintaining
the integrity of those membranes. A kinetic study of the influence
of the LPC concentration in both single bilayer vesicles (4) and
liver microsomal membranes (5) has shown that the velocity of
LPC hydrolysis by the soluble lysophospholipase increases with
increasing mol percentages of LPC in the membranes. These results
demonstrated the usefulness of single bilayer vesicles as model
systems for biomembranes in the study of the action of soluble
enzymes on membrane-bound substrates. The data also imply that
the soluble enzyme acts intracellularly, i.e. with LPC
concentrations in the subcellular membranes of about 1% of the
total phospholipids, far below its maximal activity. This
suggested, that an increased LPC concentration may lead to
enhanced activity of the lysophospholipase in an attempt to
restore low LPC concentrations.

In this respect, it was important to know whether the
enzyme can degrade LPC in both monolayers of a biomembrane or
only the LPC present in the outer monolayer of a phospholipid
bilayer. This question was first answered for model membranes.
When vesicles consisting of 5 mol % {^{14}C}-LPC and 95 mol % PC
were incubated with an excess of lysophospholipase, a rapid
degradation of about 85% of the LPC was observed (fig. 1). The
remaining LPC was not available for degradation, despite addition
of fresh enzyme and long incubation periods. This has led us to
the interpretation that about 85% of the LPC in these single
bilayer vesicles is present in the outer monolayer. In vesicles
consisting of 5 mol % LPC in an equimolar mixture of PC and
cholesterol, approximately 60% of the LPC is present in the outer
monolayer. The half-time of transbilayer movement for LPC in both
types of vesicle preparations was calculated from the slow phases

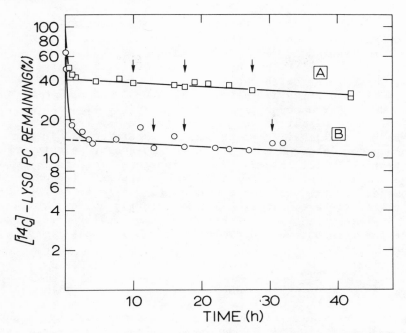

Fig. 1. Time course of vesicular LPC hydrolysis by bovine liver
         lysophospholipase I. A: Vesicles consisting of 5 mol
         % LPC, 47.5 mol % egg PC and 47.5 mol L cholesterol.
         B: Vesicles consisting of 5 mol % LPC and 95 mol % egg
         PC At the times marked by arrows, additional amounts of
         enzymes were added (for experimental details, see ref. 6).

         Membrane A   Outer/Inner 60/40   Half-time (Hr.)   93±12
                  B   85/15   100±30

of the hydrolysis to be about 100 hr.   In agreement with this
slow process of transbilayer movement of LPC, we were able to show
that LPC, introduced into the outer monolayer of PC/cholesterol
vesicles only, could be completely degraded by the lysophospholipase
(6).

    Several arguements can be provided to sustain the interpreta-
tion that the first phase of rapid hydrolysis in fig. 1 represents
only the deacylation of outer monolayer LPC. First, exactly the
same results were obtained using two different lysophospholipases
with molecular weights of 25.000 and 60.000, respectively. The
observed LPC localization is thus independent of the tool used to
determine its distribution Secondly, when multilayer liposomes
and single bilayer vesicles, both containing 10 mol % LPC, were
compared, the velocity of LPC deacylation for a given concentration
of LPC was much faster with vesicles as substrate (4). This
indicates that the enzyme does not have access to LPC in the inner

layers of liposomes. Only at high membrane concentrations, when
the enzyme became saturated with either vesicle membranes or
liposomal membranes were equal velocities measured. At this point
the rates are determined by the identical mol % LPC in the membrane.
Thirdly, experiments with vesicles containing 5 mol % {^{3}H}-LPC and
entrapped {^{14}C}-dextran demonstrated that no leakage of dextran
occurred during lysophospholipase treatment (7). If dextran, with
a mean molecular weight of 20.000 does not leak out of the
vesicles, it is unlikely that the membranes are permeable for
the lysophospholipases with still higher molecular weights. Fourthly,
the enzymatically determined LPC distributions over inner and outer
monolayers are in exact agreement with the results of NMR-
measurements on such vesicles containing {^{13}C}-enriched LPC (8).
It can therefore be concluded, that in strongly curved single
bilayer vesicles the LPC is extremely asymmetrically distributed
and that the transbilayer movement is slow, with half-times in
the order of days.

DISTRIBUTION AND RATE OF TRANSBILAYER MOVEMENT OF LYSOPHOSPHATIDYLCHOLINE IN BIOMEMBRANES

The reasons for our interest in the distribution and transbilayer movement of LPC in biomembranes is two-fold. First, there
is accumulating evidence to suggest that transbilayer movements of
diacylphospholipids in some biological membranes is much faster
than in model membranes without proteins (see refs. 9 and 10 for
reviews). In this respect no data are available for LPC transmembrane mobilities. The results with diacylphospholipids are
indicative of the fact that phospholipid vesicles, although they
can be used as an adequate model for biological membranes in
several aspects, do no represent the highly dynamic structural
organization present in biomembranes. The second reason for our
interest in the transbilayer distribution of LPC in biomembranes
is related to the stability of bilayers. It has been hypothesized
already in 1970 by Lucy (11) that fusion of biomembranes could be
facilitated by such factors as LPC which favour a micellar rather
than a bilayer configuration. It is logical to expect that fusion
is initiated at locally highly curved membrane surfaces. If our
findings about the strongly asymmetric distribution of LPC in the
outer monolayer of highly curved model membranes could be extrapolated to biomembranes, this could be of importance for the local
destabilization of the bilayer in highly curved regions of the
membrane to facilitate the fusion process. There is only one
biomembrane with a sufficiently high LPC concentration to make a
study of its distribution feasible, i.e. the chromaffin granule
membrane.

Chromaffin granule membrane. Bovine chromaffin granule
membranes contain about 17 mol % LPC and this unusual high level
has been discussed in relationship to the exocytosis process by

which catecholamines are released from these granules (12). For
such a function of the LPC one would expect this component to be
located in the outer monolayer. However, treatment of intact
granules with lysophospholipases resulted in only about 10%
hydrolysis of LPC, whereas similar treatment of broken granules
gave 65% hydrolysis (13). This indicates that little LPC is
present in the outer monolayer. The alternative explanation
that all LPC is present in the outer monolayer but cannot be
reached by the lysophospholipase, due to shielding by granule
proteins, was ruled out on the basis of the following experiments.
Pretreatment of intact granules with trypsin had no influence on
LPC availability. When a trace amount of radioactive LPC (about
2% of endogenous LPC content) was incorporated into presumably the
outer monolayer of granules, subsequent isolation of the granula
and treatment with lysophospholipase resulted in almost complete
hydrolysis of the radioactive LPC (fig.2). The concomitant
decrease in the specific radioactivity of the remaining LPC
showed that hardly any endogenous LPC was hydrolyzed. Thus, the
outer monolayer LPC in intact granules is available for hydrolysis
by lysophospholipase. Furthermore, the added radioactive LPC does
not rapidly equilibrate with the endogenous pool in the inner
monolayer. It can be concluded from these experiments that the
transbilayer movement of LPC in the granule membrane is a slow

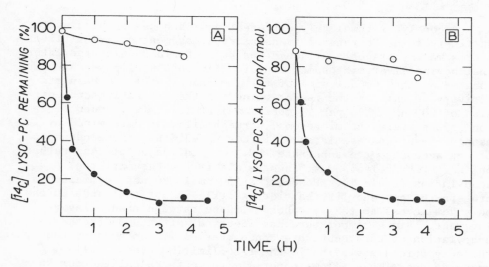

Fig. 2.   Comparison of the accessibility of added and endogenous
          lysophosphatidylcholine in chromaffin granules. Granules
          were incubated with a trace amount of {^{14}C}-LPC,
          reisolated and treated with (• - •) or without (o - o)
          lysophospholipase at 25° C. (For experimental details,
          see ref. 13).

process. The predominantly inner monolayer localization of LPC
in the granule membrane makes it unlikely that LPC plays an
important role in the initial phase of the fusion with the plasma
membrane. The possibility that initial events which trigger the
exocytosis process cause transmembrane LPC rearrangements cannot
be excluded at present.

Liver microsomal membrane. In initial experiments to
determine the transbilayer distribution and movement of LPC in
rat liver microsomal membranes, the rats were injected in the
portal vein with a synthetic radioactive LPC analog in which
the -OH at the 2-position was replaced by a H-atom to prevent
acylation by microsomal acyltransferases. Treatment of the
isolated microsomes with lysophospholipase resulted in complete
hydrolysis of the LPC analog within 30 min. Since the hydrolysis
as a function of time was not biphasic and the initial distribution
of the LPC analog was unknown it was not possible to distinguish
between the two alternatives of a complete outer monolayer
localization or a distribution over both monolayers accompanied
by a rapid transbilayer movement. Attempts to determine the
initial distribution by NMR-measurements on ${^{13}C}$-LPC enriched
microsomes in conjunction with the shift reagent Dy^{3+} (see
sarcoplasmic reticulum membranes) were unsuccessful due to
precipitation of the microsomes and complete loss of signal
intensity.

Recently, a completely different approach has enabled us to
get insight in the rate of transmembrane movement of LPC in liver
microsomal membranes. Evidence has been obtained which indicates
that bovine liver microsomes contain a lysophospholipase which is
located at the lumenal site of the membrane (14, 15). When the
activity of this enzyme is determined at the saturating concentration of 200 nmol LPC per mg microsomal protein, i.e. under
conditions where the microsomal permeability, as determined by
mannose-6-phosphatase latency, is disrupted, the enzyme has
direct access to the substrate LPC. The influence of temperature
on the LPC hydrolysis must thus be due to the enzymatic
deacylation (table 1). However, at 50 nmol LPC per mg microsomal
protein the permeability barrier is still intact (14) and LPC can
only get access to the lysophospholipase through transbilayer
movement. Since temperature has identical effects on the
deacylation at this substrate concentration it can be concluded that
the enzymatic deacylation is the rate-limiting step at all
temperatures. This allows upper limits to be calculated for the
transbilayer movement, assuming this is a first order process.
Thus, at 37º C the minimal half-time for LPC transbilayer movement
is 42 min. As pointed out, since transmembrane movement is not
the rate-limiting step in the overall deacylation process, the
half-time could in fact be much smaller. However, even the value
of 42 min. indicates that LPC transbilayer movements in liver

TABLE I

Effect of temperature on bovine liver microsomal lysophospholipase.

TEMP. ($^\circ$C.)	LYSOPHOSPHOLIPASE ACTIVITY				MAXIMAL HALF-TIME TRANSVERSE MOVEMENT (MIN.)
	50 nmol (mU)	LPC/mg (%)	200 nmol (mU)	LPC/mg (%)	
0	0.086	11	0.294	9	403
8	0.176	22	0.696	20	197
23	0.476	57	2.03	59	74
37	0.814	100	3.45	100	42

Initial velocities of {1-^{14}C} palmitoyl-LPC hydrolysis were measured at the indicated temperatures and at substrate concentrations of 50 nmol LPC/mg microsomal protein (permeability barrier intact) or 200 nmol LPC/mg microsomal protein (permeability barrier disrupted). Results are expressed as nmol LPC hydrolyzed per min. (mU) and as percentage of the rate measured at 37° C.

microsomal membranes is a 150 times faster than in single bilayer lipid vesicles.

Sarcoplasmic reticulum membrane. In contrast to the results obtained with liver microsomes it appeared to be possible to determine the equilibrium distribution of N-{Me-^{13}C} choline labelled LPC in sarcoplasmic reticulum membranes by NMR. The membranes were incubated with micellarly dispersed 1-palmitoyl lysophosphatidyl-N-{Me-^{13}C} choline for 30 min. at 20°C. and reisolated. The NMR spectrum (fig. 3A) shows only one {^{13}C} choline resonance peak, 14 ppm upfield from external 1,4-dioxane. Addition of Dy^{3+} resulted in a loss of 58% of the peak intensity (fig. 3B) and no further decrease was measured over a 7 h period at 30°C. (fig. 3C). This shows that the membrane vesicles do not become leaky for the shift reagent. The results showed that 42% of the LPC has moved to the inner monolayer and that the equilibrium distribution is attained already after the initial incubation for 30 min. at 20°C. In an attempt to slow down the transverse mobility of LPC spectra were recorded after different incubation times at 0° C. (16). The amount of LPC in the inner monolayer increases with time to reach a plateau after 5 h. At this point

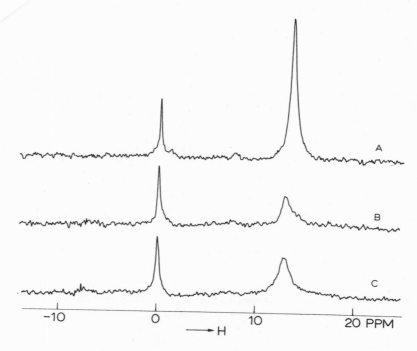

Fig. 3.   90.5 MH$_z$ ^{13}C NMR spectra of rat sarcoplasmic reticulum
membranes to which 1-palmitoyl lysophosphatidyl-N-(ME-^{13}C)
choline has been added. A: Spectrum of reisolated
membranes in the absence of D$_y$$^{3+}$. B: Spectrum in the
presence of 3mM D$_y$$^{3+}$ recorded 2.5 h after addition of LPC
to the membranes. C: As B, but after further incubation
for 7 h at 25° C. in the presence of 3mM D$_y$$^{3+}$ (for
experimental details, see ref. 16).

the same equilibrium distribution as seen in fig. 3 was reached.
Fresh membranes were then preincubated with {^{14}C}-LPC to obtain
this equilibrium distribution of 42% LPC inside and 58% LPC
outside and treated with lysophospholipase. This resulted in
complete hydrolysis of LPC (fig. 4). Thus, from the NMR experiments
it can be concluded that LPC initially added to the outer monolayer
of sarcoplasmic reticulum membranes moves for 42% to the inner
monolayer. From the lysophospholipase treatment it follows that
the LPC can move back to the outer monolayer once the LPC in this
monolayer is depleted by lysophospholipase action. Both trans
bilayer movements have half-times at 25° C. which are 30 min. or
less, in good agreement with the results for liver microsomal
membranes. Transbilayer movements of LPC in some intracellular
biomembranes is thus at least two orders of magnitude faster than
in model membranes. In this respect it is interesting to note that
the half-time of LPC transmembrane movement in phospholipid vesicles

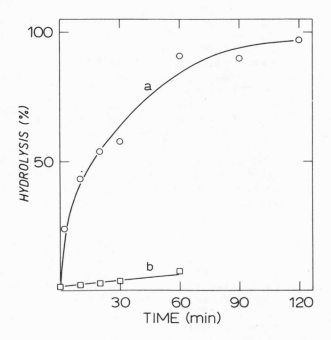

Fig. 4.   Complete hydrolysis of lysophosphatidylcholine incorporated
          in sarcoplasmic reticulum membranes. a: with enzyme,
          b: without enzyme. (For experimental details, see ref.
          16).

containing the membrane-spanning protein glycophorin has been
estimated to be about 1 h at 37° C.   (17).

DISTRIBUTION AND RATE OF TRANSBILAYER MOVEMENT OF PHOSPHATIDYL-CHOLINE IN BIOMEMBRANES

Transbilayer movement for phosphatidylcholine (PC) in
phospholipid vesicles is extremely slow and lower limits for the
half-time of this process were estimated to be in the order of
4 - 10 days (9, 10). Similar data were obtained for influenza
virus membranes. In phospholipid vesicles the rates can be
enhanced tremendously (t 1/2 in the order of 1 - 10 h) by a
variety of manipulations, such as induction of compositional
asymmetry, order-disorder transition or incorporation of
glycophorin (18). Such values are comparable to the half-times
of 2 - 5 h observed for PC transpositioning in erythrocyte membranes
(19, 20). On the other hand, an even shorter half-time in the
order of minutes, has been measured for the transmembrane movement
of phosphatidylethanolamine in growing B. megaterium (21). In
view of these results we have measured PC mobilities in microsomal
membranes using phosphatidylcholine-exchange protein (22).

plasmic reticulum membrane. In order to be able to study
transmembrane mobility of PC with PC-exchange protein as a tool,
the initial distribution of PC in the membrane has to be known.
This distribution was determined by ^{13}C-NMR of sarcoplasmic
reticulum membranes isolated from rats fed a choline-deficient
diet supplemented with N-{Me$_3$-^{13}C} choline. The choline methyl
signal in those membranes was found to be due for over 95% to
PC and under conditions of membrane vesicle intactness could be
shifted for 40% by Dy^{3+} ions (23). Knowing the equilibrium
distribution of PC in the membrane (40% in the outer - and 60% in
the inner monolayer) we asked ourselves the question how much PC
could be exchanged from ^{32}P-labelled membranes to rat liver
mitochondria by an exchange protein which is specific for PC and
only exchanges PC-molecules from the outer monolayer (22).
The results indicated a biphasic exchange process (fig. 5).
Extrapolation of the slow phase to zero time shows that over 80%
of the total PC was exchanged in the first rapid phase. With only
40% of the total PC in the outer monolayer this means that at least
70% of the PC pool in the inner monolayer must become available for
exchange through a rapid transbilayer movement. The half-time of
this process is estimated to be less than 10 min.

Liver microsomal membranes. Unfortunately, as mentioned before
the NMR-technique with Dy^{3+} as shift reagent could not be used to
determine the distribution of PC in liver microsomal membranes.
Other methods to localize phospholipids in the transverse plane
of these membranes from rat liver have yielded conflicting results.
Based on phospholipase A$_2$ degradations Nilsson and Dallner (24)
claimed that phosphatidylethanolamine was present for 92% in
the outer monolayer. In contrast, Higgins and Dawson (25) using
phospholipase C arrived at the conclusion that this phospholipid
was located for 81% in the inner monolayer. With such data it is
clear that the problem of phospholipid asymmetry in rat liver
microsomes still has to be considered unresolved. In fact, Sundler
et al (26) provided evidence which seemed to argue against the
existence of phospholipid asymmetry in those subcellular membranes.
Agreement between these three research groups exists in the fact
that not all PC is in the outer monolayer. At least 25% (25)
and probably as much as 50% (26) or 60% (24) of the PC is in the
inner monolayer. With this knowledge we asked ourselves the
question how much of the total microsomal PC could be exchanged?
As can be seen in fig. 6 at least 90% of PC can be exchanged in 20
min., strongly suggesting that part of the total microsomal PC
pool must be involved in a rapid transbilayer movement with a
half-time of at the most 10 min. (27).

At present it is not known how these rapid transbilayer
movements have to be envisaged. It has been suggested that membrane
proteins could be involved in catalyzing or facilitating this
process (9, 21). If so, the actions of such proteins is not

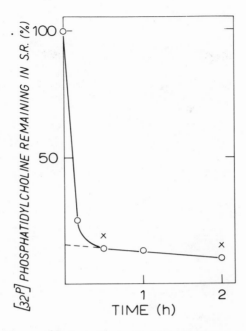

Fig. 5.   Transfer of {^{32}p} phosphatidylcholine from rat sarcoplasmic
           reticulum membranes to rat liver mitochondria. The
           experiment was carried out with 439 nmol sarcoplasmic
           reticulum (S.R.) membrane phospholipid and either 3000
           (x) or 7600 (o) nmol mitochondrial phospholipid (for
           experimental details, see ref. 23).

impaired by glutaraldehyde cross-linking (fig. 6). It is clear,
however, that the rapid transbilayer movement of PC is related to
the structure of the microsomal membrane. In vesicles prepaired
from microsomal lipids, 60% of PC is exchangeable and no rapid
transpositioning is seen (27).

     It is tempting to speculate that the rapid PC transpositioning
rates in microsomal membranes is somehow related to the occurrence
of phospholipids experiencing isotropic motion on the NMR
timescale (28, 29). In this respect it should be mentioned that
complete exchange of microsomal PC was observed at temperatures
at which isotropic motion was seen. However, below 8° C.,
where phospholipids in microsomal membranes occur in a bilayer
structure (29), exchange of PC levelled off long before
complete exchange was obtained. The exchangeable pool under these
conditions may represent the outer monolayer pool and complete
exchangeability at 25° C. may be possible because the inner monolayer pool is in rapid equilibrium with the outer monolayer pool
through the intermediary phase of phospholipid molecules
experiencing nearly isotropic motion.

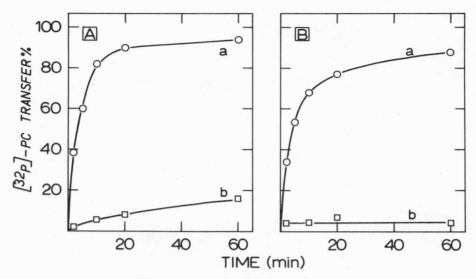

Fig. 6.   Exchange of rat liver microsomal {^{32}P} phosphatidyl-
          choline for egg phosphatidylcholine. A: Microsomes.
          B: Glutaraldehyde treated microsomes. a: plus PC-
          exchange protein, b: minus PC-exchange (for experimental
          details, see ref. 27).

     It will take some time before these hypotheses can be (in)
validated. Whatever the exact mechanisms underlying transmembrane movements, it is clear that such phospholipid mobilities
in some metabolically active intracellular membranes are much
more rapid than in previously investigated erythrocyte and virus
membranes.

REFERENCES

1. R. F. A. Zwaal, B. Roelofsen and C. M. Colley, Localization of
    red cell membrane constituents, Biochem. Biophys. Acta 300:
    159 (1973).
2. M. S. Bretscher, Phosphatidylethanolamine: Differential
    labelling in intact cells and cell ghosts of human erythrocytes
    by a membrane-impermeable reagent, J. Mol. Biol., 71:523 (1972).
3. H. van den Bosch and J. G. N. de Jong, The subcellular
    distribution of two lysolecithin-hydrolyzing enzymes in beef
    liver, Biochim. Biophys. Acta, 398:244 (1975).
4. A. M. H. P. van den Besselaar, J. H. Verheijen and H. van den
    Bosch, The action of two purified lysophospholipases from
    beef liver on membrane-bound lysophosphatidylcholine,
    Biochim. Biophys. Acta, 431:75 (1976).

5. H. Moonen, P. Trienekens and H. van den Bosch, The action of purified lysophospholipases on microsomal membrane-bound lysophosphatidylcholine, Biochim. Biophys. Acta., 489:423 (1977).

6. A. M. H. P. van den Besselaar, H. van den Bosch and L. L. M. van Deenen, Transbilayer distribution and movement of lysophosphatidylcholine in liposomal membranes, Biochim. Biophys. Acta., 465:454 (1977).

7. O. M. de Oliveira Filgueiras, A. M. H. P. van den Besselaar and H. van den Bosch, Availability of lysophosphatidylcholine in single bilayer vesicles for hydrolysis by lysophospholipase, Lipids, 13:898 (1978).

8. B. de Kruyff, A. M. H. P. van den Besselaar and L. L. M. van Deenen, Outside-inside distribution and translocation of lysophosphatidylcholine in phosphatidylcholine vesicles as determined by ^{13}C-NMR using (n-^{13}CH$_3$)-enriched lipids, Biochim. Biophys. Acta., 465:443 (1977).

9. J. E. Rothman and J. Lenard, Membrane asymmetry, Science, 195:743 (1977).

10. J. A. F. op den Kamp, Lipids asymmetry in membranes, Annu. Rev. Biochem., 48:47 (1979).

11. J. A. Lucy, The fusion of biological membranes, Nature 227:815 (1970).

12. H. Blaschko, H. Firemark, A. D. Smith and H. Winkler, Lipids of the adrenal medulla: lysolecithin, a characteristic constituent of chromaffin granules, Biochem. J., 104:545 (1967).

13. O. M. de Oliveira Filgueiras, A. M. P. H. van den Besselaar and H. van den Bosch, Localization of lysophosphatidylcholine in bovine chromaffin granules, Biochim. Biophys. Acta., (1979) in press.

14. J. H. E. Moonen and H. van den Bosch, Studies on the transverse localization of lysophospholipase in bovine liver microsomes using proteolytic enzymes, Biochim. Biophys. Acta, 573:114 (1979).

15. H. Moonen and H. van den Bosch, Studies on the transverse localization of lysophospholipase II in bovine liver microsomes by immunological techniques, Biochim. Biophys. Acta., (1979) in press.

16. A. M. H. P. van den Besselaar, B. de Kruyff, H. van den Bosch and L. L. M. van Deenen, Transverse distribution and movement of lysophosphatidylcholine in sarcoplasmic reticulum membranes as determined by ^{13}C NMR and lysophospholipase, Biochim. Biophys. Acta, 555:193 (1979).

17. E. J. J. van Zoelen, B. de Kruyff and L. L. M. van Deenen, Protein mediated transbilayer movement of lysophosphatidylcholine in glycophorin-containing vesicles, Biochim. Biophys. Acta, 508:97 (1978).

18. B. de Kruyff, E. J. J. van Zoelen and L. L. M. van Deenen, Glycophorin facilitates the transbilayer movement of phosphatidylcholine in vesicles, Biochim. Biophys. Acta, 509:537 (1978).

19. W. Renooy, L. M. G. van Golde, R. F. A. Zwaal and L. L. M. van
     Deenen, Topological asymmetry of phospholipid metabolism in
     rat erythrocyte membranes, Eur. J. Biochem., 61:53 (1976).
20. B. Bloj and D. B. Zilversmit, Asymmetry and transposition
     rates of phosphatidylcholine in rat erythrocyte ghosts,
     Biochemistry, 15:1277 (1976).
21. J. E. Rothman and E. P. Kennedy, Rapid transmembrane movement
     of newly synthesized phospholipids during membrane assembly,
     Proc. Nat. Acad. Sci. (U.S.A.), 74:1821 (1977).
22. K. W. A. Wirtz, Transfer of phospholipids between membranes,
     Biochim. Biophys. Acta., 344:95 (1974).
23. B. de Kruyff, A. M. H. P. van den Besselaar, H. van den Bosch
     and L. L. M. van Deenen, Inside- outside distribution and
     diffusion of phosphatidylcholine in rat sarcoplasmic reticulum
     as determined by ^{13}C NMR and phosphatidylcholine exchange
     protein, Biochim. Biophys. Acta., 555:181 (1979).
24. O. S. Nilsson and G. Dallner, Enzymic and phospholipid
     asymmetry in liver microsomal membranes, J. Cell Biol., 72:
     568 (1977).
25. J. A. Higgins and R. M. C. Dawson, Asymmetry of the phospho-
     lipid bilayer of rat liver endoplasmic reticulum, Biochim.
     Biophys. Acta., 470:342 (1977).
26. R. Sundler, S. L. Sarcione, A. W. Alberts and P. Roy Vagelos,
     Evidence against phospholipid asymmetry in intracellular
     membranes from liver, Proc. Nat. Acad. Sci. (U.S.A.), 74:3350
     (1977).
27. A. M. H. P. van den Besselaar, B. de Kruyff, H. van den
     Bosch and L. L. M. van Deenen, Phosphatidylcholine mobility
     in liver microsomal membranes, Biochim. Biophys. Acta.,
     510:242 (1978).
28. B. de Kruyff, A. M. H. P. van den Besselaar, P. R. Cullis,
     H. van den Bosch and L. L. M. van Deenen, Evidence for
     isotropic motion of phospholipids in liver microsomal
     membranes; A ^{31}P NMR study, Biochim. Biophys. Acta., 514:1
     (1978).
29. A. Stier, S. A. E. Finch and B. Bösterling, Non-Lamellar
     structure in rabbit liver microsomal membranes, A ^{31}P
     NMR study, FEBS Letters, 91:109 (1978).

BIOSYNTHESIS OF PROSTAGLANDINS AND THROMBOXANES

Elisabeth Granström

Department of Chemistry, Karolinska Institutet
S-104 01 Stockholm 60
Sweden

The biosynthesis of the prostaglandins, and later also the thromboxanes, from polyunsaturated fatty acids has been the subject of a vast number of studies since the mid -60's (see 1, 2 and references therein). When the identification of the precursor fatty acids was made (3,4), it became obvious that the "prostaglandin synthetase" must be a multienzyme complex. How complicated this area actually is has become increasingly evident during the last decade with the discoveries of several new compounds and pathways (2).

The following discussion will be limited mainly to the arachidonic acid family of compounds, i.e. the prostaglandins and thromboxanes of the 2 series.

The first compounds formed from arachidonic acid that are possible to isolate are the prostaglandin endoperoxides, PGG_2 and PGH_2 (5-7). They are formed by the action of an enzyme named prostaglandin endoperoxide synthase. The biosynthesis of PGH_2 consists of two steps: first, oxygenation of arachidonic acid, leading to PGG_2 and catalyzed by the enzyme fatty acid cyclooxygenase, and second, cleavage of the hydroperoxy group of PGG_2 to form PGH_2, catalyzed by a peroxidase.

Prostaglandin endoperoxide synthase has been purified to homogeneity from bovine and sheep vesicular glands (8-11). The details of the purification procedures vary, but they all involve an initial solubilization by a detergent, as the enzyme is microsomal. The enzyme was subsequently purified by ion exchange chromatography, isoelectrofocussing, molecular sieving, precipitation steps, gel electrophoresis, etc., to homogeneity. A special

15

technique was introduced by Roth and Mejerus (12), who successfully
radiolabeled the enzyme by taking advantage of the reaction of
^{3}H-aspirin with the cyclo-oxygenase.

The properties of the purified prostaglandin endoperoxide
synthase have been extensively studied. It has characteristics
of a hemoprotein (10,13) and is a membrane bound glycoprotein,
isolated as a dimer with a molecular weight of approximately
129 000 (13).

Attempts to separate the cyclo-oxygenase from the peroxidase
have not been successful, and it thus seems that both the reactions,
arachidonic acid → PGG$_2$ and PGG$_2$ → PGH$_2$, are catalyzed by the same
enzyme (8,10,14). Nevertheless it is possible to some extent to
study these two functions separately. Both reactions require heme,
either as hematin or in a protein bound form such as hemoglobin
or myoglobin (8,14). In a study on other possible metalloprotopor-
phyrins it was discovered that manganese protoporphyrin could
replace hematin. However, the endoperoxide biosynthesis then
stopped at the PGG$_2$ stage, and thus the two enzyme activities could
be discriminated (15). Furthermore, aspirin inhibits the cyclo-
oxygenase but leaves the peroxidase function intact. The latter
enzyme can also be studied separately by using PGG as substrate.
It may also be possible to use a wide variety of other hydroperoxides (14,16). The peroxidase step is stimulated by several
compounds (14), such as tryptophan (8), epinephrine (17) and
uric acid (18).

A prostaglandin endoperoxide E-isomerase has been purified
from bovine vesicular gland microsomes (19). The purification
procedure included Tween 20 solubilization, DEAE cellulose
chromatography and hydrophobic chromatography on ω-aminobutyl
Sepharose 4B. The purification was 26-fold from microsomes, and
the enzyme was very labile but could be protected from inactivation
by thiol compounds, such as reduced glutathione. This compound
also served as a cofactor for the isomerization of PGH to PGE.
Glutathione is a common oxidoreduction coenzyme, but its role in
this reaction is not clear: it was not oxidized stoichiometrically
during the reaction (19).

Both PGG and PGH were substrates for this enzyme, but PGH
was the preferred one. PGG yielded 15-hydroperoxy-PGE as product;
thus, the isomerase did not possess peroxidase activity (19).
The preferred pathway for PGE synthesis seems to be PGG → PGH →
PGE. An alternative pathway with 15-hydroperoxy-PGE as an intermediate has also been suggested (20).

The prostaglandin endoperoxide E-isomerase has recently been
purified also from sheep vesicular gland microsomes (21). This
enzyme was more difficult to solubilize than the endoperoxide

synthetase, but solubilization could be achieved with Triton X-100 or deoxycholate. The solubilized enzyme was labile, did not need phospholipids for its activity, and was possibly an SH-enzyme (21).

A group of compounds that has recently attracted some attention is the D type of prostaglandins. PGD was formerly regarded as an inactive byproduct of prostaglandin biosynthesis. This view has however changed after the identification of several important biological effects of these compounds (e.g. 22-25) and the discovery that PGD_2 is the major prostaglandin in many biological systems (26-29).

The study of PGD biosynthesis has been rather complicated, since PGD_2 is easily formed non-enzymatically together with PGE_2 from its immediate precursor, PGH_2 (5,6). Several factors can increase the PGD_2/PGE_2 ratio, such as silica gel (7) and serum albumin from several species (30,31).

Several enzymes capable of stimulating PGD_2 biosynthesis have been purified. Two glutathione requiring enzymes isolated from sheep lung were found to stimulate both PGD_2 and $PGF_{2\alpha}$ synthesis from PGH_2 (32). They were however tentatively identified as glutathione S-transferases, which evidently also have the capacity of catalyzing the conversion of PGH_2 (32).

Recently, however, two real prostaglandin endoperoxide D-isomerases have been purified, devoid of glutathione S-transferase activity. One was purified from rat spleen (33) and the other from rat brain (34). The rat spleen enzyme was cytoplasmic in contrast to all other endoperoxide isomerases. It had a molecular weight of only 30 000, was rather labile and required glutathione specifically for its action. Its cytoplasmic localization was suggested to imply a protective function: prostaglandin endoperoxide that escaped from other conversions might then be converted into the less harmful PGD_2 in the cytoplasm (33).

Also the rat brain enzyme was predominantly found in the cytosol fraction (34). However, a significant part of the enzymatic activity was also associated with small membrane fragments. The authors concluded that the enzyme might actually be membrane associated but easily dissociable during the tissue homogenization (34). This enzyme differed from the rat spleen enzyme in that it did not require glutathione. It was however stabilized by glutathione and other thiol compounds.

Of all enzymes that convert PGH_2 into end products, only one is not an isomerase: prostaglanding endoperoxide F-reductase. Very little is known about the occurrence and properties of this enzyme. In vitro studies on $PGF_{2\alpha}$ forming systems in tissues are

difficult, because PGH_2 is easily reduced non-enzymatically by
for example thiol groups and hemoproteins (21). Such compounds
are always found in crude homogenates and supernatants, and it has
even been reported that the $PGF_{2\alpha}$ forming capacity of homogenates
may increase after boiling (21). Certain metal ions exert the
same effect, and even the small amounts that may be present in
distilled water may suffice for this reduction (21).

It has sometimes been suggested that $PGF_{2\alpha}$ biosynthesis
might in fact be entirely non-enzymatic. This can however hardly
be the case: the $PGF_{2\alpha}$ production for example during luteolysis
(35-37) is evidently very rigorously controlled, which is hardly
compatible with a non-enzymatic formation.

Some proteins have been found with prostaglandin endoperoxide F-reductase activity. The microsomal fraction of guinea
pig uterus contains a reducing factor, which has several
characteristics of an enzyme: saturability at high substrate
concentration, inhibition by p-hydroxymercuribenzoate, ability to
be solubilized by Cutscum and subsequent elution with the void
volume of a Sephadex G-75 column (38). However, this factor was
very heat resistant and even survived boiling, and is thus not
likely to be an enzyme.

Two enzymes possessing endoperoxide F-reductase activity were
recently purified from sheep lung (31); however, both of them also
had D-isomerase activity. It was established, as mentioned above,
that they were actually glutathione S-transferases (31).

The thromboxane pathway was first discovered in platelets (39)
and lung tissue (40), where it represents the major pathway in
endoperoxide metabolism. Thromboxane synthesis has later been
demonstrated in a vast number of cell types and tissues (see 2 and
references therein).

Thromboxane synthase has been purified from platelets (41,42)
and lung (43). The platelet enzyme was microsomal, localized
mainly to the dense tubular system, whereas plasma membranes,
dense bodies, α-granules and the cytosol were devoid of enzymatic
activity. The enzyme catalyzing the conversion of arachidonic
acid into thromboxane was solubilized from the microsomes by
treatment with a detergent and separated into two components by a
subsequent DEAE cellulose chromatography. The first component was
prostaglandin endoperoxide synthase and the second one thromboxane
synthase, catalyzing the conversion of PGH_2 to TXA_2 (41,42).

The purified thromboxane synthase has been employed for
studies on the mechanism of the biosynthesis of TXA_2 from PGH_2.
There always seemed to be formed equal amounts of 12-hydroxy-
heptadecatrienoic acid (HHT) and TXB_2 (44). During experiments

with inhibitors of thromboxane synthesis it was observed that HHT formation was also inhibited and to the same extent as the TXB_2 formation. An almost identical inhibition of the formation of both compounds was seen with five structurally unrelated compounds, which indicated that the same enzyme was responsible for the formation of both HHT and TXB_2 (44). This enzyme may catalyze the formation of a common precursor of TXA_2 and HHT by an initial protonation of the oxygen atom at C19, followed by cleavage of the O-O bond (44). The formed cation might then rearrange in two different ways: to form either TXA_2 or HHT plus MDA, or to form only TXA_2 which will then decompose to a mixture of TXB_2 and HHT plus MDA.

The second possibility could however be ruled out from comparison between short and long time incubations (44), where the TXA_2 present in the incubation at the time of interruption was determined after its conversion into mono-O-methyl TXB_2 by excess methanol (39). A decrease of TXA_2 and a corresponding increase of TXB_2 was seen between the 10 sec and the 2 min incubations. The HHT amount was however unchanged, and thus TXA_2 cannot be an intermediate in HHT formation.

It thus seems that the initially formed cation rearranges to a mixture of TXA_2 and HHT plus MDA. As these rearrangements are thus two separate steps, malondialdehyde measurements may not always be reliable indicators of TXA_2 formation. Such measurements are frequently performed in platelet studies because of the simplicity of the method.

The above hypothesis of thromboxane formation has recently been challenged (45): in a detailed kinetic study it was demonstrated that the rate of thromboxane formation was not directly dependent of {PGH_2} but rather on {PGH_2}^{2}. This could indicate a bimecular reaction: two molecules of PGH_2 combine, and the formed complex decomposes to one molecule of TXA_2 and one molecule of HHT (plus MDA). If this is the case, thromboxane is a dismutase type of enzyme rather than an isomerase (45).

Several investigators have noticed that incubations with PGH_1 do not seem to yield TXA_1 (44,46). It is thus possible that the Δ^5 double bond is essential for the enzymatic biosynthesis of thromboxanes. To test this hypothesis, the Δ^4 analogue of PGH_2 was prepared and tried as a substrate (47). A complete conversion into the Δ^4 analogue of HHT was seen, but no Δ^4 thromboxane was formed.

Finally, it was demonstrated that PGG_2 was a good substrate for thromboxane synthase (48). This endoperoxide yielded 15-hydroperoxy-TXA_2 and 12-hydroperoxy-HHT as products.

PGI$_2$ (prostacyclin) biosynthesis was first demonstrated in aortic microsomes (49,50), but has later been demonstrated in a wide variety of tissues, such as other arteries, heart, stomach, lung, uterus, vesicular gland, inflammatory granuloma (see 3 and references therein).

The chemical events during PGI$_2$ biosynthesis from its immediate precursor, PGH$_2$ are not quite clear yet. Several mechanisms are possible. Huang and coworkers (51) proposed three different possibilities. One is a homolytic cleavage of the endoperoxide bridge, followed by attack of the 9-oxygen radical on position C-6 of the Δ^5 double bond with hydroperoxidation at C-5. PGI$_2$ would then be formed by subsequent elimination of this hydroperoxy or hydroxyl group. A second possibility involves the formation of an oxonium ion at C-9, which upon addition to the Δ^5 double bond results in the formation of a carbonium ion at C-5. This unstable intermediate may then either lose the C-6 proton directly to form PGI$_2$, or may be converted into the corresponding 5-hydroxy compound which subsequently forms PGI$_2$ upon enzymic elimination of water. Thirdly, a 5, 6-epoxy compound may be formed from the endoperoxide, followed by a concerted attack of the 9-oxygen on C-6 with concomitant opening of the endoperoxide to generate the 5-hydroxy-6(9α)-oxido cyclic ether (51). As such a 5-hydroxy intermediate would be involved in most of these pathways, two of the four possible isomers of this compound were synthesized. However, it was shown that none of them could be enzymatically converted into PGI$_2$ (51).

PGI$_2$ synthase has been partially purified from pig aorta (52) and rabbit aorta (53). The microsomal fraction was solubilized by Triton X-100 and was further purified by ion exchange chromatography. The purified protein was used for studies on the conversion of PGH$_1$ or PGH$_2$ into different products (52,53). The simultaneous formation of PGI$_2$ and HHT was studied under different conditions (52). It was proposed that if PGI$_2$ biosynthesis starts with protonation of the oxygen at C-11 of PGH$_2$, the formed intermediate might undergo cleavage to give HHT and malondialdehyde, in analogy with the events during thromboxane biosynthesis. However, it was demonstrated by the use of enzyme inhibitors and protein denaturing agents that PGI$_2$ synthase did not enzymatically form HHT (52).

15-Hydroperoxy-eicosatetraenoic acid, 15-HPETE, is an inhibitor of PGI$_2$ synthesis (54). This inhibitor was tested using the purified PGI$_2$ synthase as a substrate (52): strong inhibition of PGI$_2$ formation was found, whereas the compound did not have any effect on the HHT formation. It was concluded from these and other experiments that PGI$_2$ synthase did not enzymatically form HHT.

On the other hand when PGH_1 was employed (53), which cannot be converted into PGI_1, the sole product of the reaction was HHD, and HHD production was strongly inhibited by 15–HPETE. These authors concluded that HHD formation was catalyzed by their preparation of PGI synthase. It was suggested that PGH_1 might interact but misfit the active site of the enzyme, thus resulting in a side reaction leading to HHD.

REFERENCES

1. B. Samuelsson, E. Granström, K. Green, M. Hamberg and S. Hammarström, Prostaglandins. Ann. Rev. Biochem., 44:669 (1975).
2. B. Samuelsson, M. Goldyne, E. Granström, M. Hamberg, S. Hammarström and C. Malmsten, Prostaglandins and thromboxanes. Ann. Rev. Biochem. 47:997 (1978).
3. D. A. Van Dorp, R. K. Beerthuis, D. H. Nugteren and H. Vonkeman, The biosynthesis of prostaglandins. Biochim. Biophys. Acta, 90:204 (1964).
4. S. Bergström, H. Danielsson and B. Samuelsson, The enzymatic formation of prostaglandin E2 from arachidonic acid. Biochim. Biophys. Acta, 90:207 (1964).
5. M. Hamberg and B. Samuelsson, Detection and isolation of an endoperoxide intermediate in prostaglandin biosynthesis Proc. Natl. Acad. Sci. USA, 70:899 (1973).
6. D. H. Nugteren and E. Hazelhof, Isolation and properties of intermediates in prostaglandin biosynthesis. Biochim. Biophys. Acta, 326:448 (1973).
7. M. Hamberg, J. Svensson, T. Wakabayashi and B. Samuelsson, Isolation and structure of two prostaglanding endoperoxides that cause platelet aggregation. Proc. Natl. Acad. Sci. USA, 71:345 (1974).
8. T. Miyamoto, N. Ogino, S. Yamamoto and O. Hayaishi, Purification of prostaglandin endoperoxide synthetase from bovine vesicular gland microsomes. J. Biol. Chem., 251:2629 (1976).
9. M. Hemler, W. E. M. Lands and W. L. Smith, Purification of the cyclo-oxygenase that forms prostaglandins: Demonstration of two forms of iron in the holoenzyme. J. Biol. Chem., 251: 5575 (1976).
10. F. J. van der Ouderaa, M. Buytenhek, D. H. Nugteren and D. A. van Dorp, Purification and characterization of prostaglandin endoperoxide synthetase from sheep vesicular glands. Biochim. Biophys. Acta., 487:315 (1977).
11. G. J. Roth, M. Stanford, J. W. Jacobs and P. W. Majerus, Acetylation of prostaglandin synthetase by aspirin. Purification and properties of the acetylated protein from sheep vesicular gland. Biochemistry, 16:4244 (1977).

12. G. J. Roth and P. W. Majerus, The mechanism of the effect of
     aspirin on human platelets. I. Acetylation of a particulate
     fraction protein. J. Clin. Invest., 56:624 (1975).
13. F. J. van der Ouderaa, M. Buytenhek. F. J. Slikkerveer and
     D. A. van Dorp, On the haemoprotein character of prosta-
     glandin endoperoxide synthetase. Biochim. Biophys. Acta.,
     572:29 (1979).
14. S. Okhi, N. Ogino, S. Yamamoto and O. Hayaishi, Prostaglandin
     hydroperoxides, an integral part of prostaglandin endoperoxide
     synthetase from bovine gland microsomes. J. Biol. Chem.,
     254:829 (1979).
15. N. Ogino, S. Ohki, S. Yamamoto and O. Hayaishi, Prostaglandin
     endoperoxide synthetase from bovine vesicular gland micro-
     somes. Inactivation and activation by heme and other metallo-
     porphyrins. J. Biol. Chem. 253 5061 (1978).
16. R. W. Egan, P. H. Gale and F. A. Kuehl, Jr., Reduction of
     hydroperoxides in the prostaglandin biosynthetic pathway
     by a microsomal peroxidase. J. Biol. Chem. 254:3295 (1979).
17. C. J. Sih, C. Takeguchi and P. Foss, Mechanism of prostaglandin
     biosynthesis. III. Catecholamines and serotonin as coenzymes.
     J. Am. Chem. Soc., 92:6670 (1970).
18. N. Ogino, S. Yamamoto, O. Hayaishi and T. Tokuyama, Isolation
     of an activator for prostaglandin hydroperoxidase from bovine
     vesicular gland cytosol and its identification as uric acid.
     Biochem. Biophys. Res. Commun. 87:184 (1979).
19. M. Ogino, T. Miyamoto, S. Yamamoto and O. Hayaishi, Prost-
     glandin endoperoxide E-isomerase from bovine vesicular gland
     microsomes, a glutathione-requiring enzyme. J. Biol. Chem.,
     252:890 (1977).
20. A. Raz, M. Schwartzman and R. Kenig-Wakshal, Chemical and
     enzymatic transformations of prostaglandin endoperoxides:
     Evidence for the predominance of the 15-hydroperoxy pathway.
     Eur. J. Biochem., 70:89 (1976).
21. D. H. Nugteren and E. Christ-Hazelhof, Chemical and enzymic
     conversion of the prostaglandin endoperoxide H_2. In:
     "Advances in Prostaglandin and Thromboxane Research" B.
     Samuelsson, P. Ramwell and R. Paoletti, eds., Raven Press,
     New York. In press (1980).
22. J. B. Smith, M. J. Silver, C. M. Ingerman and J. J. Kocsis,
     Prostaglandin D_2 inhibits the aggregation of human platelets.
     Thromb. Res., 5:291 (1974).
23. M. Hamberg, P. Hedqvist, K. Strandberg, J. Svensson and B.
     Samuelsson, Prostaglandin endoperoxides IV. Effects on smooth
     muscle. Life Sci. 16:451 (1975).
24. M. A. Wasserman, D. W. Ducharme, R. L. Griffin, G. L. de Graaf
     and F. G. Robinson, Bronchopulmonary and cardiovascular
     effects of prostaglandin D_2 in the dog. Prostaglandins,
     13:255 (1977).

25. M. O. Whitaker, P. Needleman, A. Wyche, F. A. Fitzpatrick and
     H. Sprecher, PGD_3 is the mediator of the antiaggregatory
     effects of the trienoic endoperoxide PGH_3. In: "Advances in
     Prostaglandin and Thromboxane Research" B. Samuelsson, P.
     Ramwell and R. Paoletti, eds., Raven Press, New York. In
     press (1980).

26. M. S. Abdel-Halim, M. Hamberg, B. Sjöqvist and E. Änggård,
     Identification of prostaglandin D_2 as a major prostaglandin
     in homogenates of rat brain. Prostaglandins, 14:633 (1977).

27. L. J. Roberts, R. A. Lewis, J. A. Lawson, B. J. Sweetman,
     K. F. Austen and J. A. Oates, Arachidonic acid metabolism
     by rat mast cells. Prostaglandins, 15:717 (1978).

28. H. R. Knapp. O. Oelz, B. J. Sweetman and J. A. Oates,
     Synthesis and metabolism of prostaglandins E_2, $F_{2\alpha}$ and
     D_2 by the rat gastrointestinal tract. Stimulation by a
     hypertonic environment in vitro. Prostaglandins, 15:751
     (1978).

29. F. A. Fitzpatrick and D. A. Stringfellow, Prostaglandin D_2
     formation by malignant melanoma cells correlates inversely
     with cellular metastatic potential. Proc. Natl. Acad. Sci.
     USA, 76:1765 (1979).

30. M. Hamberg and B. Fredholm, Isomerization of prostaglandin
     H_2 into prostaglandin D_2 in the presence of serum albumin.
     Biochim. Biophys. Acta, 431:189 (1976).

31. E. Christ-Hazelhof, D. H. Nugteren and D. A. van Dorp,
     Conversion of prostaglandin endoperoxides by glutathione
     S-transferases and serum albumins. Biochim. Biophys. Acta,
     450 450 (1976).

32. D. A. van Dorp, M. Buytenhek, E. Christ-Hazelhof, D. H.
     Nugteren and F. J. van der Ouderaa, Isolation and properties
     of enzymes involved in prostaglandin synthesis. Acta Biol.
     Med. Germ., 37:691 (1978).

33. E. Christ-Hazelhof and D. H. Negteren, Purification and
     characterization of prostaglandin endoperoxide D-isomerase,
     a cytoplasmic glutatione-requiring enzyme. Biochim. Biophys.
     Acta, 572:43 (1979).

34. T. Shimizu, S. Yamamoto and O. Hayaishi, Purification and
     properties of prostaglandin D synthetase from rat brain.
     J. Biol. Chem., 254:5222 (1979).

35. J. A. McCracken, J. C. Carlson, M. E. Glew, J. R. Godin,
     D. T. Baird, K. Green and B. Samuelsson, Prostaglandin $F_{2\alpha}$
     identified as a luteolytic hormone in sheep. Nature (New
     Biol.) 238:129 (1972).

36. G. D. Thorburn, R. I. Cox, W. B. Currie, B. J. Restall and W.
     Schneider, Prostaglandin F concentration in the utero-
     ovarian venous plasma of the ewe during the estrus cycle.
     J. Endocrinol., 53:325 (1972).

37. H. Kindahl, L.-E. Edqvist, A. Bane and E. Granström, Blood
    levels of progesterone and 15-keto-13,14-dihydro-prosta-
    glandin $F_{2\alpha}$ during the normal oestrous cycle and early
    pregancy in heifers. Acta Endocrin. (Kbh.) 82:134 (1976).
38. P. Wlodawer, H. Kindahl and M. Hamberg, Biosynthesis of
    prostaglandin $F_{2\alpha}$ from arachidonic acid and prostaglandin
    endoperoxides in the uterus. Biochim. Biophys.. Acta.,
    431:603 (1976).
39. M. Hamberg, J. Svensson and B. Samuelsson, Thromboxanes:
    A new group of biologically active compounds derived from
    prostaglandin endoperoxides. Proc. Natl. Acad. Sci. USA,
    72:2994 (1975).
40. M. Hamberg and B. Samuelsson, Prostaglandin endoperoxides
    VII. Novel transformations of arachidonic acid in guinea
    pig lung. Biochem. Biophys. Res. Commun., 61:942 (1974).
41. T. Yoshimoto, S. Yamamoto, M. Okuma and O. Hayaishi,
    Solubilization and resolution of thromboxane synthesizing
    system from microsomes of bovine blood platelets. J. Biol.
    Chem., 252:5871 (1977).
42. S. Hammarström and P. Falardeau, Resolution of prostaglandin
    endoperoxide synthase and thromboxane synthase of human
    platelets. Proc. Natl. Acad. Sci. USA, 74:3691 (1977).
43. P. Wlodawer and S. Hammarström, Thromboxane synthase from
    bovine lung-solubilization and partial purification. Biochem.
    Biophys. Res. Commun., 80:525 (1978).
44. U. Diczfalusy, P. Falardeau and S. Hammarström, Conversion
    of prostaglandin endoperoxides to C_{17}-hydroxy acids catalyzed
    by human platelet thromboxane synthase. FEBS Lett., 84:271
    (1977).
45. M. W. Anderson, D. J. Crutchley, B. E. Tainer and T. E.
    Eling, Kinetic studies on the conversion of prostaglandin
    endoperoxide PGH_2 by thromboxane synthase. Prostaglandins,
    16:563 (1978).
46. P. Needleman, M. Minkes and A. Raz, Thromboxanes:
    Selective biosynthesis and distinct biological properties.
    Science, 193:163 (1976).
47. U. Diczfalusy and S. Hammarström, A structural requirement
    for the conversion of prostaglandin endoperoxides to
    thromboxanes. FEBS Lett., 105:291 (1979).
48. S. Hammarström, Enzymatic synthesis of 15-hydroperoxy-
    thromboxane A_2 and 12-hydroperoxy-5, 8, 10-heptadecatrienoic
    acid. J. Biol. Chem., in press (1979).
49. S. Moncada, R. J. Gryglewski, S. Bunting and J. R. Vane, An
    enzyme isolated from arteries transforms prostaglandin
    endoperoxides to an unstable substance that inhibits platelet
    aggregation. Nature, 263:663 (1976).
50. R. J. Gryglewski, S. Bunting, S. Moncada, R. J. Flower and
    J. R. Vane, Arterial walls are protected against deposition
    of platelet thrombi by a substance (prostaglandin X) which
    they make from prostaglandin endoperoxides. Prostaglandins
    12:685 (1976).

51. F. C. Huang, M. Zmijewski, G. Girdaukas and C. J. Sih, Concerning the biosynthesis of prostaglandin I_2. Bioorganic Chem., 6:311 (1977).

52. P. Wlodawer and S. Hammarström, Some properties of prostacyclin synthase from pig aorta. FEBS Lett., 97:32 (1979).

53. K. Watanabe, S. Yamamoto and O. Hayaishi, Reactions of prostaglandin endoperoxides with prostaglandin I synthetase solubilized from rabbit aorta microsomes. Biochem. Biophys. Res. Commun., 87:192 (1979).

54. S. Moncada, R. J. Gryglewski, S. Bunting and J. R. Vane, A lipid peroxide inhibits the enzyme in blood vessel microsomes that generates from prostaglandin endoperoxides the substance (prostaglandin X) which prevents platelet aggregation. Prostaglandins, 12:715 (1976).

PHOSPHOLIPASES AND THEIR RELEVANCE TO PROSTAGLANDIN BIOSYNTHESIS

Roderick J. Flower

Department of Prostaglandin Research
Wellcome Research Laboratories, Langley Court
Beckenham, Kent, U.K.

In this chapter I will briefly outline the experimental evidence which suggests an important role for phospholipase enzymes in the initiation and regulation of prostaglandin biosynthesis. The effect of corticosteroids on phospholipase activity is described elsewhere in this book.

WHAT ARE PHOSPHOLIPIDS AND PHOSPHOLIPASES?

Before embarking upon a discussion of the possible role of phospholipases in initiating prostaglandin biosynthesis, I will briefly review the basic biochemistry of phospholipids (sometimes called phosphatides) and phospholipases.

The phosphatides we shall be most concerned about are derivatives of the 3-carbon compound glycerol (see Fig. 1). Glycerol can be regarded as a "backbone" to which other components of the phospholipid molecule are linked. As far as we are concerned the 1' and 2' positions are occupied by fatty acids and the third by a phosphorylated nitrogenous "base". Generally speaking the 1'-position is occupied by a saturated fatty acid (i.e. palmitic) whereas the 2'-position (which is assymetric) is occupied by an unsaturated fatty acid (i.e. arachidonic or dihomo-γ-linolenic acid). The most common bases found are ethanolamine, choline, inositol and serine (see Figures 1 & 2).

Phospholipases are ubiquitously distributed enzymes which hydrolyse phospholipids, Many such enzymes exist, some differ in their positional specificity others vary in their pH optimum, subcellular location, requirements for Ca^{2+} etc. We have not room here to catalogue all the phospholipases that have been found,

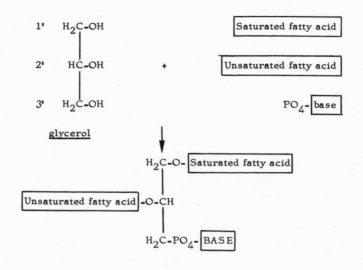

POSSIBLE BASES

Choline $CH_3 CH_2 - \overset{+}{N}(CH_3)_3$

Ethanolamine $CH_3 CH_2 - \overset{+}{N} H_3$

Serine $CH_3 - CH(\overset{+}{N}H_3)COOH$

Inositol

Fig. 1. A highly simplified scheme showing the principal phospholipids and their precursors.

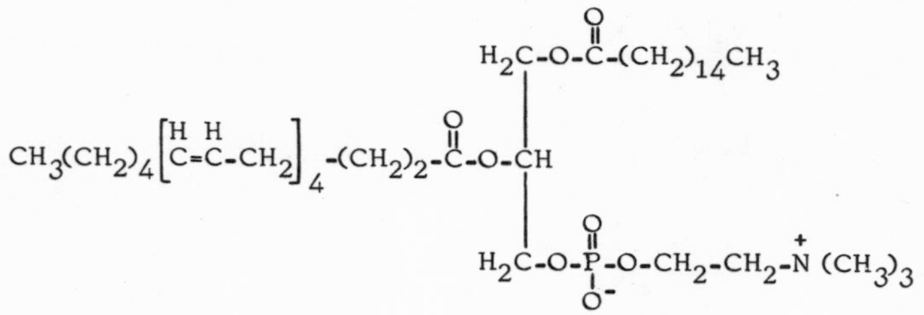

$$H_2C-O-\overset{\overset{O}{\|}}{C}-(CH_2)_{14}CH_3$$

$$CH_3(CH_2)_4\left[\overset{H\ H}{\underset{}{C=C-CH_2}}\right]_4-(CH_2)_2-\overset{\overset{O}{\|}}{C}-O-\overset{|}{C}H$$

$$H_2C-O-\overset{\overset{O}{\|}}{\underset{\underset{O^-}{|}}{P}}-O-CH_2-CH_2-\overset{+}{N}(CH_3)_3$$

Fig. 2. Example of a phospholipid: full structure of 1'
palmitoyl, 2' arachidonyl phosphatidylcholine.
Phosphatidylcholines are sometimes called "lecithin".

instead we will concentrate on those which seem most applicable
to prostaglandin biosynthesis. Figure 3 shows the sites at which
the known phospholipases act, and the resultant products of their
hydrolytic activity. It would be a mistake to regard phospholipases
as only being "destructive" enzymes. The phospholipids (especially
those in the membrane) of many (but not all) cells are in a
constant state of turnover and phospholipases are undoubtedly
important for this task.

Figure 3 shows that there are basically four sites for attack
on the phospholipid molecule. Phospholipase A_1 hydrolyses the
1'-fatty acid from the glycerol backbone giving a 1'-lysophosphatide.
Similarly phospholipase A_2 hydrolyses the 2'-fatty acids giving a
2'-lysophosphatide. These lysophosphatides are generally cytotoxic,
causing haemolysis in RBCS and membrane damage to other cells or
organelles, and they are usually quickly disposed of in the cell
either by lysophospholipases or by re-acylation to phosphatides.
Two other sorts of phospholipase are known, a phospholipase C which
removes the phosphorylated base leaving a diglyceride, and
phospholipase D which removes only the base leaving phosphatidic
acid. Phospholipase D has only been detected in plants and therefore has little relevance to our present discussion. It will not
be referred to again.

Why we think phospholipases are important for prostaglandin biosynthesis

PGs, and by implication other cyclo-oxygenase products, are
not stored within cells (23) and so biosynthesis must immediately
precede release. The substrates must be in a nonesterified form
(15, 32) for synthesis of the products to occur, and yet the level
of such substrates in cells - as free acids at least - is
extremely low (14, 11, 26). However, these acids are present in
high concentrations in cells as esters, mainly in the form of
phospholipids. In an analysis of sheep vesicular gland phospholipids

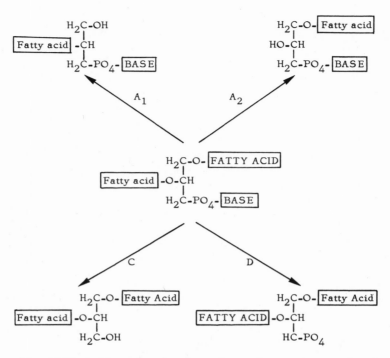

Fig. 3.   Simplified diagram showing the points of attack of the
          various phospholipase enzymes.

for example, Samuelsson (25) found high concentrations of dihomo-
γ-linolenic acid in both the phosphatidylcholine (17.5 moles %)
and ethanolamine (21.8 mol %) fractions. Arachidonic acid was
also present in other phosphatides but in 7-11 fold less
concentration. This situation appears to be a typical and in most
tissues it is arachidonic, rather than dihomo-γ-linolenic acid
which appears to be the major substrate (8), even though the
latter is apparently an intermediate in the preferred pathway for
synthesis of arachidonic acid - at least in the rat (28, 18).
It seems that the presence of the precursors of dihomo-γ-linolenic
(linolenic and γ-linolenic) increase the final desaturation step
- perhaps explaining why dihomo-γ-linolenic acid (as the ethyl
ester) to rats caused a rise not only in tissue and plasma ester
levels of dihomo-γ-linolenate, but that in most tissues, it also
caused a rise in esterified arachidonate as well. Two interesting
exceptions to this were the platelets and the renal medulla where
a rise in dihomo-γ-linolenate occurred without a rise in arachidonic
acid.

     It seems from the foregoing discussion that the vast majority
of the cyclo-oxygenase substrate is present in tissues in an

esterified form. Clearly, before synthesis can occur the substrate must first be released. These precursor acids could arise from a number of intracellular lipid pools; cholesterol esters, phosphatides, mono, di or triglycerides might all contain sufficient substrate to support biosynthesis. Thus, several enzymes are potentially capable of mobilising fatty acid substrates. The suggestion which has received most attention, however, is that the free substrate originates from the phospholipid fraction of the cell, under the influence of the hydrolytic enzyme phospholipase A_2.

The implication of this idea is that the appearance of substrate is a rate limiting step in cyclo-oxygenase activity and that phospholipase A_2 is a regulatory enzyme. Some of the early experimental evidence which supported this important concept may be summarised thus:

1. Phospholipids can act as stores of precursor fatty acid (15,32).

2. Infusion of arachidonic acid through frog intestine (3) or lungs (30,20), results in a release of PGs.

3. Perfusion of guinea pig lungs or frog intestine with phospholipase A leads to a rapid release of large quantities of PGs (31,3).

4. Infusion of arachidonic acid or bradykinin through guinea pig lungs leads to an appearance of PGs in the perfusate, mepacrine, a phospholipase inhibitor, blocks the releasing action of bradykinin but not of arachidonic acid (30). These results are consistent with the idea that bradykinin releases PGs by stimulating phospholipase, whereas arachidonic acid is converted to PGs directly.

5. Thyroid stimulating hormone apparently increases the synthesis of PGs in the thyroid by stimulating the activity of an endogenous phospholipase (11).

6. When incubated with labelled arachidonic acid, slices of guinea pig spleen incorporated the substrate into neutral lipid and phosphatide pools. The majority is incorporated into the 2' position of a phosphatide with the chromatographic mobility of lecithin. During mechanical vibration, homogenisation or immunological stimulation, radioactive arachidonic acid is released from the lecithin fraction and converted into PGs. No release of arachidonate is observed from the neutral lipid pools at any time (10).

7.   Experiments similar to these (6) were performed using platelets
     which depend upon the generation of TXA$_2$ for aggregation.
     Platelets, like spleen slices, incorporate labelled arachi-
     donic acid into the 2' position of phosphatides – chiefly
     choline and inositol phosphatides. During exposure of the
     platelets to aggregating agents, significant losses of
     arachidonic acid from the phosphatidylcholine, phosphatidy-
     linositol and phosphatidylethanolamine fractions are observed,
     with the concomitant generation of cyclo-oxygenase products.
     The experiments have been repeated using gas chromatography
     to estimate the arachidonate content of platelet phosphatides.
     Again, a striking fall in the phosphatidylcholine and
     phosphatidylinositol and phosphatidylethanolamine arachidonate
     content is seen after the addition of collagen (6).

     Although the foregoing evidence in favour of phospholipase A$_2$
as the regulator of cyclo-oxygenase activity is as yet incomplete,
it is highly suggestive. Recently some evidence has been provided
by two laboratories (24,4) that the main mechanism whereby
platelets obtain their arachidonic acid during the aggregation
process is by the combined action of a phospholipase C specific
for phosphatidylinositol and a digylceride lipase (see Figure 4).
The net result of these two enzymes would be to liberate the 1' and
2' fatty acid making it difficult, in many experimental instances,
to distinguish the final result from an attack by phospholipase
A$_2$. This mechanism is obviously important but it is not yet known
whether it operates in tissues other than platelets.

     The possibility that lipid pools other than phosphatides are
important for cyclo-oxygenase activity cannot be ruled out at
this stage, but nonetheless the possibility of a regulatory
mechanism involving phospholipase A$_2$ is certainly very attractive.
Because the cellular membrane system to a large extent controls
the integrity of the cell (the cyclo-oxygenase is also membrane
bound), its function as a storehouse of fatty acid substrates
and as a regulator of permeability are intimately linked. Thus,
damage to a section of membrane resulting in a turnover of
phosphatides could not only release fatty acids but also result in
an increased diffusion of those precursors into the cyclo-oxygenase
compartment. Audet et al (1) investigated the activity of
phospholipase A in three different strains of E.coli. Very little
activity was found in two of the strains which had rigid cell
envelopes and were thus relatively resistant to lysis. The other
strain, however, had high phospholipase activity, was easily
lysed and during growth released lipid, protein and polysaccharide
material into the medium. There was also production of free
fatty acids. Other workers have also noticed that the activity
of this enzyme is greater in cells subjected to adverse conditions
(27,5,21). On the basis of this evidence, it is attractive to
speculate that a primary lesion in cell damage is disruption of the

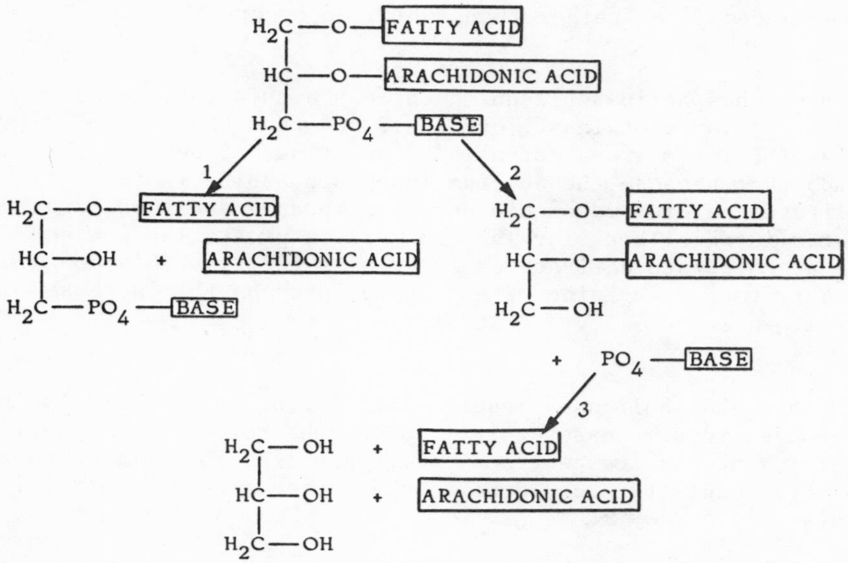

Fig. 4. Two pathways by which arachidonic acid can be liberated from phospholipids. 1. phospholipase A_2; 2. phospholipase C; 3. diglyceride lipase. The phospholipase C (a phosphatidylinositol phosphodiesterase) from platlets which catalyses this reaction is specific for phosphatidlinositol.

cellular membrane system leading to a release of fatty acids and an increase in permeability which enables the liberated fatty acids to reach the cyclo-oxygenase enzyme, culminating in a release of PGs and other lipid mediators.

Of course, as one might expect, the type of PGs produced by a cell depends upon the type of fatty acid present in the phospholipid stores. Such an idea has been used as the basis of an ingenious experiment by Willis and his coworkers (29). Utilising the fact that E_1 blocks platelet aggregation, these authors fed rats with oral dihomo-γ-linolenate, a precedure which results in increased ratios of this acid to arachidonic acid in the phospholipid fraction. Platelets from these rats were much less suceptible to the aggregating activity of several agents, which normally act by generation arachidonate oxidation products such as TXA_2.

Regulation of phospholipase activity

Not a great deal is known about the way in which phospholipases are regulated (i.e. rather than inhibited by drugs).

Many phospholipases require Ca^{2+} as a cofactor and so on a
superficial level at least, one could say that the intracellular
levels of calcium are a potential regulating influence. This may
be important because the calcium ionophore A23187 (which
facilitates calcium movements across membranes and therefore
elevates intracellular levels) can release prostaglandins and
other arachidonate derivatives from cells (22,2): This could be
secondary to a triggering of a phospholipase by the increased
calcium.

Other phospholipases require "activation" before catalysis
can proceed in some cases this involves the removal of a peptide
protecting the active centre by a trypsin-like enzymatic attack
(9). Presumably this could be another site at which control is
exercised.

Phospholipase A_2 (in platelets) seems to be under the control
of cAMP. Lapetina and his colleagues (16) found that cAMP prevents
the deacylation of platelet phospholipids induces by thrombin.
In another cell line however (cultured mouse fibroblasts),
Lindgren and coworkers (17) reported exactly the reverse - that
cAMP could stimulate prostaglandin production and that this was
secondary to an increase in acylhydrolase activity.

Many agents - some of them·physiological, other pathological
have been shown to stimulate phospholipase activity in vitro by
unknown mechanisms. These include RCS-RF, bradykinin, antigen,
histamine, angiotensin II, vasopressin and mechanical trauma
(7,13). Whether or not these agents have a stimulating effect
under normal physiological conditions remains to be seen.

With regard to other mechanisms of control, it is probably
safe to say that stimuli which require an increase in membrane
turnover, i.e. phagocytosis, pinocytosis etc. probably result in
an increase in phospholipase activity. In secretory cells, one
particular phospholipid pool - phosphatidylinositol seems to be
exquisitely sensitive to a variety of agents including some
neurotransmitters, all of which produce a rapid "turnover"
of phosphatidylinositol presumably secondary to an increased
phospholipase activity (12,19). The significance of this turnover
for prostaglandin biosynthesis is not known at the moment, and it
will be up to the ingenuity of future investigators to solve this
problem.

REFERENCES

1. A. Audet, G. Nantel and P. Prolx, Phospholipase A activity
    in growing Escherichia coli cells. Biochim. Biophys. Acta.
    348:334-343 (1974).
2. M. K. Bach, J. R. Brashier, and R. R. Gorman, On the structure
    of slow reacting substance of anaphylaxis: Evidence of
    biosynthesis from arachidonic acid. Prostaglandins,
    14:21-38 (1977).
3. J. Bartels, H. Kunze, W. Vogt and G. Willis, Prostaglandin:
    liberation from and formation in perfused frog intestine.
    Naunyn-Schmiedebergs Arch. Pharmacol., 266:207 (1970).
4. R. L. Bell, D. A. Kennedy, N. Stanford, and P. W. Majerus,
    Diglyceride lipase: a pathway for arachidonate release from
    human platelets. Proceedings of IV Int. Conference on
    Prostaglandins, Washington, (1979).
5. J. Bennett, J. Glavenovich, R. Liskay, D. L. Wullf, and
    J. E. Cronan Jr., Phospholipid hydrolysis in Escherichia coli
    infected with rapid lysis mutants of phage T_4. Virology,
    43:516-518 (1971).
6. G. J. Blackwell, G. J. Duncombe, R. J. Flower, M. F. Parsons
    and J. R. Vane. The distribution and metabolism of arachidonic
    acid in rabbit platelets during aggregation and its modification
    by drugs. Br. J. Pharmacol., 59:353-366 (1977).
7. G. J. Blackwell, R. J. Flower, F. P. Nijkamp, and J. R. Vane,
    Phospholipase A_2 activity of guinea pig isolated perfused
    lungs: stimulation and inhibition by anti-inflammatory steroids.
    Br. J. Pharmac., 62:79-89 (1978).
8. A. Danon, M. Heimberg, and J. A. Oates, Enrichment of rat
    tissue lipids with fatty acids that are prostaglandin
    precursors. Biochim. Biophys. Acta, 388:318-330 (1975).
9. J. Drenth, C. M. Enzing, K. H. Kalk, and J. C. A. Wessies,
    Structure and function of phospholipases. An x-ray study
    of phospholipase A_2. In: "advances in Prostaglandin and
    Thromboxane Research", ed. C. Galli, et al. Raven Press,
    New York, pp.23-30 (1978).
10. R. J. Flower and G. J. Blackwell, The importance of
    phospholipase A_2 in prostaglandin biosynthesis. Biochem.
    Pharmacol., 25:285-291 (1976).
11. B. Haye, S. Champion and C. Jacquemin, Control of TSH of a
    phospholipase A_2 activity, a limiting factor in the bio-
    synthesis of prostaglandins in the thyroid. FEBS Lett.,
    30:253-260 (1973).
12. L. E. Hokin, Functional activity in glands and synaptic
    and the turnover of phosphatidylinositol. Ann. N.Y. Acad.
    Sci., 165:696-709 (1969).
13. P. C. Isakson, A. Raz, W. Hsueh and P. Needleman, Lipases and
    prostaglandin biosynthesis. In: "Advances in Prostaglandin
    and Thromboxane Research", Vol. 3, ed. C. Galli et al.
    Raven Press, New York, pp.113-120 (1978).

14. H. Kunze and W. Vogt. Significance of phospholipase A for
     prostaglandin formation. Ann. N.Y. Acad. Aci. 180:123-125
     (1971).
15. W. E. M. Lands, and B. Samuelsson, Phospholipid precursors
     of prostaglandins. Biochim. Biophys. Acta., 164:426-429
     (1968).
16. E. G. Lapetina, C. J. Schmitges, K. Chandrabose and P.
     Cuatrecasas, Regulation of phospholipase activity in platelets,
     In: "Advances in Prostaglandin and Thromboxane Research,"
     Vol. 3, ed. C. Galli et al., Raven Press, New York, pp.127-
     136 (1978).
17. J. A. Lindgren, H. E. Claesson and S. Hammarstrom, Stimulation
     of arachidonic acid release and prostaglandin production in
     3T3 fibroblasts by adenosine 3:5' monophosphate, In:
     "Advances in Prostaglandin and Thromboxane Research", Vol.3,
     ed. C. Gall, et al., Raven Press, New York, pp.167-174
     (1978).
18. Y. L. Marcel, K. Christiansen and R. T. Holman, The preferred
     metabolic pathway from linolenic acid to arachidonic acid in
     vitro. Biochem. Biophys. Acta., 164:25-34 (1968).
19. R. H. Michell, Inositol phospholipids and cell surface receptor
     function. Biochim. Biophys. Acta., 415:81-147 (1975).
20. M. A. Palmer, P. J. Piper and J. R. Vane, Release of rabbit
     aorta contracting substance (RCS) and prostaglandins induced
     by chemical or mechanical stimulation of guinea pig lungs.
     Br. J. Pharmcol., 49:226-242 (1972).
21. P. Patriarca, S. Beckerdite and P. Elsbach, Phospholipases
     and phospholipid turnover in Escherichia coli spheroplasts.
     Biochim. Biophys. Acta., 260 593-600 (1972).
22. W. C. Pickett, R. L. Jesse and P. Cohen, Initiation of
     phospholipase activity in human platelets by the calcium
     ionohore A23187. Biochim. Biohphys. Acta., 486:209-213
     (1977).
23. P. J. Piper and J. R. Vane, The release of prostaglandins
     from lung and other tissues. Ann. N.Y. Acad. Sci., 180:
     363-385 (1971).
24. S. Rittenhouse-simmons, Production of diglyceride from
     phosphatidylinositol in activated human platelets. J. Clin.
     Invest., 63:580-587 (1979).
25. B. Samuelsson, Biosynthesis of prostaglandins. Progr. Biochem.
     Pharmacol., 5:109-128 (1969).
26. B. Samuelsson, Biosynthesis of prostaglandins. Fed. Proc.
     31:1442-1450 (1972).
27. J. Scandella and A. Kornberg, A membrane bound phospholipase
     A_1 purified from Escherichia coli. Biochemistry, 10:4447-
     4456 (1971).
28. H. Sprecher and C. J. Lee, The absence of an 8-desaturase in
     rat liver: a re-evaluation of optional pathways for the
     metabolism of linoleic and linolenic acids. Biochem.
     Biophys. Acta., 388:113-125 (1975).

29. A. L. Willis, K. Comai, D. C. Kuhn and J. Paulsrud,
     Dihomo-γ-linolenate suppresses platelet aggregation when
     administered in vitro or in vivo. Prostaglandins, 8:
     509-519 (1974).

30. B. B. Vargaftig and N. Dao Hai, Selective inhibition by
     mepacrine of the release of "rabbit aorta contracting
     substance evoked by the administration of bradykinin.
     J. Pharm. (Lond.), 24:159-161 (1972).

31. W. Vogt, U. Meyer, H. Kunze, E. Lufft and S. Babilli,
     Entstehung von SRSC in der durchstromten Meerschweinchenlunge
     durch Phospholipase A. Identifizierung mit Prostaglandin.
     Naunyn-Schmiedebergs Arch Exp. Path. Pharmak., 262:124-134
     (1969).

32. H. Vonkeman and D. A. Van Dorp, The action of prostaglandin
     synthetase on 2-arachidonyl-lecithin. Biochim. Biophys.
     Acta., 164:430-432 (1968).

METABOLISM OF PROSTAGLANDINS AND THROMBOXANES

Elisabeth Granström

Department of Chemistry, Karolinska Institutet
S-104 01 Stockholm
Sweden

Around 15 years ago the first metabolic steps in the inactivation of prostaglandins were elucidated. It was demonstrated that PGs of the E and F type were extensively taken up by many organs and tissues in the body (see (1) and references therein), mainly by the liver, kidney and lungs, and were inactivated by a few metabolic steps.

The first step is dehydrogenation at C-15 which leads to a 15-keto-PG, in most cases a biologically inactive product. The enzyme catalyzing this step is 15-hydroxy prostanoate dehydrogenase (PGDH), which has a very wide-spread occurrence (see p.00, this volume). The formed 15-keto metabolite may then be reduced by the enzyme Δ^{13} reductase to a 15-keto-13,14-dihydro PG. These two reactions have been shown to take place with a large number of compounds in this field, and the 15-keto-13,14-dihydro compounds are now recognized as the major plasma metabolites of many prostaglandins (1).

The ubiquitous occurrence of the two enzymes, 15-PGDH and Δ^{13} reductase, results in an extremely short biological half-life in the circulation of their substrates. The half-life of the primary PGs for example is probably less than 30 sec, whereas on the other hand that of their 15-keto-13,14-dihydro metabolites is around 10 min (2,3). Consequently, these latter occur in much larger amounts in the circulation than the parent PGs (1). Thus, in quantitative measurements of PG production the major circulating metabolites should be monitored rather than their short-lived parent compounds. In addition, the artifactual formation of primary PGs during the blood sampling further distorts the picture, if these compounds are measured as such in blood (1).

39

Since this concept became well-known and accepted, a large number of studies on the role of $PGF_{2\alpha}$ in the body have been successfully carried out using 15-keto-dihydro-$PGF_{2\alpha}$ as the target for measurements in blood plasma. Surprisingly, this has not been the case with the corresponding PGE_2 metabolite, 15-keto-dihydro-PGE_2. The reason is the pronounced chemical instability of this compound, with several different side reactions decreasing its concentration (4). In analogy with other PGE compounds, this metabolite can occur in two forms, epimeric at C-8 (5,6). Furthermore, dehydration to the corresponding PGA_2 metabolite occurs rapidly, after which water soluble adducts easily can form, probably as the result of the so called Michael addition of nucleophilic groups at the activated C-11 (cf. 7). Sulfhydryl groups of amino acids, peptides or proteins are likely reactants in this reaction, and as a consequence the chemical half-life of 15-keto-13,14-dihydro-PGE_2 is considerably shortened in for example plasma samples.

The formation of water-soluble adducts with sulfhydryl containing compounds, such as glutathione, is known to occur also with 15-keto prostaglandins (8). These compounds also have an α,β unsaturated keto structure in their molecules. This reaction may occur either non-enzymatically or enzymatically, catalyzed by glutathione S-transferases. It is not known to what extent this reaction occurs in vivo. The PGs following this pathway escape detection by common assay methods.

A 15-keto-13,14-dihydro metabolite may in some cases undergo a reduction at C-15 to give a dihydro-PG (1,9). The importance of this reaction is not well understood: the reactions described so far lead to extensive inactivation of potent compounds, but this lastmentioned step again yields a biologically active compound.

The further fates of the prostaglandins include β-oxidation to dinor or tetranor compounds, ω-hydroxy or ω-keto compounds or dioic acids, and sometimes also β-oxidation from the ω end (1). All these reactions lead to more water-soluble compounds which are easily excreted into urine. The metabolic pattern in urine for each pathway is invariably very complex, with a multitude of breakdown products formed by various combinations of the above-mentioned metabolic pathways (1,10-13).

The knowledge of these pathways is of great importance. In many types of in vivo studies where it is necessary to measure the total daily production of a certain PG, the best approach is to quantify a major, typical urinary metabolite from this particular pathway (14).

The prostaglandins may undergo several other metabolic fates, PGE compounds can for example be reduced into PGFs (6,11,15,16) by a 9-keto reductase. This reaction may be of biological significance, as PGs of the E and F type often have opposite biological effects,. The opposite reaction, viz, dehydrogenation of PGF to form PGE, may also take place (17), although this reaction may occur somewhat better at the metabolite stage (18,19). A recent, very interesting finding is the efficient hepatic conversion of 6-keto-$PGF_{1\alpha}$ into 6-keto-PGE_1 by this pathway: 6-keto-PGE_1 was shown to be equipotent with PGI_2 as an inhibitor of platelet aggregation (20).

Detailed knowledge of the metabolic reactions, involved in the biologic inactivation of PGs, has provided the bases for the synthesis of a great number of potent and long-acting PG analogues, which are more or less resistant to metabolic degradation. Most of these are modified at or near C-15 to prevent the initial dehydrogenation of the hydroxyl group at this carbon (eg. 21-26). An additional advantage may be obtained if also the carboxyl side chain is modified to inhibit degradation by β-oxidation (27,28).

A group of compounds that has recently attracted some attention is the D type of PGs, however, virtually nothing has been known about their metabolism until recently (13). About half of the identified urinary metabolites of PGD_2 in the monkey had retained the PGD structure, and were formed by various combinations of all the abovementioned metabolic reactions. A very interesting and somewhat disturbing finding was the identification of a number of $PGF_{2\alpha}$ compounds, including $PGF_{2\alpha}$ itself, formed from the injected PGD_2. In fact, the greater part of the break-down products in urine was in the form of PGF_{α} metabolites, The major metabolite was dinor-$PGF_{2\alpha}$, which was believed to be a specific PGD_2 metabolite (13). This is however not the case: it is formed in great yield also from $PGF_{2\alpha}$ (cf. 1), The implications of these findings are, first, that measurements of a biological response to PGD compounds may be very uncertain, as the compound may be partially converted into PGF, which may increase or reverse the action of PGD. Second, all quantitative measurements of PGF metabolites should be viewed in the light of these findings, as it is now obvious that measured levels may reflect not only PGF production, but PGE and PGD production as well.

Thromboxane metabolism has evoked great interest ever since the thromboxane pathway was discovered 5 years ago (29). The potent TXA_2 was already then known to be rapidly hydrolyzed into the almost inactive TXB_2 with a $t_{1/2}$ of about 30 sec in aqueous solution. It was then erroneously assumed that this hydrolysis of TXA_2 always occurred to completion under all circumstances, and most studies of TXA_2 metabolism have thus dealt with the further transformation of TXB_2 (30-34).

Metabolic studies were first undertaken to find an alternate compound to TXB_2 for monitoring, particularly in the circulation. A stable, major plasma metabolite, such as 15-keto-13,14-dihydro-TXB_2 was looked for, in analogy with the PG transformations, however, in vitro studies using crude 15-PGDH preparations from kidney, liver and lungs indicated that TXB_2 does not seem to be a substrate for this enzyme. Furthermore, i.v. injection of ^3H-TXB_2 into monkeys did not reveal any analogous conversion into 15-keto-dihydro-TXB_2 (30). ^3H-TXB_2 itself remained for a long time as the dominating compound in the blood stream. This precludes simple measurements of thromboxane production in vivo by monitoring a compound in plasma: it is obvious that TXA_2 formation and release in vivo cannot be studied by measuring TXB_2 itself in plasma. The problem is the same, or rather worse, than with the primary prostaglandins: a very large artifactual formation of TXB_2 occurs during the sample collection which completely over-shadows the low, endogenous levels.

Measurements of a urinary metabolite instead would overcome these difficulties. In several species the major urinary metabolite was dinor TXB_2 (30-34). A number of other metabolites were also found which had been formed by various combinations of the common metabolic reactions described above (32). Several metabolites, however, had the saturated keto structure in the side chain: it is possible that some of the break-down products are better substrates for 15-PGDH than TXB_2 itself. In addition to the common metabolic pathways, dehydrogenation at C-11 had also taken place in many metabolites (32). These 11-dehydro compounds are in fact δ-lactones of dioic acids.

For quantitation of thromboxane formation in vivo, it seemed possible to monitor the major urinary metabolite, dinor-TXB_2. A mass spectrometric method for this compound was developed and used for a quantative study in the guinea pig (34). The basal excretion of this metabolite was very low, and a total TXB_2 production of 500 ng/day was calculated. Surprisingly, when then guinea pigs were sensitized and anaphylaxis was induced by challenge with the immunogen, no increase at all was seen in the excretion of dinor-TXB_2. This was difficult to explain, as anaphylactic lungs are known to produce large amounts of TXA_2 (35,36). Thus, it was possible that the released TXA_2 was metabolized by a different pathway than by hydrolysis into TXB_2 and later β-oxidation to dinor-TXB_2. This has also been supported by findings from perfusion experiments with anaphylactic guinea pig lungs (37-39). The anticipated thromboxane metabolites, 15-keto-13,13-dihydro-TXB_2, was identified in the perfusate and later also quantitated together with several other products (39). In non-sensitized lungs it occurred in small amounts, but the importance of this metabolic pathway increased after sensitization, and after repeated challenges 15-keto-dihydro-TXB_2 was by far the major metabolite. The explanation for the different results in these two quantitative studies on sensitized guinea pigs may thus be that the wrong compound was monitored in the former study. TXA_2 is hydrolyzed to TXB_2 in aqueous medium in vitro, but this reaction may in vivo be preceded by the action of 15-PGDH and Δ^{13} reductase. Whether the 15-keto-dihydro metabolite is normally a major circulating metabolite of TXA_2 in vivo, and thus the proper target for plasma measurements, is not known yet.

TXA_2 metabolism has been shown to be unexpectedly complicated also in simpler systems, such as in platelet rich plasma (PRP) in vitro. In such a system TXB_2 was supposed to be the only end product, as no metabolizing enzymes are present. In studies on PGH_2 induced platelet aggregation in PRP it was however found that the method of interruption of the reaction in removed aliquots was of great importance for the measured TXB_2 levels (40,41). When acetone was used, the normal increase to a high and constant level was seen. On the other hand, when acid was used to quench the reaction, a rapid burst of thromboxane formation was seen, which was followed by an apparent decrease in detected TXB_2 levels; the final level was about the same as in the acetone experiment. The explanation is that released TXA_2 is quickly and extensively trapped by proteins, mainly albumin (41), and only when acid was added did the hydrolysis to TXB_2 become sufficiently rapid to compete efficiently with the reaction with proteins.

Albumin binding by TXA_2 has been noticed earlier (42,43), but in those studies a different phenomenon was seen: the half-life of this very unstable compound was considerably prolonged in the presence of albumin. This was apparently caused by the common, non-covalent binding by albumin, which for a considerable time protected the compound against hydrolysis. Thus, albumin seems to exert opposite actions: one protective and one destructive action. The relative importance of these two and their function in vivo is not known at present.

The metabolic fates of TXA_2 thus seem to be very complicated. A few years ago, TXB_2 was almost automatically considered the end product of TXA_2 formation and a reliable indicator. Now it has become clear that under many circumstances it is only a minor and insignificant product. TXA_2 seems to be metabolized partially via different pathways and form covalent derivatives with proteins, or be metabolized via the 15-PGDH pathway. The further fates of these products are not known.

The metabolism of PGI_2 has been the subject of several studies during the last few years (44-61). In analogy with the studies on thromboxane metabolism, the first studies were not carried out with PGI_2 itself but with its non-enzymatically formed hydrolysis product, 6-keto-$PGF_{1\alpha}$. When ^3H-labeled 6-keto-$PGF_{1\alpha}$ was administered to rats only β- and ω-oxidized products of this compound

could be found in urine; the metabolites had not undergone dehydrogenation at C-15 (44). That 6-keto-$PGF_{1\alpha}$ was a poor substrate
for 15-PGDH was also confirmed in several in vitro studies (46,51,
52).

However, later some other metabolites were identified, which
were either endogenous products or were derived from labeled PGI_2
(45-48, 50154). These new metabolites were in the normal way
dehydrogenated at C-15, and sometimes also the Δ^{13} double bond
had been reduced. Several in vitro studies using homogenates
from various organs have also confirmed that PGI_2 is an excellent
substrate for 15-PGDH, whereas 6-keto-$PGF_{1\alpha}$ is a poor one. The
mode of administration of the compound in in vivo experiments seems
of great importance: when 6-keto-$PGF_{1\alpha}$ was given by continous i.v.
infusion instead of bolus injection, even this compound was
extensively dehydrogenated at C-15 (48).

The identity of the major circulating compound from the PGI_2
pathway has not yet been conclusively established, and thus
plasma measurements for studies on PGI_2 production are still somewhat uncertain. PGI_2 has been postulated as a circulating hormone
(49,51,55,56), and then either PGI_2 itself of 6-keto-$PGF_{1\alpha}$ may be
the major plasma product. It has been demonstrated that PGI_2 is
not a substrate for the uptake system in the lung (51). However,
PGI_2 may be extensively taken up by other organs, such as the
liver, kidney etc. (53,57,58). It was recently shown (59) that
2 min after an i.v. bolus injection of labeled PGI_2 into a rat,
40% of the plasma radioactivity was in the form of a less polar
metabolite (behaving like 6,15-diketo-$PGF_{1\alpha}$), a situation
strikingly similar to the fate of the classical prostaglandins.

There is also the possibility of a spontaneous hydrolysis
of PGI_2 into 6-keto-$PGF_{1\alpha}$ in the blood stream, followed by
dehydrogenation at C-9 to yield the powerful antiaggregatory
agent, 6-keto-PGE_1(20). This may influence the on-line bioassay
designed for the detection of circulating PGI_2 (60).

PGI_2 has also recently been demonstrated to undergo an
uncommon metabolic fate: a one-carbon degradation of the carboxyl
side chain, which in combination with two steps of β-oxidation
yields pentanor-$PGF_{1\alpha}$ (61).

REFERENCES

1. B. Samuelsson, E. Granström, K. Green, M. Hamberg and S.
    Hammarström, Prostaglandins. Ann. Rev. Biochem., 44:669 (1975).
2. M. Hamberg and B. Samuelsson, On the metabolism of prosta-
    glandins E_1 and E_2 in man. J. Biol. Chem., 246:6713 (1971).
3. E. Granström and B. Samuelsson, On the metabolism of prosta-
    glandin $F_{2\alpha}$ in female subjects: structures of two metabolites
    in blood. Eur. J. Biochem. 27:462 (1972).

4. E. Granström and H. Kindahl, Radioimmunologic determination
    of 15-keto-13,14-dihydro-PGE_2: a method for its stable
    degradation product, 11-deoxy-13,14-dihydro-15-keto-11β,16-
    cyclo-prostaglandin E_2. In: "Advances in Prostaglandin and
    Thromboxane Research", Vol.6, Eds. B. Samuelsson, P. Ramwell,
    R. Pooletti,Raven Press, New York (1980) p.181.
5. E. Daniels, W. Krueger, F. Kupiecki, J. Pike and W. Schneider,
    Isolation and characterization of a new prostaglandin isomer.
    J. Amer. Chem. Soc., 90:5849 (1968).
6. M. Hamberg and U. Israelsson, Metabolism of prostaglandin E_2
    in guinea pig liver. Identification of seven metabolites.
    J. Biol. Chem., 245:5107 (1970).
7. L. Cagen, J. Pisano, J. Ketley, W. Habig and W. Jakoby, The
    conjugation of prostaglandin A_1 and glutathione catalyzed
    by homogenous glutathione S-transferases from human and rat
    liver. Biochim. Biophys. Acta, 398:205 (1975).
8. A. Chaudhari, M. Anderson and T. Eling, Conjugation of 15-keto
    prostaglandins by glutathione S-transferases. Biochim.
    Biophys. Acta, 531:56 (1978).
9. M. Hamberg and B. Samuelsson, Metabolism of prostaglandin
    E_2 in guinea pig liver. Pathways in the formation of the
    major metabolites. J. Biol. Chem., 246:1073 (1971).
10. E. Granström, Structures of C_{14} metabolites of prostaglandin
    $F_{2\alpha}$. Adv. Biosci. 9:7 (1973).
11. M. Hamberg and M. Wilson, Structures of new metabolites of
    Prostaglandin E_2 in man. Ibid, p.39 (1973).
12. F. Sun and J. Stafford, Metabolism of prostaglandin $F_{2\alpha}$ in
    Rhesus monkeys. Biochim. Biophys.Acta, 369:95 (1974).
13. C. Ellis, M. Smigel, J. Oates, O. Oelz and S. Sweetman,
    Metabolism of prostaglandin D_2 in the monkey. J. Biol. Chem.,
    254:4152 (1979).
14. E. Granström and B. Samuelsson, Quantitative measurement of
    prostaglandins and thromboxanes: General considerations. In:
    "Advances in Prostaglandin and Thromboxane Research".
    Vol. 5, Ed. J. Frölich, Raven Press, New York, (1978), pp.
    1-13.
15. C. Leslie and L. Levine, Evidence for the presence of a
    prostaglandin E_2 9-ketoreductase in rat organs. Biochem.
    Biophys. Res. Commun. 52:717 (1973).
16. K. Stone and M. Hart, Prostaglandin E_2-9-ketoreductase in
    rabbit kidney. Prostaglandins 10:273 (1975).
17. C. Pace-Asciak and D. Miller, Prostaglandins during develop-
    ment. II. Identification of prostaglandin 9-hydroxydehydro-
    genase activity in adult rat kidney. Experientia 30:590
    (1974).
18. C. Pace-Asciak, Prostaglandins during development. III.
    Prostaglandin 9-hydroxydehydrogenase activity in the adult
    rat kidney. Identification, assay, pathway and some
    properties. J. Biol. Chem., 250:2789 (1975).

19. P. Moore and J. Hoult, Distribution of four prostaglandin-metabolising enzymes in organs of the rabbit. Biochem. Pharmacol., 27:1839 (1978).

20. P. Wong, K. Malik, F. Sun, W. Lee and J. McGiff, Hepatic metabolism of PGI_2 in the rabbit: Formation of a potent inhibitor of platelet aggregation. Abstr. IV International Prostaglandin Conference, Washington D.C., May 1979.

21. J. Weeks, D. Ducharme, W. Magee, W. Miller, The biological activity of the (15s)-15-methyl analogs of prostaglandins E_2 and $F_{2\alpha}$. J. Pharmacol. Exp. Ther., 186:67 (1973).

22. B. Magerlein, D. Ducharme, W. Magee, W. Miller, A. Robert and J. Weeks, Synthesis and biological properties of 16-alkyl-prostaglandins. Prostaglandins, 4:143 (1973).

23. B. Magerlein and W. Miller, 16-Fluoroprostaglandins. Prostaglandins, 9:527 (1975).

24. H. Ohno, Y. Morikawa and F. Hirata, Studies on 15-hydroxy-prostaglandin dehydrogenase with various prostaglandin analogues. J. Biochem., 84:1485 (1978).

25. M. O. Pulkkinen, Pregnancy termination with the PGE_2 analogue SHB 286 Prostaglandins, 15:161 (1978).

26. D. Binder, J. Bowler, E. Brown, N. Crossley. J. Hutton, M. Senior, L. Slater, P. Wilkinson and N. Wright, 16-Aryloxy-prostaglandins: a new class of potent luteolytic agents. Prostaglandins, 6:87 (1974).

27. K. Green, B. Samuelsson and J. Magerlein, Decreased rate of metabolism induced by a shift of the double bond in prosta-glandin $F_{2\alpha}$ from the Δ^5 to the Δ^4 position. Eur. J. Biochem. 62:527 (1976).

28. G. Tarpley and F. Sun, Metabolism of cis-Δ^4-15(S)-15-methyl-prostaglandin $F_{1\alpha}$ methyl ester in the rat. J. Med. Chem., 21:288 (1978).

29. M. Hamberg, J. Svensson and B. Samuelsson, Thromboxanes: A new group of biologically active compounds derived from prostaglandin endoperoxides. Proc. Natl. Acad. Sci. USA, 72:2994 (1975).

30. H. Kindahl, Metabolism of thromboxane B_2 in the cynomolgus monkey. Prostaglandins 13:619 (1977).

31. J. Roberts II, B. Sweetman, J. Morgan, N. Payne and J. Oates, Identification of the major urinary metabolite of thromboxane B_2 in the monkey. Prostaglandins, 13:631 (1977).

32. J. Roberts II, B. Sweetman and J. Oates, Metabolism of thromboxane B_2 in the monkey. J. Biol. Chem., 253:5305 (1978).

33. J. Roberts II, B. Sweetman, N. Payne and J. Oates, Metabolism of thromboxane B_2 in man. Identification of the major urinary metabolite. J. Biol. Chem., 252:7415 (1977).

34. J. Svensson, Structure and quantitative determination of the major urinary metabolite of thromboxane B_2 in the guinea pg. Prostaglandins 17:351 (1979).

35. P. Piper and J. Vane, Release of additional factors in anaphylaxis and its antagonism by anti inflammatory drugs, Nature, 223:29 (1969).

36. M. Hamberg, J. Svensson, P. Hedqvist, K. Strandberg and B. Samuelsson, Involvement of endoperoxides and thromboxanes in anaphylactic reactions. In: "Advances in Prostaglandin and Thromboxane Research", B. Samuelsson and R. Paoletti, eds., Raven Press, New York, Vol. 1, pp.495-501 (1976).

37. W. Dawson, J. Boot, A. Cockerill, D. Mallen and D. Osborne, Release of novel prostaglandins and thromboxanes after immunological challenge of guinea pig lung. Nature, 262:699 (1976).

38. J. Boot, W. Dawson, A. Cockerill, D. Mallen and D. Osborne, The pharmacology of prostaglandin like substances released from guinea pig lungs during anaphylaxis. Prostaglandins, 13:927 (1977).

39. J. Boot, A. Cockerill, W. Dawson, D. Mallen and D. Osborne, Modification of prostaglandin and thromboxane release by immunological sensitisation and successive immunological challenges from guinea-pig lung. Int. Arch. Allergy Appl. Immunol. 57:159 (1978).

40. F. Fitzpatrick and R. Gorman, Platelet rich plasma tranforms exogenous prostaglandin H_2 into thromboxane A_2. Prostaglandins 14:881 (1977).

41. J. Maclouf, H. Kindahl, E. Granström and B. Samuelsson, Thromboxane A_2 and prostaglandin endoperoxide H_2 form covalently linked derivatives with human serum albumin. In: "Advances in Prostaglandin and Thromboxane Research", Vol. 6, Eds. B. Samuelssen, P. Ramwell, R. Pooletti, Raven Press, New York (1980) p.283.

42. G. Folco, E. Granström and H. Kindahl, Albumin stabilizes thromboxane A_2. FEBS Lett, 82:321 (1977).

43. J. Smith, C. Ingerman and M. Silver, Persistence of thromboxane A_2-like material and platelet release-inducing activity in plasma. J. Clin. Invest. 58:1119 (1976).

44. C. Pace-Asciak, M. Carrara and Z. Domazet, Identification of the major urinary metabolites of 6-keto-prostaglandin $F_{1\alpha}$ (6K-PGF$_{1\alpha}$) in the rat. Biochem. Biophys. Res. Commun. 78:115 (1977).

45. C. Pace-Asciak, Z. Domazet and M. Carrara, Catabolism of 6-keto-prostaglandin $F_{1\alpha}$ by the rat kidney cortex. Biochim. Biophys. Acta, 487:400 (1977).

46. J. McGuire and F. Sun, Metabolism of prostacyclin. Oxidation by rhesus monkey lung 15-hydroxyl prostaglandin dehydrogenase. Arch. Biochem. Biophys. 189:92 (1978).

47. F. Sun and B. Taylor, Metabolism of prostacyclin in rat. Biochemistry, 17:4096 (1978).

48. F. Sun, B. Taylor, D. Sutter and J. Weeks, Metabolism of prostacyclin. III. Urinary metabolite profile of 6-keto PGF$_{1\alpha}$ in rat. Prostaglandins, 17:753 (1979).

49. G. Dusting, S. Moncada and J. Vane, Recirculation of prostacyclin (PGI$_2$) in the dog. Br. J. Pharmac., 64:315 (1978).

50. P. Wong, J. McGiff, F. Sun and K. Malik, Pulmonary metabolism
     of prostacyclin (PGI$_2$) in the rabbit. Biochem. Biophys. Res.
     Commun., 83:731 (1978).
51. H. Hawkins, J. Smith, K. Nicolaou and T. Eling, Studies of
     the mechanisms involved in the fate of prostacyclin (PGI$_2$)
     and 6-keto-PGF$_{1\alpha}$ in the pulmonary circulation. Prostaglandins,
     16:871 (1978).
52. P. Wong, F. Sun and J. McGiff, Metabolism of prostacyclin in
     blood vessels. J. Biol. Chem., 253:5555 (1978).
53. P. Wong, J. McGiff, L. Cagen, K. Malik and F. Sun, Metabolism
     of prostacyclin in the rabbit kidney. J. Biol. Chem., 254:
     12 (1979).
54. A. Cockerill, D. Mallen, D. Osborne, J. Boot and W. Dawson,
     The identification of two novel prostaglandins and a
     thromboxane. Prostaglandins, 13:1033 (1977).
55. S. Moncada, R. Korbut, S. Bunting and J. Vane, Prostacyclin
     is a circulating hormone. Nature, 273:767 (1978).
56. H. Waldman, I. Alter, P. Kot, J. Rose and P. Ramwell, Effect
     of lung transit on systemic depressor responses to arachidonic
     acid and prostacyclin in dogs. J. Pharmacol. Exp. Ther.
     204:289 (1978).
57. B. Taylor and F. Sun, Hepatic metabolism of prostacyclin in
     the rat. Abstr. IV. International Prostaglandin Conference,
     Washington D.C., May 1979.
58. P. Needleman, S. Bronson, A. Wycke, M. Sivakoff and K. Nicolaou,
     Cardiac and renal prostaglandin I$_2$. Biosynthesis and
     biological effects in isolated perfused rabbit tissues. J.
     Clin. Invest. 61:839 (1978).
59. C. Pace-Asciak and A. Rosenthal, Comparison between the in
     vivo rates of matabolism of PGI$_2$ and its blood pressure
     lowering effect after intravenous administration in the rat.
     Abstr. IV International Prostaglandin Conference, Washington
     D.C., May 1979.
60. R. Gryglewski, R. Korbut, A. Ocetkiewicz and T. Stachwa,
     In vivo method for quantitation of anti-platelet potency
     of drugs. Naunyn-Schmiedebergs Archs.Pharmacol, 302:25
     (1978).
61   F. Sun, K. Malik, J. McGiff and P. Wong, Evidence for a one
     carbon degradation pathway in the metabolism of PGI$_2$ by
     rabbit kidney. Abstr. IV International Prostaglandin
     Conference, Washington D.C., May 1979.

BASIC BIOCHEMISTRY OF PROSTAGLANDIN METABOLISM WITH ESPECIAL

REFERENCE TO PGDH

Roderick J. Flower

Department of Prostaglandin Research
Wellcome Research Laboratories Langley Court
Beckenham, Kent, U.K.

The mammalian organism possesses extremely efficient mechamisms for the catabolism of PGs and hence their biological inactivation. The effeciency of certain vascular beds – for example, the lung – in inactivating PGs is well illustrated by the observations of Ferreira and Vane (18), who found that more than 95% of infused PGE_2 was inactivated during one circulation through the lungs and by those of Hamberg and Samuelsson (26), who showed that only 3% of an intravenous bolus injection of tritiated PGE_2 remained in the plasma after 90 s. After 4.5 min there was no detectable PGE_2 at all.

Tissue or blood concentrations of PGs must therefore be regarded as a net result of the activity of two sorts of enzymes: those which biosynthesise and those which inactivate PGs. If PGs are important in physiological or pathological responses then it is clear that the activity of the catabolic enzymes could have a crucial effect on the duration and intensity of any such response.

In this chapter we will consider the basic biochemistry of what is arguably the most important prostaglandin metabolising enzyme: NAD^+-dependent prostaglandin 15-dehydrogenase. Other metabolising enzymes will also be briefly mentioned, and the physiological regulation of these enzymes discussed.

A GENERAL OVERVIEW OF PROSTAGLANDIN CATABOLISM

Enzymic mechanisms exist (at least for PGs of the E or F series) whereby the biological activity of the PG molecule is rapidly destroyed, the metabolite being excreted in the urine after successive modifications of the native structure. Broadly

speaking, these reactions are of two types: an initial (relatively
rapid) step, catalyzed by PG specific enzymes, whereby PGs lose
most of their biological activity, and a second (relatively slow)
step in which those metabolites are oxidised by enzyme (probably)
identical to those responsible for the β- and γ-oxidation of
fatty acids in general. This sequence of reactions has been
investigated in man (26) and the degradation of PGE_2 is summarised
in Figure 1a and b.

      The initial step in this degradation is the oxidation of the
15-hydroxyl group to the corresponding ketone under the influence
of the enzyme PGDH (3,26). The 15-keto compound is then transformed
into the 13,14-dihydro compound, a reaction catalyzed by the
enzyme prostaglandin Δ^{13}-reductase (3,4,2). The first two reactions
occur very rapidly, but subsequent steps are probably slower.
These consist of oxidation of the β- and ω-side chains of the PGs
giving rise to a more polar product (a dicarboxylic acid) which is
excreted in the urine as the major metabolite both PGE_1 and PGE_2.
A similar situation obtains with PGs of the F series: Thus, in
man the major plasma metabolites of $PGF_{2\alpha}$ and PGE_2 are the
corresponding 13,14-dihydro-15-keto compounds whilst 5_α 7_α-dihydroxy
-11-keto-tetranor-prostane-1, 16-dioic acid (PGF-MUM) and 7_α-
hydroxy-5,11-diketo-prostane-1, 16-dioic acid (PGE-MUM) are the
main urinary metabolites (MUM) of PGF and PGE respectively. The
di-acid metabolite of PGF may also exist as a ᶴ-lactone. Several
other products of metabolism of prostaglandins in primates have
been identified (22-24, 21, 28, 75). The kinetics of
these reactions are of interest; in the experiments of Hamberg
and Samuelsson (26) only 3% of an original tritiated PGE_2
injection was present in the blood after 90s, the bulk of
the radioactivity in the plasma being present as the 13,14-dihydro-
15-keto metabolite; this metabolite itself only had a half-life
of some 8 min in the circulation. Samuelsson et al (67)
administered tritiated $PGF_{2\alpha}$ to human subjects and measured the
excretion rate of tritium (present mainly as the dioic
metabolite) into the urine. Approximately 40% was excreted during
the first 30 min, almost 80% after 2 h had maximal excretion,
about 90% had occurred after 4 h. Similar studies have also
been performed in the rat (25,72) and guinea pig (27). In each
case, the initial transformations (i.e. oxidation of the C-15
hydroxy group and saturation of the 13,14 double bond) were
observed but the final product of the ω- and β-oxidising systems,
whilst similar to that in man, was not identical.

      PGD_2 is not a substrate for PGDH (74) and consequently this
prostaglandin has longer biological half life than PGE or
PGF. PGA is a substrate for PGDH in vitro but it appears to
traverse the lungs without deactivation presumably because it is
not a substrate for the uptake mechanism (46).

PGI$_2$, itself, is a relatively good substrate for PGDH but the breakdown product, 6-keto-PGF$_{1\alpha}$ was metabolised at only 10% the rate of PGE$_2$ (74,55). 6-keto-PGF$_{1\alpha}$ is also a poor substrate for prostaglandin Δ^{13}-reductase (55), thus, 6,15-diketo-PGF$_{1\alpha}$ may be expected to be the major circulating metabolite. Pace-Asciak, et al. (54) demonstrated that a considerable amount (ca 30%) of

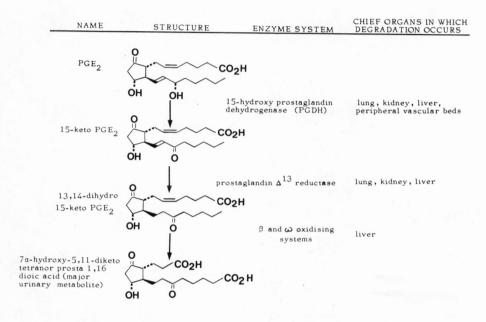

Fig. 1a. Metabolism of prostaglandin E$_2$ in man.

the 6-keto-PGF$_{1\alpha}$ administered to rats was excreted unchanged; these investigators also identified dinor-6-keto-PGF$_{1\alpha}$ as urinary metabolites. Sun et al. (74) reported that the urinary metabolites of PGI$_2$ have a 15-keto group (whereas metabolites of 6-keto-PGF$_{1\alpha}$ have a 15-hydroxy group) thus implying that PGI$_2$ is metabolised under the influence of 15-PGDH although 6-keto-PGF$_{1\alpha}$ is not. However, prostacyclin and 6-keto-PGF$_{1\alpha}$ appear to be metabolised at approximately the same rate in vivo, since plasma levels obtained during infusion of both compounds at the same rate were very similar but were approximately ten times higher than the plasma

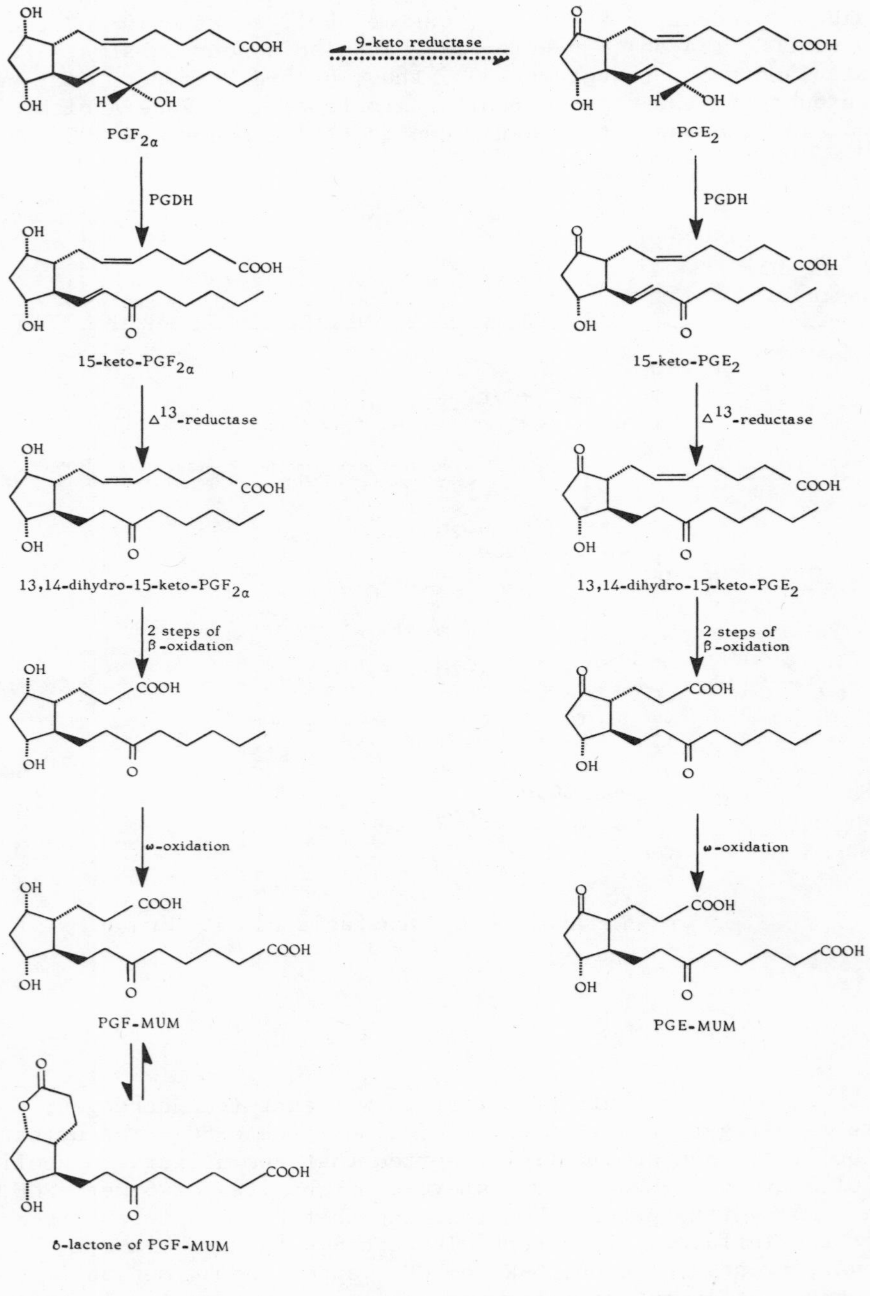

Fig. 1b. Summary of the main metabolite transformations of $PGF_{2\alpha}$
and PGE_2.

level of $PGF_{2\alpha}$ obtained after a comparable infusion into dogs (17).

A novel compound believed to be a metabolite of TXB_2 was identified as 13,14-dihydro-15-keto-TXB_2 by Dawson et al (14). The compound was obtained during infusion of arachidonic acid through antigen-challenged guinea pig lungs. The major urinary metabolite of TXB_2 in man was identified as 2,3-dinor-TXB_2 (63).

The presence of a specific enzyme, 9-keto reductase, which causes the 9-keto group of PGE to be reduced to the corresponding hydroxyl compound (i.e. to PGF), has been demonstrated in kidney of monkey (37), pig (38) and rabbit (71).

Enzymes in plasma have also been described which cause dehydration of PGE to PGA (39) isomerisation of PGA to PGC (33) and isomerisation of PGC to PGB (62). However, these enzymatic conversions appear to be of minor importance. In fact, the observation of dehydrase activity may be suspect and the formation of PGA could arise as an artifact of the extraction techniques employed.

Tissue Distribution of Catabolising Enzymes

Enzymes which catalyse PG degradation are widely distributed throughout the animal body, being present in the kidney of several species (4,52,53,44,45,50) and intestine (4), isolated rat liver and testicle (16,49,50), as well as guinea pig lung (3). Anggard et al. (2) studied the distribution of PGDH and PG-Δ^{13} reductase in swine tissue and found that both of the enzymes were located in the 100.1000 g supernatant of cell-free homogenates. The tissues with the highest reductase activity was found in the spleen, liver, kidney, adrenals and small intestine. The highest activity of PGDH per g of tissue, however, was found in adipose tissue.

The enzymes responsible for β- or ω-oxidation are found in the liver (66-67), in lung and kidney (48) and intestine (59). The liver is probably the major site of side chain oxidation.

The lungs are a rich source of both the PGDH and the Δ^{13}-reductase enzyme. Because of the reduction of biological activity, which is a consequence of metabolism as well as the unique position of the lungs between venous and arterial circulation, the pulmonary circulation constitutes an important barrier through which many PGs which have potent smooth muscle stimulating, cardiovascular or other actions cannot normally pass and are thus prevented from reaching target organs via the arterial circulation.

The significance of the pulmonary vascular bed as a site of PG inactivation in vivo was first demonstrated by Ferreira and

Vane (18). Although stable in blood, greater than 95% of infused
PGE_1 or PGE_2 (0.5-1 µg/min) were removed during one passage
through cat lungs, as determined by bioassay. Similar effects
were observed when the experiment was repeated in dogs and
rabbits. Other vascular beds such as those of liver and hind
quarters also inactivated PGs although not so effectively. The
same year, McGiff et al. (43), using changes in dog renal blood
flow as an index of PG concentration in the arterial blood,
confirmed that PGE_1 and PGE_2 were rapidly inactivated by the lung,
whereas PGA_1 and PGA_2 were not. This finding was in qualitative
if not quantitative agreement with the kinetic data obtained
in vitro (4). The authors thus speculated that the A-series are
the only PGs likely to act as circulating hormones. Horton and
Jones (30) have confirmed that a single passage through the
pulmonary circulation of the cat or dog causes substantial losses
of the vasodilator activity of PGE_1 but not of PGA_1. Perfused
lungs in vitro can also inactivate PGs, an effect which seems
to be due to the action of PGDH (61).

Loss of Biological Activity with Metabolism

Because PGs possess extremely potent pharmacological activity,
an important consideration is the stage of the metabolic sequence
at which this loss occurs; Anggard and Samuelsson (5) and Anggard
(1) synthetised the 13,14-dihydro-PGE_1, 15-keto-13,14-dihydro-PGE_1
and compared the biological activity (smooth muscle contractile
and vasodepressor effects in the guinea pig and rabbit) with
that of the parent molecule. Figure 2 shows the loss of
biological activity in the guinea pig which occurs on successive
modifications of the PGE_1 molecule. After saturation of the 13,14
double bond the molecule still retains a significant proportion of
its biological activity, indeed, the vasodepressor effect is
somewhat greater. Biological activity is, however, greatly
attenuated when the 15-hydroxyl group is oxidized, and virtually
disappears when both modifications are introduced. Qualitatively
similar results were seen when the metabolites were tested for
smooth muscle contractile and vasodepressor activity in the
rabbit. Nakano (46) reported that the vasodilator actions of
13,14-dihydro-E_1, 15-keto-E_1 and 15-keto-13,14-dihydro-PGE_1
were approximately 1/4, 1/80 and 1/100 of PGE_1 in dog hind limb
preparations. As inhibitors of platelet aggregation, Kloeze (35)
found that the 13,14-dihydro derivative of PGE_1 had an activity
of 0.64 relative to the parent molecule and that the 15-keto
compound was inactive. The 15-keto-13,14-dihydro-PGE_2 has
been shown by Pike et al. (60) to have little spasmogenic activity
on many smooth muscle preparations. 15-keto-$PGF_{2\alpha}$, however, has
up to ten times the contractile activity of the parent molecule
on smooth muscle preparations including human bronchial muscle
and guinea pig trachea (15) and is also a more potent pressor
agent (34).

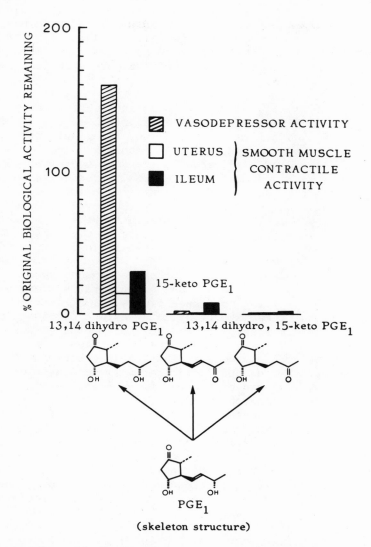

Fig. 2.   Loss of vasodepressor and smooth muscle contracting activity
(guinea pig), after metabolic transformation. This information is based on data published by Anggard (1966).
Biological activity was assayed in the guinea pig.

Biochemistry of PGDH

As the enzyme which initiates the inactivation of compounds of high biological activity such as prostaglandins, PGDH has been compared in its importance by Marazzi and Andersen (40) to enzymes such as cholinesterase and phosphodiesterase. Of all the metabolising enzymes PGDH has received the most attention from biochemists.

Anggard and Samuelsson (4) were also the first workers to isolate and purify PGDH and used swine lung as a source. Using ammonium sulphate and column chromatography (TEAE-cellulose, Sephadex G100, hydroxyapatite, and DEAE Sephadex), they were able to isolate an enzyme that was shown to be NAD^+ dependent and specific for the C-15 hydroxyl group of PGs. Prostaglandin E_1 was the best substrate tested, the relative reaction rates of PGE_2 and PGE_3 being 0.97 and 0.6, respectively ($PGE_1 = 1$). The reaction rate of 13,14-dihydro PGE_1 was 0.2 compared to PGE_1. Among the F series, $PGF_{1\alpha}$ had a relative reaction rate of 0.75, $F_{2\alpha}$ and $F_{3\alpha}$, 0.62. Dehydration products of PGEs had the following relative reaction rates, PGA_1, 0.45 and PGA_2 0.33; PGB_1 or B_2 were not substrates for the enzyme. Several other compounds, such as steroids, alcohols, hydroxy acids, and carbohydrates, were not oxidized at all, indicating good specificity. The reaction rate rose with increasing temperatures up to a maximum of 55°C after which denaturation occurred; little dependence on pH between 6 and 8 was noted. Vonkeman et al. (76) have extended this work on the specificity of the enzyme to include several PGs that do not occur naturally and concluded that a fixed length of carboxyl and/or alkyl chain of PGs was unimportant for oxidation. Thus PGs, which are biologically active yet not known to occur naturally, are metabolized and lose biological activity in the same way as do the native compounds. Shio et al. (69) have published data on the specificity of the swine lung enzyme. They noted that the enzyme was stereospecific for the C-15 (S)-configuration, thus confirming the observations of Nakano et al. (47). The latter authors also noted that while the constituents of the cyclopentane ring were relatively unimportant, the nature of the carboxyl side chain was.

Marrazzi and Matschinsky (41) published a careful study of the PGDH from swine lung and elucidated its structural requirements for substrate binding as well as for inhibition by substrate and cofactor analogs. Unlike that of Anggard and Samuelsson their enzyme preparation was very sensitive to changes of pH between 6 and 8. Marrazzi et al. (42) found that swine lung PGDH was reversible and could catalyze the reduction of 15-keto PGE_1. During the reaction, however, an inhibitor accumulated, which rendered the reaction quasi-irreversible.

Purified PGDH has been isolated from beef lungs by Saeed and Roy (65) who reported an increased specific activity over the swine lung enzyme. Shannahan et al. (1974), quoted in Marazzi and Andersen, (40) have also reported purification of a beef lung enzyme. Table 1 gives a brief resume of the biochemical properties of some lung PGDH enzymes.

Inhibition of PGDH

Obvious candidates for inhibitors of all enzymes are substrate analogs. Nakano et al. (1969) found that swine lung PGDH was noncompetitively inhibited by a synthetic epimer of PGE_1, 15-R-PGE_1 and that the B-type PGs (though not substrates) were also non-competitive inhibitors; dihydro PGE_1 and 8-iso PGE_1 were inactive. Fried et al. (20) found that several PG analogs were active against the dehydrogenase from human placenta. Marrazzi and Matschinsky (41), using swine lung, found that a derivative of $PGF_{1\alpha}$, 7-oxa $PGF_{1\alpha}$ (oxygen substituted at C-7), had the same V_{max} as the original substrate (but much lower affinity), and various stereoisomers of this derivative (15-epimer, the optical antipode, and an analog with both of these modifications) all showed mixed inhibitors of PGDH, as did several fatty acids (arachidonic, linolenic, and oleic, and their respective coenzyme A derivatives). Polyphloretin phosphate (PPP), a high molecular weight polymer of phloretin (which antagonizes some of the actions of PGs on smooth muscle, (8) was also a competitive inhibitor of the enzyme but SC19222, another antagonist, (8) was not.

The foregoing compounds were inhibitors at the substrate site of the enzyme. With regard to the cofactor site, Marazzi and Matschinsky (41) found that certain NAD^+ analogues or derivatives were inhibitory and a range of substituted pyridines were noncompetitive inhibitors. Several nucleosides and nucleotides, in concentrations of 3 to 10 mM, were also active, as were the methylxanthines, caffeine, and theophylline as well as amino-phylline. Among compounds inactive against the preparation were the barbiturates.

The aspirin-like drugs are inhibitors of PG synthesis (see above), and it has been subsequently found that indomethacin inhibits the NAD^+ dependent destruction of PGE_1 or E_2 by the high-speed supernatant of dog spleen (19). Cheung and Cushman (unpublished observations 1972) found that some other aspirin-like drugs inhibited the rabbit lung dehydrogenase. Indomethacin, in concentrations of 1 mM, gave a 93% inhibition of PGE_2 metabolism, niflumic acid in a concentration inhibited 14%. Aspirin, naproxen, ibuprofen, phenylbutazone, and benzydamine were inactive. Hansen (29) reported inhibition of a purified bovine lung PGDH by indomethacin($K_i = 1.4 \times 10^{-4}M$) and aspirin. Indomethacin inhibition was noncompetitive.

TABLE 1

Some Properties of Lung PGDH

Parameter	Source			
	Swine lung[a]	Swine lung[b]	Beef lung[c]	Beef lung[d]
pH optimum	8.5-9.0	>8.0	$\approx$9.0	–
Approximate molecular weight (Daltons)	$60\text{-}70 \times 10^3$	20×10^3	20×10^3	40×10^3
Specific activity (nmole) NAD$^+$ reduced/min/mg protein)	$0.13\text{-}0.65 \times 10^{-3}$	4.2	1.0	1.4 mU/mg[e]
K_m PGE$_1$ (μm)	$\approx$10.0	1.14	4.0	3.4
K_m NAD$^+$ (μm)	200.0	60.0	–	110.0

[a]Anggard 1971

[b]Marazzi and Matschinsky 1972

[c]Shanahan et al. quoted in Marazzi and Anderson 1974

[d]Hansen 1974

[e]1 unit here is identified as the amount of enzyme that oxidized 1 μmol PGE$_1$/min at saturating PGE$_1$ and NAD$^+$ concentrations.

One study supports the concept that aspirin-like drugs can inhibit lung dehydrogenase in vivo. Jackson and associates (32) studied the pulmonary inactivation of PGF$_{2\alpha}$ during one passage through the pulmonary circulation of dogs. In these experiments the mean inactivation of PGF$_{2\alpha}$ on passage through the lungs (6 dogs) was 91.9%. After treatment with aspirin, 50 mg/kg repeated hourly, there was a small but statistically highly significant decrease (almost 10%) in the inactivation. When the same experiment was performed in sheep, however, aspirin was inactive, indicating perhaps a species difference. Against these results one must balance the results of Hamberg and Samuelsson (27) who found that administration of indomethacin (50 mg/day) to guinea pigs did not change the metabolism of tritiated PGE_2 in vivo.

It is not known how aspirin-like drugs inhibit PGDH. However, the salicylates are known to inhibit several dehydrogenases (70), probably by competing for the cofactor site, so possibly a similar action could account for the inhibition of PGDH. It seems, from what limited data are available, that the concentrations required to inhibit the synthetase are considerably less than those that produce a corresponding inhibition of the dehydrogenase.

Crutchley and Piper (12) performed parallel investigations on the inhibition of pulmonary removal of prostalgandins by isolated guinea pig lungs and the inhibition of prostaglandin metabolism by a crude enzyme preparation from guinea pig lung homogenates. Polyphloretin phospate as well as diphloretin phosphate (DPP), in doses of 0.1 to 5 µg/ml of the perfusing fluid, inhibited the inactivation of PGE_2, $F_{2\alpha}$ and $F_{2\beta}$ and therefore increased the amount of PGs surviving passage through the lungs. Both agents also inhibited the crude enzyme preparation. Polyphloretin phosphate had no effect on the pulmonary inactivation of bradykinin or 5-hydroxytryptamine by isolated guinea pig lungs. A number of metabolic inhibitors and sulphydryl binding reagents were also tested: 2,4 dinitrophenol was inactive at doses of 0.5 mM, whereas iodoacetate was inactive at 0.25 mM but showed weak activity (about 10.) at 0.5 mM. In doses of 3 mM 2:3-dimercaptopropanol was inactive; disulfiram showed no significant inhibition at 6 µM. Two suphydryl binding agents sodium p-chloromercuriphenylsulphonate and N-ethylmaleimide were, however, active, having an ID_{50} of 0.6 mM and 70 µM, respectively. Both these agents were also active against the crude enzyme preparation. The same authors also tried some anti-inflammatory agents: phenylbutazone (50 µg/ml) and indomethacin(20 µg/ml) showed slight activity (a reduction of 40% and 10%. respectively) but aspirin, paracetamol, ibuprofen and meclofenamic acid were inactive.

In a later paper the same authors (13) investigated the actions of one of these agents (DPP) in the rabbit in vivo. By infusing PGE_2 and $PGF_{2\alpha}$ into the superior vena cava and comparing the response with that of an infusion into the aorta, a measure of pulmonary inactivation was obtained. Diphloretin phosphate potentiated, 25 to 100 times, the depressor effects of the PGs and also the effects on gastrointestinal motility, as measured by a balloon in the jejunum.

More recently Hoult and Moore (31) have demonstrated that sulphasalazine is a potent inhibitor (ID_{50} = 50 µM) of rabbit colon PGDH.

Uptake of Prostaglandins into Cells Prior to Metabolism

The exact mechanics of PG metabolism by the lungs are not entirely clear. It seems very likely that the hydrolytic enzymes responsible for the metabolism of AMP, angiotensin I, bradykinin, and ATP (64) are located close to the luminal surface of the pulmonary vascular endothelium. Sander and Huggins (68) have suggested that the angiotensin I converting enzymes are located on the external surface of the plasma membrane. As mentioned before, PGDH resists sedimentation at 100,000 x g and is therefore presumably a soluble cytoplasmic enzyme. This being the case, it would seem that at least three steps are involved in the metabolism of PGs by the lung: (a) entry of PGs into the cell cytoplasm, (b) metabolism per se, and (c) release of metabolites from the cell. Because of the complexity of this process, one might anticipate a delay in the clearance of PGs and their metabolites from the lung when compared, for example, to the passage of a high molecular weight compound unlikely to leave the vascular space. Ryan et al. (64) have shown that such delay does indeed occur in the washout of labelled PG metabolites from rat lungs. Exactly how PGs enter the cells and PG metabolites leave is not clear. Transport mechanisms for PGs are thought to exist in some tissues (9), but while metabolism is a temperature-dependent process (61), it is not sensitive to metabolic poisons (12) so presumably the transport process (if there is one) is not directly energy linked.

Regulation of PGDH

Although few accurate details are known concerning the physiological regulation of PGDH activity there are clues in the literature strongly suggesting that the cellular levels of PGDH do indeed vary in response to physiological events, and that this effect may well be mediated by hormones.

Actually, PGDH is apparently quite a short lived enzyme within the cell, the replacement of which depends on continual protein synthesis (11). This fact suggests that the enzyme is under fairly tight control. It is known that the levels of PGDH in the lung of guinea pigs falls dramatically after exposure of the animals to 100% oxygen (58).

There are also reports that the levels of PGDH (and the Δ^{13} reductase) in the lung and kidneys of rats changes with age (56). Perhaps the most well studied effect is the increase in PGDH activity seen during pregnancy – especially near term – in rats and rabbits (7,10,73). Since the uterus is especially sensitive to prostaglandins during pregnancy this could be regarded as a safety mechanism to prevent uterotropic substances from reaching the uterus. Blackwell and Flower (10) found that the levels of

PGDH in the rat lung could be changed by steroid treatment: oestradiol depressed PGDH activity whereas ovariectomy or progesterone elevated enzyme levels, possibly accounting for the fluctuations seen during pregnancy.

Pathological conditions may also alter enzyme levels: acute hydration of dehydrated rats led to a decrease in PGDH in the loop of Henle (52). Endotoxin shock in rats also reduces PGDH levels (51) perhaps partially accounting for the high prostaglandin levels in such animals.

Two interesting cases of "inborn errors of metabolism" have been reported in connection with PGDH. Labrum et al. (36) noted the case of a woman with "hyperprostaglandinemia" thought to be secondary to a deficiency of PGDH. Secondly, genetic hypertension in rats is accompanied by abnormally low renal PGDH levels and this could explain the genesis of the hypertension (6).

REFERENCES

1. E. Anggard, The biological activities of three metabolites of prostaglandin E_1. Acta physiol. scand., 66:509-511 (1966).
2. E. Anggard, C. Larsson and B. Samuelsson, The distribution of 15-hydroxyprostaglandin dehydrogenase and prostaglandin Δ^{13} reductase in tissues of the swine. Acta Physiol. Scand., 81:396-404 (1971).
3. E. Anggard and B. Samuelsson, Prostaglandins and related factors. 28. Metabolism of prostaglandin E_1 in guinea pig lungs: the structures of two metabolites. J. biol. Chem., 239:4087-4102 (1964).
4. E. Anggard and B. Samuelsson, Purification and properties of a 15-hydroxy prostaglandin dehydrogenase from swine lung. Prostaglandins and related factors 55. Ark. kemi, 25:293-300 (1966).
5. E. Anggard and B. Samuelsson, The metabolism of prostaglandins in lung tissue. In: "Prostaglandins", Nobel Symposium 2, New York, Interscience, pp.97-105 (1967).
6. J. M. Armstrong, G. J. Blackwell, R. J.Flower, J. C. McGiff, K. M. Mullane and J. R. Vane, Genetic hypertension in rats is accompanied by a defect in renal prostaglandin catabolism. Nature, 260:582-586 (1976).
7. J. R. Bedwani and P. B. Marley, Increased inactivation of prostaglandin E_2 by the rabbit lung during pregnancy. Br. J. Pharmcol., 50:459P (1974).
8. A. Bennett, Prostaglandin antagonists. In: "Advances in Drug Research", A. B. Simmonds, ed. Academic Press, London pp.83-118 (1975).

9. L. Z. Bito, Accumulation and apparent active transport of
    prostaglandins by some rabbit tissues in vitro. J. Physiol.,
    221:371-387 (1972).

10. G. J. Blackwell and R. J. Flower, Effects of steroid hormones
    on tissue levels of prostaglandin 15-hydroxydehydrogenase in
    the rat. Br. J. Pharmac., 56:343P (1976).

11. G. J. Blackwell, R. J. Flower and J.R. Vane, Rapid reduction
    of prostaglandin 15-hydroxydehydrogenase activity in rat
    tissues after treatment with protein synthesis inhibitors.
    Br. J. Pharmac., 55:233-238 (1975).

12. D. J. Crutchley and P. J. Piper, Prostaglandin inactivation
    in guinea pig lung and its inhibition. Br. J. Pharmac.,
    52:197-203 (1974).

13. D. J. Crutchley and P. J. Piper, Inhibition of the pulmonary
    inactivation of prostaglandins in rabbit in vivo. Br. J.
    Pharmac., 53:467P (1975).

14. W. Dawson, J. R. Boot, A. F. Cockerill, D. N. B. Mallen and
    D. J. Osborne, Release of novel prostaglandins and thromboxanes
    after immunological challenge of guinea-pig lung, Nature, Lond.,
    262:699 (1976).

15. W. Dawson, R. L. Lewis, R. E. Macmahone and W. J. F. Sweatman,
    Potent bronchoconstrictor activity of 15-keto prostaglandin
    $F_{2\alpha}$. Nature (Lond.), 250:331-332 (1974).

16. W. Dawson, P. W. Ramwell and J. Shaw, Metabolism of prosta-
    glandins by rat isolated liver. Br. J. Pharmac., 34:668-
    669 (1968).

17. J. A. Salmon, G. Dusting, S. Moncada, K. Mullane and J. R.
    Vane, Elimination of prostacyclin (PGI_2) and 6-oxo-$PGF_{1\alpha}$ in
    anaesthetized dogs. J. Pharm. Pharmac., 31:529-532 (1978).

18. S. H. Ferreira, and J. R. Vane, Prostaglandins: their
    disappearance from and release into the circulation.
    Nature (Lond.) 216:868-873 (1967).

19. R. J. Flower, Drugs which inhibit prostaglandin biosynthesis.
    Pharmac. Rev., 26:33-67 (1974).

20. J. Fried, M. M. Mehrer and B. J. Gaede, Novel selective
    inhibitors of human placental PG-15-dehydrogenase. In:
    Supplement to "Advances in the Biosciences", vol.9.
    International Conference on Prostaglandins, S. Bergstrom and
    S. Bernhard, eds., Vienna, Pergamon Press, Viewig,
    Braunschweig, p.18 (1973).

21. E. Granström, On the metabolism of prostaglandin $F_{2\alpha}$ in
    female subjects. Structures of two C14 metabolites. Eur. J.
    Biochem., 25:581-589 (1972).

22. E. Granström and B. Samuelsson, On the metabolism of
    prostaglandin $F_{2\alpha}$ in female subjects. J. biol. Chem., 246:
    5254-5263 (1971a).

23. E. Granström and B. Samuelsson, On the metabolism of
    prostaglandin $F_{2\alpha}$ in female subjects II. Structures of
    six metabolites. J. biol. Chem., 246:7470-7485 (1976).

24. E. Granström and B. Samuelsson, Structure of a deoxy-
    prostaglandin in man. J.Am.Chem.Soc., 94:4380-4381 (1972).

25. K. Green and B. Samuelsson, Quantitative studies on the synthesis in vivo of prostaglandins in the rat. Cold stress induced stimulation of synthesis. Eur. J. Biochem., 22: 39 1-395 (1971).

26. M. Hamberg and B. Samuelsson, On the metabolism of prostaglandins E_1 and E_2 in man. J. biol. Chem., 246:6713-6721 (1971).

27. M. Hamberg and B. Samuelsson, On the metabolism of prostaglandins E_1 and E_2 in the guinea pig. J. biol. Chem., 247: 3495-3502 (1972).

28. M. Hamberg and M. Wilson, Structures of new metabolites of postaglandin E_2 in man, In: "Advances in the Biosciences", S. Bergstrom ed., Vol.9, Pergamon Press, Oxford, p.39 (1973).

29. H. S. Hansen, Inhibition by indomethacin and aspirin of 15-hydroxy prostaglandin dehydrogenase in vitro. Prostaglandins, 8:95-105 (1974).

30. E. W. Horton and R. L. Jones, Prostaglandins A_1 A_2 and 19-hydroxy A_1; their actions on smooth muscle and their inactivation of passage through the pulmonary and hepatic portal vascular beds. Br. J. Pharmacol., 37:705-722 (1969).

31. J. R. S. Hoult and P. K. Moore, Sulphasalazine is a potent inhibitor of prostaglandin 15-hydroxydehydrogenase: Possible basis for therapeutic action in ulcerative colitis. Br. J. Pharmac., 64:6-8 (1968).

32. H. R. Jackson, R. D. Hall, R. L. Hodge, E. L. Gibson, F. P. Katik and M. Stevens, The effect of aspirin on the pulmonary extraction of $PGF_{2\alpha}$ and the cardiovascular response to $PGF_{2\alpha}$. Aust. J. Exp. Biol. Med. Sci., 51:837-846 (1973).

33. R. L. Jones, 15-hydroxy-9-oxoprosta-11, 13-dienoic acid as the product of a prostaglandin isomerase. J. Lipid. Res., 13: 511-518 (1972).

34. R. L. Jones, Actions of prostaglandins on the arterial system of the sheep: some structure-activity relationships. Br. J. Pharmac., 53:464P (1975).

35. J. Kloeze, Relationship between chemical structures and platelet-aggregation activity of prostaglandins. Biochim. biophys. Acta., 187:285-292 (1969).

36. A. H. Labrum, M. Lipkin Jr., and F. Dray, Hyperprostaglandinaemia a previously unrecognised syndrome. In: "Advances in Prostaglandin and Thromboxane Research," Samuelsson and Paoletti",eds., Raven Press, New York, pp.888-889 (1976).

37. S-C. Lee and L. Levine, Prostaglandin metabolism. I. cytoplasmic reduced nicotinamide adenine dinucleotide phospate - dependent and microsomal reduced nicotinamide adenine dinucleotide - dependent prostaglandin E 9-keto reductase activities in monkey and pigeon tissues. J. biol. Chem., 249:1369-1375 (1974).

38. S-C. Lee, S-S Pong, D. Katzen, K-Y Wu and L. Levine, Distribution of prostaglandin E 9-keto reductase and types I and II 15-hydroxy dehydrogenase in swine kidney, medullar and cortex. Biochemistry, 14:142-145 (1975).

39. L. Levine, R. M. Gutierrez-Cernosek and H. Van Vunakis,
     Advances in the Biosciences (S. Bergstrom, ed.) Vol. 9,
     Pergamon Press, Oxford, p.71 (1973).
40. M. A. Marrazzi and N. H. Andersen, Prostaglandin dehydrogenase.
     In: "The Prostaglandins," P. Ramwell, ed., Vol 2, Plenum Press,
     New York, pp.99-155 (1974).
41. M. A. Marrazzi and F. M. Matschinsky, Properties of 15-hydroxy-
     prostaglandin dehydrogenase: structural requirements for
     substrate binding. Prostaglandins, 1:373-388 (1972).
42. M. A. Marrazzi, J. E. Shaw, F. T. Tao and F. M. Matschinsky,
     Reversibility of 15-hydroxy prostaglandin dehydrogenase from
     swine lung. Prostaglandins, k:389-395 (1972).
43. J. C. McGiff, N. A. Terragno, J. C. Strand, J. B. Lee, A. J.
     Lonigro and K. K. F. Ng, Selective passage of prostaglandins
     across the lung. Nature (Lond.), 223:742-745 (1969).
44. J. Nakano, Metabolism of prostaglandin E_1 in dog kidneys.
     Br. J. Pharmac., 40:317-325 (1970a).
45. J. Nakano, Metabolism of prostaglandin E_1 (PGE_1) in kidney
     and lung. Fed. Proc., 29:746 (1970b).
46. J. Nakano, Effects of the metabolites of prostaglandin E_1
     of the systemic and peripheral circulation in dogs. Proc.
     Soc. exp. Biol. (N.Y.), 136:1265-1268 (1971).
47. J. Nakano, E. Angggard and B. Samuelsson, 15-hydroxy
     prostanoate dehydrogenase. Prostaglandins as substrates and
     inhibitors. Eur. J. Biochem., 11:386-389 (1969).
48. J. Nakano and N. H. Morsy, Beta-oxidation of prostaglandins
     E_1 and E_2 in rat lung and kidney homogenates. Clin. Res.,
     19:142 (1971).
49. J. Nakano. B. Montague and B. Darrow, Metabolism of
     prostaglandin E_1 in human plasma, uterus and placenta in
     swine ovary and rat testicle. Biochem. Pharmacol., 20:2512-
     2514 (1971).
50. J. Nakano and A. V. Prancan, Metabolic degradation of
     prostaglandin E_1 in the rat plasma and in the rat brain, heart,
     lung, kidney and testicle homogenates. J. Pharm. (Lond.),
     23:231-232 (1971).
51. J. Nakano and A. V. Prancan, Metabolic degradation of
     prostaglandin E_1 in the lung and kidney of rats in endotoxin
     shock. Proc. Soc. exp. Biol. (N.Y.), 144:506-508 (1973).
52. H. M. Nissen, and H. Andersen, On the localization of a
     prostaglandin dehydrogenase activity in the kidney.
     Histochemie, 14:189:200 (1968).
53. H. M. Nissen and H. Andersen, On the activity of prostaglandin
     dehydrogenase system in the kidney. A histo-chemical study
     during hydration-dehydration and salt-repletion-depletion.
     Histochemie, 17:241-247 (1969).
54. C. R. Pace-Asciak, M. C. Carrara and Z. Domazet, 1977a,
     Identification of the major urinary metabolites of 6-keto
     prostaglandin $F_{1\alpha}$ (6k-$PGF_{1\alpha}$) in the rat. Biochem. biophys.
     Res. Commun., 78:115-121 (1977a).

55. C. R. Pace-Asciak, Z. Domazet and M. Carrara, Catabolism of 6-keto prostaglandin $F_{1\alpha}$ by the rat kideny crotex. Biochim. biophys. Acta., 487:400-404 (1977b).

56. C. Pace-Asciak and D. Miller, Prostaglandins during development. I. age dependent activity profiles of prostaglandin 15-hydroxy-dehydrogenase and 13,14-reductase in lung tissue from late pre-natal, early post-natal and adult rats. Prostaglandins, 4:351-362 (1973).

57. D. G. Parkes and T. E. Eling, Characterization of prostaglandin synthetase in guinea pig lung. Isolation of a new prostaglandin derivative from arachidonic acid. Biochemistry, 13:2598:2604 (1974).

58. D. G. Parkes and T. E. Eling, The influence of environmental agents on prostaglandin dehydrogenase in vitro. Prostaglandin biosynthesis and metabolism in the lung. Biochem. J., 146:549-556 (1975).

59. T. M. Parkinson and J. C. Schneider, Absorption and metabolism of prostaglandin E_1 by perfused rat jejunum in vitro. Biochim. biophys. Acta., 176:78 (1969).

60. J. E. Pike, F. P. Kupiecki and J. R. Weeks, Biological activity of the prostaglandins and related analogies, In:"Prostaglandins", Nobel Symposium, Vol.II, New York, Interscience, pp.161-171 (1967).

61. P. J. Piper, J. R. Vane and J. H. Wyllie, Inactivation of prostaglandins by the lungs. Nature, 225:600-604 (1970).

62. H. Polet and L. Levine, Serum prostaglandin A isomerase. Biochem. biophys. Res. Commun., 45:1169-1176 (1971).

63. L. J. Roberts, B. J. Sweetman, N. A. Payne and J. A. Oates, Metabolism of thromboxane B_2 in the monkey,. J.biol. Chem. 252:7415-7417 (1977).

64. J. W. Ryan, R. S. Niemeyer and D. W. Goodwin, Metabolic rates of bradykinin, angiotensin I, adenine nucleotides and prostaglandins E_1 and $F_{1\alpha}$ in the pulmonary circulation. Adv. Exp. Med. Biol., 21:259-265 (1972).

65. S. A. Saeed and A. C. Roy, Purification of 15-hydroxy prostaglandin dehydrogenase from bovine lung. Biochem. Biophys. Res. Commun., 47:96-102 (1972).

66. B. Samuelsson, Structures, biosynthesis and metabolism of prostaglandins. In:"Lipid Metabolism," New York-London, Academic Press, pp.107-153 (1970).

67. B. Samuelsson, E. Granstrom, K. Green and M. Hamberg, Metabolism of prostaglandins. Ann.N.Y.Acad.Sci., 180:138-163 (1971).

68. G. E. Sander and C. G. Huggins, Subcellular localization of angiotensin I converting enzyme in rabbit lung. Nature, New Biol., 230:27-29 (1971).

69. H. Shio, P. W. Ramwell, N. A. Andersen and E. J. Corey, Stereospecificity of the prostaglandin 15-dehydrogenase from swine lung. Experientia, 26:335-357 (1970).

70. M. J. H. Smith and P. D. Dewkins, Salicylate and enzymes.
     J. Pharm. Pharmacol., 23:729-744 (1971).
71. K. J. Stone and M. Hart, Prostaglandin-E_2-9-Ketoreductase in
     rabbit kidney, Prostaglandins, 10:273 (1975).
72. D. D. Sun, Metabolism of prostaglandin $F_{2\alpha}$ in the rat.
     Biochem. Biophys. Acta., 348:249-262 (1974).
73. F. F. Sun and S. B. Armour, Prostaglandin 15-hydroxy
     dehydrogenase and 13 reductase levels in the lungs of
     maternal fetal, and neonatal rabbits. Prostaglandin, 7:327-
     338 (1974).
74. F. F. Sun, J. C. McGuire and B. M. Taylor, Presentation at the
     Winter Meeting on Prostaglandins at Sarasota, Florida, USA,
     January, 1978.
75. F. F. Sun and J. E. Stafford, Metabolism of $PGF_{2\alpha}$ in rhesus
     monkey. Biochim. Biophys. Acta., 369:95-110 (1974).
76. H. Vonkeman, D. H. Nugteren and D. A. Van Dorp., The action
     of prostaglandin 15-hydroxy dehydrogenase on various
     prostaglandins. Biochim. Biophys. Acta., 187:581-583 (1969).

ASSAY METHODS FOR PROSTAGLANDINS AND THROMBOXANES: GAS CHROMATOGRAPHIC - MASS SPECTROMETRIC METHODS AND RADIOIMMUNOASSAY

Elisabeth Granström

Department of Chemistry, Karolinska Institutet
S-104 01 Stockholm
Sweden

The metabolites of polyunsaturated fatty acids constitute a large and steadily growing family of compounds, with the classical prostaglandins as the first identified members, and the thromboxanes, prostacyclins and leukotrienes as more recently discovered products. Most kinds of studies in this increasingly complicated area involve detection and often also quantitation of these compounds, which generally occur in extremely small amounts. Thus, sensitive and specific assay methods are needed.

Some of the compounds in this field are biologically active, and for those some type of bioassay may be suitable. Others are however essentially inactive, such as the major break-down products from each pathway: 15-keto-13,14-dihydro compounds (major circulating metabolites), dioic tetranor metabolites (major urinary products), etc. As many kinds of studies necessitate the monitoring of such inactive metabolic end products (see (1) and reference therein), different types of assay methods must be employed. Radioimmunoassay (RIA) and the gas chromatography - mass spectrometry methods (GC/MS) are the most commonly used ones.

The GC/MS methods are based on the addition of a comparatively large amount of the deuterium labelled compound to a sample, and mass spectrometric analysis of the resulting mixture of the deuterium and protium (natural) forms of the compound in the sample. Knowledge of the added amount of the deuterium form, and the measured proportion between the protium and the deuterium form in the mixture allows the calculation of the amount of prostaglandin or thromboxane originally present in the sample. This method was originally introduced for PGE_1 (2), but similar assays now exist for a large number of compounds: prostaglandins, thromboxanes, and metabolites and analogs of these compounds (3).

The GC/MS methods are highly specific and often allow the simultaneous analysis of several compounds in one sample. The deuterium labeled substance does not only act as an internal standard during the final MS analysis, but also as a carrier for the minute amounts of the natural PG during the purification procedure, protecting it against degradation and adsorption. The analytical procedure involves an extensive purification of the compounds, followed by derivatization prior to gas chromatography. This purification requires a small amount of radioactive tracer, which is added together with the deuterium carrier.

The final MS analysis consists of either multiple ion detection (MID fragmentography) or repetitive scanning during gas chromatography of the prostaglandin derivative. In the former case one or a few ions are selected, characteristic of the mass spectrum of the analyzed PG derivative, and the mass spectrometer records the intensities of only these fragments and the corresponding heavier fragments of the deuterated standard. The specificity of the MID method can be increased by monitoring several characteristic ions for each compound; thus confusion with other substances with the same retention time becomes unlikely. The second method consists of repetitive scans of the magnetic field over a narrow mass range, involving several characteristic ions. A computer is necessary for the evaluation of data in this case. This method is less commonly used than the MID method; it is mainly employed for qualitative analysis of samples.

Many different types of deuterium labeled carriers have been used in the past. Today most carriers are labeled with four deuterium atoms in the carboxylic side chain at carbons 3 and 4. In these positions the deuterium atoms are stable and are retained in many of the most characteristic ions. These deuterium atoms are introduced during the chemical synthesis of the compound (cf. (4)); if a synthetic method is not available, e.g. with a newly discovered compound, it may be possible to prepare a deuterium labeled carrier by biosynthetic methods from {5,6,8,9,11, 12,14,15-$^2H_8$} - arachidonic acid (3).

The greatest advantage with the GC/MS methods is their very high specificity. Confusion with interfering substances is highly unlikely. Though there are sources of error also in this type of methodology, the GC/MS assays may almost be regarded as reference methods. The sensitivity of the assays is also high: the limit of detection of published GC/MS methods is generally 50-250 pg. The sample capacity is however very low, due to the necessary and very time-consuming purification of the samples.

Radioimmunoassay is probably the most commonly employed

quantitative method in prostaglandin research today (for review articles, see Refs. 5-7). The method is based on the competition between radiolabeled and unlabeled molecules of a certain compound for the binding sites of an antibody directed against this substance. The concentrations of labeled compound and antibody are kept constant in all the tubes, whereas the concentration of the unlabeled compound is either known and varied (standard tubes) or unknown (sample tubes). When the concentration of the unlabeled molecules increases, a corresponding amount of the radiolabeled molecules will be displaced for the antibodies, and thus the radio-activity of the antibody-bound fraction decreases. After a certain incubation time the antibody-bound and the free fraction are separated, and the radioactivity in either of the fractions is measured. The amount of the prostaglandin in question in an unknown sample is then obtained from comparison with a standard curve.

Several steps are involved in the development of a RIA: production of an antiserum (a prostaglandin - or thromboxane-protein conjugate is generally used as the antigen), preparation of a radio-labeled ligand of high specific activity, development of a method to separate the bound and the free fractions, in some cases the development of a suitable purification procedure for the samples, and finally, evaluation of the assay. As these steps are time-consuming and perhaps beyond the capacity of many laboratories, many investigators prefer to obtain the necessary reagents and methods from commercial or other sources.

Radioimmunoassays are often extremely sensitive. Many PG or TX assays can detect as little as a few picograms of the substance in question. If proper precautions are taken the method may also be very specific. The greatest advantages of the method are however that it is simple and has a large sample capacity: if no prior purification of the samples is required, it may be possible to analyse several hundred samples per week.

The specificity of radioimmunoassay may however be doubtful, and in many cases very low. Many common and serious sources of error may influence the results, and for the correct interpretation of data it is essential that the scientist is thoroughly familiar with the method. For example, one must keep in mind that all that RIA does is to give information about the degree of inhibition of the binding between the antibody and the labeled antigen. In the ideal case this inhibition is identical with the normal displacement of the labeled molecules, caused by unlabeled molecules of the substance under study. However, an antigen-antibody binding can also be extensively inhibited, not only by cross-reacting compounds of similar structures, but by a large number of totally unrelated compounds. If not aware of this, the scientist will interpret the data as high PG levels.

Such non-specific interfering factors may be of very different nature: proteins, lipids, changes in pH, ionic strength, etc. Some of these disturbing factors may be removed by extraction and purification of the samples; on the other hand such procedures may introduce other and worse interfering compounds. For example, Fig. 1 shows the RIA results from three different assays when the effluent of an empty Amberlite XAD-2 column was analyzed. The strongly interfering substance that is eluted from the column with the methanol is not structurally related to prostaglandins or thromboxanes; it is a degradation product of the XAD-2 polymer.

Similar findings may be obtained when impurities from solvents, adsorbents or other chemicals are introduced. Unfortunately, these very serious sources of error are not well known, and radioimmunoassay is commonly regarded as a "kit type" of assay, which, even in the hands of an inexperienced scientist, automatically will give reliable results, if only the instructions are carefully followed. This is a most unfortunate attitude, which is no doubt responsible for the sometimes quite unrealistic RIA data that have been published in the past, with "prostaglandin levels" often 100-1000 times higher than the true amounts.

One possible way to avoid this problem is to avoid measuring single samples, and instead aim at following changes in the prostaglandin concentration: the analysis is then carried out with a series of samples taken during a time period when an increase or decrease in the PG production is expected. Even if the measured amounts are not quite accurate using RIA, such an experimental design is likely to give reliable information about the changes in the PG levels (see (7) for discussion).

Both GC/MS and RIA require a considerable chemical stability of the measured compound. Thus, some of the most interesting substances in this field are difficult or impossible to measure as such: the potent and highly unstable $PG G_2$, PGH_2, TXA_2 and PGI_2. It is however possible to quantify them using these methods after conversion of these labile compounds into stable derivatives. The prostaglandin endoperoxides may be reduced by stannous chloride into $PGF_{2\alpha}$ (8): $PG G_2/PGH_2$ levels are thus measured as the differences in $PGF_{2\alpha}$ levels before and after treatment with stannous chloride (9). Thromboxane A_2 may be converted by excess methanol into mono-O-methyl TXB_2 (two epimers) (10), which also may be reliably quantitated by either GC/MS or RIA (11).

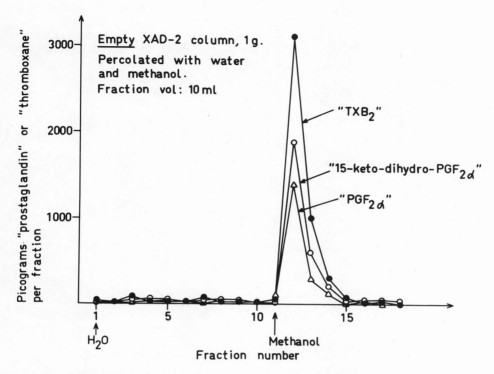

Fig. 1. Fractions from a blank column of Amberlite XAD-2
analyzed by three different radioimmunoassays. The
"sample" applied to the column was 1 ml distilled
H_2O. Elution was done with water, followed by
methanol. Fraction vol: 10ml.

REFERENCES

1. E. Granström and B. Samuelsson, Quantitative measurement of
    prostaglandins and thromboxanes: General considerations.
    In: "Advances in Prostaglandin and Thromboxane Research,"
    Vol. 5, J. C. Frölich ed., Raven Press, New York, (1978),
    pp. 1-13.
2. B. Samuelsson, M. Hamberg and C. Sweeley, Quantitative gas
    chromatography of prostaglandin E_1 at the nanogram level:
    Use of deuterated carrier and multiple-ion analyzer. Anal.
    Biochem., 38:301 (1970).
3. K. Green, M. Hamberg, B. Samuelsson, M. Smigel and J. C.
    Frölich, Measurement of prostaglandins, thromboxanes,
    prostacyclin and their metabolites by gas-liquid chromatography
    - mass spectrometry. In: "Advances in Prostaglandin and

Thromboxane Research", Vol. 5. J. C. Frölich ed., Raven Press,
New York, (1978), pp. 39-94.

4. K. Green, E. Granström, B. Samuelsson and U. Axen, Methods
    for quantitative analysis of $PGF_{2\alpha}$, PGE_2, 9α, 11α-dihydroxy-
    15-keto-prost-5-enoic acid and $9\alpha,11\alpha,15$-trihydroxyprost-5-
    enoic acid from body fluids using deuterated carriers and
    gas chromatography - mass spectrometry. Anal. Biochem.
    54:434 (1973).

5. B. Samuelsson, M. Goldyne, E. Granström, M. Hamberg, S.
    Hammarström and C. Malmsten, Prostaglandins and thromboxanes.
    Ann. Rev. Biochem., 47:997 (1978).

6. E. Granström, Radioimmunoassay of prostaglandins. Prostaglandins,
    15:3 (1978).

7. E. Granström and H. Kindahl, Radioimmunoassay of prostaglandins
    and thromboxanes. In: "Advances in Prostaglandin and
    Thromboxane Research", Vol. 5. J. C. Frölich ed., Raven Press,
    New York (1978), pp. 119-210.

8. M. Hambers, J. Svensson, T. Wakabayashi and B. Samuelsson,
    Isolation and structure of two prostaglandin endoperoxides
    that cause platelt aggregation. Proc. Natl. Acad. Sci. USA,
    71:345 (1974).

9. M. Hamberg, J. Svenssen and B. Samuelsson, Prostaglandin
    endoperoxides. A new concept concerning the mode of action
    and release of prostaglandins. Proc. Natl. Acad. Sci. USA,
    71:3824, (1974).

10. M. Hamberg, J. Svensson and B. Samuelsson, Thromboxanes:
    A new group of biologically active compounds derived from
    prostaglandin endoperoxides. Proc. Natl. Acad. Sci. USA,
    72:2994 (1975).

11. E. Granström, H. Kindahl and B. Samuelsson, A method for
    measuring the unstable thromboxane A_2: Radioimmunoassay of
    the derived mono-O-methyl-thromboxane B_2. Prostaglandins,
    12:929 (1976).

BIOASSAY OF PROSTACYCLIN AND THROMBOXANE A$_2$

Ryszard J. Gryglewski,

Department of Pharmacology,
Copernicus Academy of Medicine,
31-531 Cracow, 16 Grzegorzecka, Poland

INTRODUCTION

Bioassay of the products of cyclo-oxygenation of arachidonic acid (AA) is not only a laboratory technique, it is also a way of biological thinking. Unlike phychicochemical techniques bioassay offers a continuous monitoring of changes in concentration of prostaglandins (PGs), prostacyclin (PGI$_2$) and thromboxane A$_2$ (TXA$_2$) in blood of anesthetized animals or in the perfusate from isolated organs. The price which is paid for the devotion to bioassay is uncertainty about the real chemical nature of a substance which is assayed. The approximation is sometimes very near to the certainty but it never reaches this point. Therefore, we frequently refer to PGI$_2$-like or TXA$_2$-like substances instead of the firm statement – this is PGI$_2$ and that is TXA$_2$. However, this handicap may appear as an advantage of bioassay. A rabbit aorta contracting substance (RCS) had been described as an unstable metabolite of AA before cyclic endoperoxides (PGG$_2$ and PGH$_2$) and TXA$_2$ were discovered. The existance of PGI$_2$ was discovered only because of its "peculiar" behaviour in the bioassay system. Bioassay, when mastered, stimulates research because of its yet unexploited possibilities. Bioassay was created by pharmacologists and thus a number of pharmacological "tricks" are available to increase its specifity and sensitivity.

PGI$_2$ and TXA$_2$ are unstable metabolites of AA with t 1/2 (pH 7,4, 37°C) of 5 min and 0.5 min, respectively. Therefore bioassay is the only technique which can be used for their direct detection, characterization and quantification. An ideal situation arises when the presence of PGI$_2$-like and TXA$_2$-like activities in a bioassayed fluid may be occasionally confirmed by mass spectrometric analysis as the presence of 6-oxo-prostaglandin $F_{1\alpha}$ (6-oxo-$PGF_{1\alpha}$) or thromboxane B_2 (TXB_2).

BIOASSAY OF PROSTACYCLIN (PGI_2)

Bioassay of PGI_2 is based on its vasodilator, anti-aggregatory or dis-aggregatory properties. Thus the most important biological properties of PGI_2 - vasodilatation of coronary arteries, inhibition of platelet aggregation and dispersion of platelet clumps - are used as the indices of its presence in biological fluids. The instability of PGI_2 may be of a help for its identification. When PGI_2-like activity disappears from a biological fluid after 10 min of incubation at 37°C, pH 7,4 then it is a strong indication that we are really dealing with PGI_2. In aqueous solution the stability of PGI_2 depends on pH and on temperature. In a buffer solution of pH 10.5 PGI_2 can be stored for several days at a temperature of + 4°C without appreciable loss of biological activity.

Relaxation of Vascular Strips by PGI_2

In the first two pioneering papers on the discovery of PGI_2 (1,2) it has been described that PGI_2 relaxes a strip of rabbit mesenteric artery (RbMA) or rabbit coeliac artery (RbCA). Unfortunately this property PGI_2 shares with PGE_2 which is 5 - 10 times stronger than PGI_2 in this respect (3). PGI_2 has no effect on strips of rabbit aorta and vena cava. PGI_2 relaxes strips of human, bovine and dog coronary artery. The spirally cut strips of bovine coronary artery (BCA) are the most frequently used as the assay tissue for PGI_2. PGI_2 at low concentrations (2 - 5 ng/ml) invariably relaxes BCA (4), whereas PGE_2 and TXA_2 contract BCA. $PGF_{2\alpha}$ and PGD_2 have no effect on BCA. PGG_2 and PGH_2 usually cause a transient contraction followed by a relaxation of BCA. High concentrations of AA (50 - 100 μg/ml) relax BCA. The endoperoxide-induced relaxation of BCA may be abolished by specific inhibitors of PGI_2 synthetase i.e. by 15-hydroperoxy-arachidonic acid or by tranylcypromine (1) and AA-induced relaxation of BCA may be abolished by indomethacin. Thus prepared BCA will selectively detect PGI_2.

Effects of PGI_2 on Other Smooth Muscle Organs

PGI_2 contracts strips of rat and hamster stomach (3) as well as a transverse-cut strip of rabbit stomach (5). Guinea pig trachea and rat uterus are also contracted by PGI_2 (3). Chick rectum is contracted by PGI_2, while rat colon is not. The suppression of the spontaneous movements of rat colon is an additional indicator for the presence of PGI_2 in the assayed fluid, however, in our hands the above mentioned organs have not been sufficiently selective for detection of PGI_2.

A Cascade of Smooth Muscle Organs for Detection of PGI_2

Vane has developed (6) an assay system in which several smooth muscle organs are superfused in cascade either with blood or with Krebs solution. When a proper choice of members of the "Vane's cascade" is made – then the obtained "fingerprints" – enable us to differentiate between PGs, PGI_2 and TXA_2. For the detection of PGI_2 we recommend (7) the following assembly. A spirally cut strip of bovine coronary artery (BCA), a strip of rabbit mesenteric artery (RbMA) and a rat colon (RC) are superfused with Krebs solution which is composed of the following in mM: NaCl, 118; KCl, 4.7; $CaCl_2$, 2.5; KH_2PO_4, 1.2; $MgSO_4$, 1.17; $NaHCO_3$, 25, glucose, 5.6 and additionally contains a mixture of antagonists of biogenic amines (μg/ml): atropine, 0.1; propranolol, 2.0; phenoxybenzamine, 0.1; mepyramine, 0.2; and metysergid, 0.2. Intramural inhibition of cyclo-oxygenase (indomethacin, 1 – 2 μg/ml) and of PGI_2 synthetase (15 hydroperoxyarachidonic acid, 0.5 – 2 μg/ml or tranylcypromine, 10 – 25 μg/ml) is advisable.

Krebs' solution (at 37°C, pre-gassed with 95% O_2 and 5% CO_2) is allowed to superfuse the assay organs in cascade at speed of 2 – 5 ml/min. The threshold sensitivity of the assay tissues to PGI_2 is inversely proportional to the speed of superfusion, however, at a low rate of superfusion the PGI_2-induced relaxation is a long-lasting one and therefore it is difficult to quantify. Tone of the assay organs is registered through auxotonic levers by electromagnetic transducers (e.g. Harvard, type 386) connected to a multichannel recorder (paper speed 2.5 – 5 mm/min). The initial tension on the organs is adjusted to 1.0 – 1.5 g. Overall amplification of the changes in length is usually 5 – 50 times. The assay organs need at least 3 hours of "preincubation" before they are ready for bioassay.

The choice of these three assay organs enables us to differentiate between PGI_2 (relaxation of BCA and RbMA, supression of spontaneous movements of RC), PGE_2 (contraction of BCA and RC, relaxation of RbMA), $PGF_{2\alpha}$ (contraction of RC, no effect on BCA and RbMA) and TXA_2 (contraction of RbMA, BCA and a small contraction of RC). When a mixture of PGI_2, PGE_2 and TXA_2 is assayed there is sometimes a possibility of detection of the components of the mixture. A usual trick is the arrangement of pairs of organs in line with a delay coils of various length in between them. Thus one can get rid of TXA_2, next of PGI_2 and the PGs are left. PGA_2, PGB_2, PGD_2, 6-oxo-$PGF_{1\alpha}$ and TXB_2 have no effect on the assay organs. PGG_2 and PGH_2 may partially mimick the action of PGI_2 on vascular strips. This interference of

endoperoxides is abolished by PGI_2 synthetase inhibitors. The
above statements refer to the doses of AA metabolites at a range
of 2 - 100 ng given as a single injection at the top of the cascade.
Even higher threshold sensitivity than that can be obtained when
infusion of PGI_2 is administered.

The presented system is used to assay PGI_2 in samples which
contain PGI_2 (e.g. arterial microsomes incubated with PGH_2) or
synthetic PGI_2 analogues (7). A more interesting approach
constitutes a continuous monitoring of the concentration of PGI_2
in the effluent from a perfused organ. In this case an isolated
organ (e.g. lungs or heart) is placed at the top of the cascade
and perfused with Krebs' solution. The total amount of the
effluent or of its portion is allowed to superfuse the assay
organs in cascade. The spontaneous release of PGI_2-like activity
is measured by a rapid change of superfusing fluid - from plain
Krebs' solution to the organ perfusate. The stimulated release
can be observed after an infusion of a stimulating agent into
the perfused organ. The same assay organs may be used in
experiments with anaesthetized animals. Then blood is used for
superfusion of biological detectors, and after this is done blood
returns to the circulation (6). The examples of bioassay of
PGI_2 are presented below.

Examples of PGI_2 Bioassay by Relaxation of BCA

We have recently shown (8) that angiotensin I and II release
PGI_2 from perfused lungs of four animal species. Fig. 1 shows
that perfused cat lungs release spontaneously a PGI_2-like
substance and that angiotensin II increases this release. In the
experiment PGI_2 was bioassayed by relaxation of BCA and after that
the pulmonary effluent was used for mass spectrometric analysis.
Although there is a discrepancy between quantification of PGI_2
by bioassay and by multiple ion detection (MID) mass fragmentography, there still exists an extremely good correlation between
the readings by both techniques as far as the fluctuation of PGI_2
concentration in the effluent is concerned.

Fig. 2 shows that angiotensin II also releases PGI_2 _in vivo_
into the circulating blood. Moreover, this experiment
demonstrates that _in vivo_ angiotensin II stimulates the secretion
of PGI_2 not only from lungs, but also from kidney.

Bioassay of PGI_2 by Reversal of Platelet Aggregation

We have described (9) an _in vivo_ method for quantification
of anti-platelet potency of drugs. The principle of this method
is that blood is withdrawn from an anesthetized and heparinized
animal and superfuses a collagen strip which is gradually covered

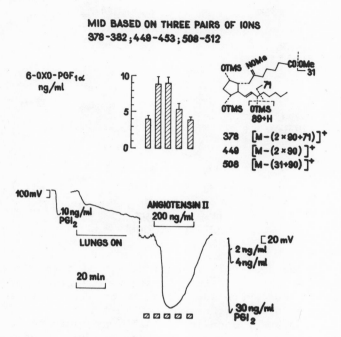

Fig. 1. Confirmation of bioassay by multiple ion detection (MID) mass fragmentography. The effluent from perfused cat lungs superfused an indomethacin-treated strip of bovine coronary artery and was collected (squares) for mass spectrometric analysis. A change of plain Krebs' solution for the lung perfusate (lung on) resulted in relaxation of the assay organ, the relaxation was still enhanced by angiotensin II which was infused into pulmonary artery. On the basis of reactions of the assay organ to synthetic PGI_2 we concluded that cat lungs release spontaneously 15 ng/ml of a PGI_2-like substance and that this amount is doubled during the stimulation with angiotensin II. MID detected in the effluent of non-treated lungs 6-oxo-$PGF_{1\alpha}$ at concentration of 4 ng/ml and this concentration was doubled by angiotensin II infusion. From now on, we can leave out a descriptive term "PGI_2-like activity" and refer to PGI_2 which is released from cat lungs.

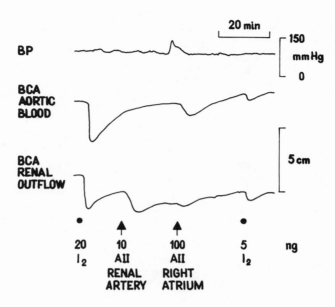

Fig. 2.   The release of PGI$_2$ by angiotensin II into circulation of
          an anaesthetized cat.   Two strips of bovine coronary
          artery (BCA) were superfused in parallel with aortic
          blood or blood withdrawn from left renal vein (renal
          outflow).   Angiotensin II (AII) was administered as a
          bolus injection into left renal artery (10 ng) or into
          right atrium (100 ng).   The bioassay tissues were
          calibrated with synthetic prostacyclin (I$_2$) at doses
          20 and 5 ng.

with platelet clumps.   The weight of collagen strip is
continuously monitored.   The pretreatment of the animal with
cyclo-oxygenase inhibitors (e.g. aspirin) or thromboxane synthetase
inhibitors (e.g. nictindole) prevents the platelet deposition on
collagen surface and therefore a rise in weight of a strip is
suppressed.   Later we have learned that PGI$_2$ infused either locally
over the collagen strip or intravenously dis-aggregates the
preformed platelet clumps and thus causes a loss in weight of a
collagen strip in a dose-dependent manner (10,11,12).   This
property of PGI$_2$ is a basis for an excellent method to quantify
PGI$_2$ in circulating blood.

The experimental set up is as follows.   Cats or rabbits are
anaesthetized with sodium pentobarbitone at a dose of 40 ∹ 60 mg/kg

and heparinized (2.500 units/kg). Mixed venous blood from right
atrium and/or arterial blood from ascending aorta is withdrawn
through appropriate cannulas by a roller pump at a speed of
3 ml/min. Blood superfusion collagen strips made out the tendons
of Achilles of rabbits (30 x 5 mm) and returns by gravity into
the venous system. The weight of blood-superfused collagen strips
is continuously monitored by a Harvard Transducer type 364.
Its lever is additionally supplied with an adjustable watch
spring which is able to counterbalance the resting weight of the
tendon. A gain in weight of the blood-superfused strips reflects
the intensity of the formation of platelet clumps on the surface
of strips and this increase in weight is recorded by a polygraph
(9). The maximal deposition of platelet clumps (200 - 500 mg)
occurs after 25 - 35 min of superfusion and no further gain in
weight is observed all over the experiment (Fig. 3). When this
plateau is reached the dis-aggregatory action of PGI_2 can be
observed. In mixed venous blood of cats a dose response curve is
obtained for local infusion of PGI_2 at a range of concentrations
from 1 to 30 ng/ml. A similar dose response curve is obtained
when PGI_2 is injected intravenously at a range of doses from 1 to
20 ug/kg (12). The dis-aggregatory action of PGI_2 is stronger
in aortic blood, than that in mixed-venous blood thus giving a
basis for an assumption that the lungs are continuously producing
PGI_2 and secreting this hormone into arterial circulation
(10,11,13). The same experimental set up can be used in clinical
investigation, however, the superfusing blood is not returned to
circulation but discarded. We have observed a profound clinical
effects of PGI_2 in healthy volunteers when the synthetic hormone
was infused intravenously at a range of doses from 2 to 20 ng/kg/
min (14). In these subjects the IC_{50} for the dis-aggregatory
effect of PGI_2 on collagen strips is approximately 15 ng/kg/min,
i.v.

   The rate of increase in weight of superfused collagen strips
as well as their maximal rise in weight depend on the amount of
circulating PGI_2. Slow rate or increase in weight and low plateau
of maximal rise indicate high levels of circulating PGI_2 and
vice versa. Binding of circulating PGI_2 by a specific antiserum
(13) or inhibition of renin-angiotensin system at the level of
converting enzyme (SQ 14225) (8) diminishes the concentration of
circulating PGI_2 and thus accelerates a rate of increase and
stimulates a maximal increase in weight of blood superfused
tendons.

   Our technique of bioassay of PGI_2 in circulation is not only
sensitive but also a specific method. Dis-aggregation is not
induced by cyclo-oxygenase inhibitors and thromboxane synthetase
inhibitors. Among other metabolites of AA only PGD_2 and PGE_1
dis-aggregate platelet clumps. These two PGs are weaker than
PGI_2 and they are stable in circulating blood. A simple

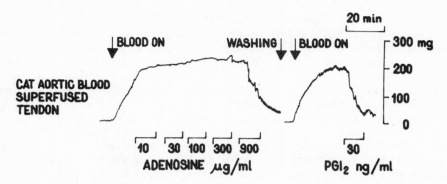

Fig. 3.   Comparison of dis-aggregatory potency of PGI_2 and
           adenosine. A tendon of Achilles of a rabbit was super-
           fused with aortic blood of anaesthetized, heparinized
           cat. (blood on). A rise in weight is recorded.
           Adenosine dis-aggregated platelet clumps on the surface
           of the tendon only at a concentration as high as 900
           μg/ml. After washing with saline the same tendon was
           again superfused with blood (blood on). PGI_2 needed
           only 30 ng/ml to induce the dis-aggregation.

arrangement of two collagen strips superfused in line with a 10
min delay coil in between them clearly differentiates between
PGE_1, PGD_2 and PGI_2. Only in case of PGI_2 the lower strip will
not respond to the dis-aggregatory action of a compound in
question. Adenosine is also a dis-aggregatory agent, however,
it is several thousand times less potent than PGI_2 (Fig. 3) and
there is no need to remember about adenosine in our assay system.

Bioassay of PGI_2 by Inhibition of Platelet Aggregation

         This is a typical in vitro method. Human or rabbit platelet
rich plasma (PRP) is prepared from citrated blood (trisodium
citrate 3.15% w/v : blood = 1 : 10) by centrifugation (400 g
for 10 min). PRP is aggregated in a 0.5 - 1.0 ml cuvette using
a Born optical aggregometer or a Flower electronic aggregometer.
Aggregation is induced by adenosine diphosphate (ADP) at a
concentration just sufficient to induce the second phase of
aggregation (usually 0.5 - 10 μM). Synthetic PGI_2 at known
concentrations or an unknown sample are added in volumes smaller
than 20 μl to 1 ml aliquots of PRP, 1 min prior to their ADP-
induced aggregation. Percent of inhibition of platelet
aggregation is registered and dose-response curves for synthetic
PGI_2 and for an unknown solution containing a PGI_2-like activity
are calculated. The reported IC_{50} for inhibitory action of PGI_2
is 0.5 ± 0.1 ng/ml and 2.8 ± 0.5 ng/ml for human PRP and rabbit
PRP, respectively (15). The concentration of a PGI_2-like activity

in an unknown solution is calculated. The only simple way to check the identity of PGI_2-like activity is to boil a sample for 1 min or to leave it for 10 min at $37^{\circ}C$ (pH 7.4). Then the anti-aggregatory activity should disappear.

BIOASSAY OF THROMBOXANE A_2 (TXA_2)

Bioassay of TXA_2 is more difficult than bioassay of PGI_2 because TXA_2 is highly unstable (t 1/2 = 30 sec at $37^{\circ}C$) and synthetic TXA_2 is not available as a reference compound. The only biological activity of TXA_2 which became useful for its bioassay is the powerful contractile action of TXA_2 on vascular strips. Originally a strip of rabbit aorta was used to assay TXA_2. This bioassay organ has a disadvantage of being also contracted by cyclic endoperoxides. Although the contractile action of TXA_2 is more potent than that of endoperoxides it is still a weak basis for differentiation between endoperoxides and TXA_2. In our hands the most suitable assay organ for TXA_2 is a strip of rabbit mesenteric artery.

Bioassay of TXA_2 by Contraction of RbMA

A strip of rabbit mesenteric artery (RbMA) is contracted by TXA_2, while other products of AA metabolites either relax or have no effect on this vascular tissue. The bioassay system is arranged in the same manner as it has been described in above paragraph (A cascade of smooth muscle organs for detection of PGI_2). TXA_2-induced contractions of RbMA are matched by contractions evoked by a reference compound, i.e. by (15 S)-hydroxy-11A,9A-(epoxymethane) prosta-5Z,13E-dienoic acid (Upjohn Co. U 46619, EMA) (16). Although EMA is a synthetic analogue of PGH_2, it behaves like TXA_2, at least in our biological system, rendering a parallel dose-response curve to that for extracted TXA_2. TXA_2 is 5 - 10 times more potent vasoconstrictor on RbMA than EMA. The amount of TXA_2 in an investigated sample is calculated by four-point assay and expressed in equivalents of EMA (ng/ml).

Examples of TXA_2 Assay

TXA_2 is formed in PRP during aggregation induced by AA, collagen and ADP (17). Aliquots of aggregating PRP (2 - 50 µl) are rapidly transferred from an aggregometer over a superfused RbMA. It is advisable to increase the concentration of methysergide in Krebs' solution up to 0.5 µg/ml (see paragraph " a cascade of smooth muscle organs for detection of PGI_2")since 5-hydroxytryptamine released from platelets may interfere with assay of TXA_2. A control experiment is to pass PRP through a millipore filter and then after 10 min to check contractile potency of the filtrate. It should be devoid of any contractile action.

A single dose of aspirin (600 mg) given orally suppresses the AA-induced generation of TXA_2 in human PRP for a couple of days. The reappearance period of TXA_2 in PRP of aspirin-treated subjects has been proposed as a measure of life span of platelets (16).

A study of the capacity of thromboxane synthetase in platelets to generate TXA_2 in response to increasing concentrations of AA has revealed that in 40% survivals from myocardial infarction this capacity is increased in comparison to the control group (15).

TXA_2 is bioassayed as the product of thromboxane synthetase in isolated biochemical systems. The most popular system is an incubation mixture consisting of horse platelet microsomes (HPM) and PGH_2, which when incubated on ice during 1 - 2 min form TXA_2 (18). This and other similar systems are used to detect thromboxane synthetase inhibitors (19).

TXA_2 is released from perfused organs, such as lungs or spleen when these are stimulated with antigens, high concentrations of AA, bradykinin or catecholamines. A typical bank of tissues superfused in cascade (paragraph - "a cascade of smooth muscle organs for detection of PGI_2") allows to detect TXA_2 and other metabolites of AA which are released from the perfused organs.

CONCLUSION

Bioassay is the only technique which can be used for a direct and continuous detection, characterisation and quantification of unstable metabolites of arachidonic acid such as prostacyclin and thromboxane A_2. The confirmation of chemical nature of bioassayed substances by mass spectrometric analysis is highly desirable.

REFERENCES

1. R. J. Gryglewski, S. Buntin S. Moncada, R. J. Flower and J. R. Vane, Arterial walls are protected against deposition of platelet thrombi by a substance (prostaglandin X) which they make from prostaglandin endoperoxides. Prostaglandins 12:685 (1976).
2. S. Moncada, R. J. Gryglewski, S. Bunting and J. R. Vane, An enzyme isolated from arteries transform prostaglandin endoperoxides to an unstable substance than inhibits platelet aggregation. Nature, 263:663 (1976).
3. C. Omini, S. Moncada and J. R. Vane, The effects of prostacyclin (PGI_2) on tissues which detect prostaglandins (PGs). Prostaglandins, 14:625 (1977).

4. G. J. Dusting, S. Moncada and J. R. Vane, Prostacyclin (PGX) is the endogenous metabolite responsible for relaxation of coronary arteries induced by arachidonic acid. Prostaglandins, 13:3 (1977).

5. S. Moncada, K. G. Mugridge and B. J. R. Whittle, The differential response of a novel bioassay tissue, the rabbit transverse stomach-strip to prostacyclin (PGI_2) and other prostaglandins. Brit. J. Pharmacol., 61:451P (1977).

6. J. R. Vane, The use of isolated organs for detection of active substances in circulating blood. Brit. J. Pharmacol. 23:360 (1964).

7. R. J. Gryglewski and K. C. Nicolaou, A triple test for screening biological activity of prostacyclin analogues. Experientia, 34:1336 (1978).

8. R. J. Gryglewski, R. Korbut and J. Splawinski, Endogenous mechanisms which regulate prostacyclin release. Washington Conference on Prostaglandins, 29 May - 3 June 1979, in press.

9. R. J. Gryglewski, R. Korbut, A. Ocetkiewicz and J. Stachura, In vivo method for quantitation of anti-platelet potency of drugs. Naunyn-Schmiedeberg's Arch. Pharmacol., 302:25 (1978).

10. R. J. Gryglewski, R. Korbut, A. Ocetkiewicz, J. Splawinski, B. Wojtaszek and J. Swiens, Lungs as generator or prostacyclin-hypothesis on physiological significance. Naunyn-Schmiedeberg's Arch. Pharmacol., 304:45 (1978).

11. R. J. Gryglewski, R. Korbut and A. Ocetkiewicz, Generation of prostacyclin by lungs in vivo and its release into the arterial blood. Nature, 273:765 (1978).

12. R. J. Gryglewski, R. Korbut and A. Ocetkiewicz, Reversal of platelet aggregation by prostacyclin. Pharmacol. Res. Commun., 10:185 (1978).

13. S. Moncada, R. Korbut and J. R. Vane, Prostacyclin is a circulating hormone. Nature, 273:767 (1978).

14. R. J. Gryglewski, A. Szczeklik and R. Nizankowski, Anti-platelet action of intravenous infusion of prostacyclin in man. Thromb. Res., 13:153 (1978).

15. B. J. R. Whittle, S. Moncada and J. R. Vane, Comparison of the effects of prostacyclin (PGI_2), prostaglandins E_1 and D_2 on platelet aggregation in different species. Prostaglandins, 16:373 (1978).

16. A. Szczeklik and R. J. Gryglewski, Thromboxane A_2 synthesis by platelets of patients with coronary heart disease. In: "International Conference on Atherosclerosis". L. A. Carlson, R. Paoletti, C. R. Sirtori and G. Weber, eds. (Raven Press, New York, (1978)).

17. E. Marcinkiewicz, L. Grodzinska and R. J. Gryglewski, Platelet aggregation and thromboxane A_2 formation in cat platelet rich plasma. Pharmacol. Res. Commun., 10:1 (1978).

18.   P. Needleman, S. Moncada, S. Bunting, J. R. Vane, M. Hamberg
      and B. Samuelsson, Identification of an enzyme in platelet
      microsomes which generates thromboxane A_2 from prostaglandin
      endoperoxides. Nature, 261:558 (1976).
19.   R. J. Gryglewski, A. Zmuda, R. Korbut, E. Krecioch and K.
      Bieron, Selective inhibition of thromboxane A_2 biosynthesis
      in blood platelets. Nature, 267:627 (1977).

PHARMACOLOGICAL INTERFERENCE IN ARACHIDONIC ACID CASCADE

Ryszard J. Gryglewski

Department of Pharmacology,
Copernicus Academy of Medicine in Cracow
31-531 Cracow, 16 Grzegorzecka, Poland

PHOSPHOLIPASES

In order to be metabolized by oxidative tissue enzymes arachidonic acid (AA) has to be liberated from the cellular phospholipids by phospholipase A_2 (1). In certain cells, e.g. in platelets, phospholipase requires calcium ions for its optimal biochemical activity (2), and therefore Ca^{2+} ionophors activate AA cascade (3), while the drugs which rise intracellular cAMP levels sequestrate Ca^{2+}, and thus inhibit AA liberation and its subsequent metabolism (4). Mepacrine and bromophenacetyl bromide are direct inhibitors of phospholipase A_2 (5). We have proposed (6,7) that the liberation of AA from intact tissues is hindered by gluco-corticosteroids as well as by anti-inflammatory steroids, eg. dexymethasone. Other authors since have confirmed our hypothesis (8,9,10), and Flower and Blackwell (11) demonstrated that glucocorticosteroids induce the endogenous synthesis of a phospholipase A_2 inhibitor.

LIPOXYGENASES

The first step of metabolism of AA is its lipoxygenation to various hydroperoxy eicosatetranoic acids (HPETEs) (Fig. 1). 12-HPETE and 15-HPETE are good substrates for peroxidases and the corresponding hydroxy acids (HETE) are formed. 5-HPETE gives a rise to the family of leukotriens (LTs), one of which (Leucotrien C) is supposed to be identical with slow reacting substance A (12). We are lacking in potent and selective inhibitors of these early enzymatic reactions, although eicosatetraynoic acit (TYA) and several other chemicals (13) inhibit both lipoxygenation and cyclo-oxygenation steps.

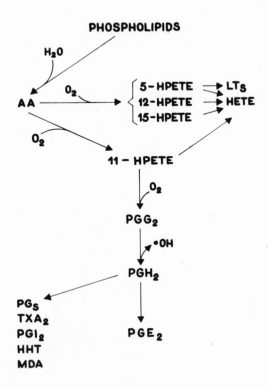

Fig. 1.   Arachidonic acid cascade. Arachidonic acid (AA) is
          liberated from phospholipids by phospholipase A_2. Free
          AA is the substrate for a number of lipoxygenases giving
          rise to hydroperoxy eicosatetranoic acids (HPETE).
          These can be reduced to corresponding hydroxy acids
          (HETE), transformed into leukotriens (LTs) or in case
          of 11–HPETE cyclo–oxygenized to prostaglandin endo-
          peroxide (PGG_2). PGG_2 is the substrate for peroxidase
          and a 15–hydroxy prostaglandin endoperoxide (PGH_2) is
          formed. This last is isomerized to prostaglandin E_2
          and other primary prostaglandins (PGs). PGH_2 is also
          the substrate for thromboxane synthetase and TXA_2 is
          formed along with a 17C hydroxy acid (HHT) and
          malondialdehyde (MDA). Prostacyclin synthetase
          isomerizes PGH_2 to prostacyclin (PGI_2).

CYCLO-OXYGENASE

The most known route of a further enzymatic transformation of AA leads through cyclo-oxygenation of 11-HPETE to a prostaglandin endoperoxide PGG_2. The activity of microsomal cyclo-oxygenase is selectively and irreversibly inhibited by aspirin, indomethacin and by other non-steroidal anti-inflammatory drugs (14,15,16,17).

PGG_2/PGH_2 PEROXIDASE

The PGG_2/PGH_2 peroxidase is stimulated by phenol and 2-aminomethyl-4-t-butyl-6-iodophenol (MK 447) (18). This last compound stimulates the generation of primary prostaglandins and yet it has an anti-inflammatory properties. Kuehl et al. (18) explain anti-inflammatory action of MK 447 through its ability to scavange free radicals. This ability - the authors postulate - is responsible for the stimulation of the conversion PGG_2 to PGH_2. The overall synthesis of primary prostaglandins is stimulated, but PGG_2 with its 15-hydroperoxy radical is quickly removed from the site of inflammation. The final conclusion is that primary prostaglandins are not important pro-inflammatory mediators. The inflammation is mediated by an unstable PGG_2. This can be done either by non-prostaglandin products which are formed from this endoperoxide or by free radicals, such as hydroxy radical, formed in the metabolism of PGG_2. Another potent stimulator of oxygen consumption, prostaglandin formation and malondialdehyde (MDA) generation from AA in ram seminal vesicle microsomes (RSVM) is chloropromazine (Fig. 2, our unpublished data). Chloropromazine was reported to be a cyclo-oxygenase inhibitor (19,20), however, in these experiments, unlike in ours, cofactors were added to the incubation mixture. Some cofactors such as hydroquinone are free radical scavengers and mask a true face of the investigated drug. It is frequently overlooked that chloropromazine has a modest but distinct anti-inflammatory action comparable to that of aspirin (carrageenin edema of rat paw is inhibited by 50% by oral doses of aspirin and chloropromazine of 65 and 80 mg/kg, respectively). The most obvious explanation would be that chloropromazine by scavenging hydroxy radicals accelerates the generation of primary prostaglandins and removes pro-inflammatory PGG_2 according to the concept of Kuehl et al. (18). However, we investigated the other two compounds which in a similar way to MK 447 and chloropromazine stimulated oxygen consumption and prostaglandin generation from AA in RSVM - these were p-acetamidophenol and 6-(phenyl)-3-hydroxy-pyrazol(3,4b)-pyridine (PHP). p-Acetamido-phenol had a weak anti-inflammatory action, while PHP actually promoted inflammation (Fig. 3). Our conclusion is that no single biochemical test <u>in vitro</u> is useful for prediction of biological activity <u>in vivo</u>, and also that possibly other metabolites of AA, apart from primary prostaglandins or PGG_2 may play a role in inflammatory response.

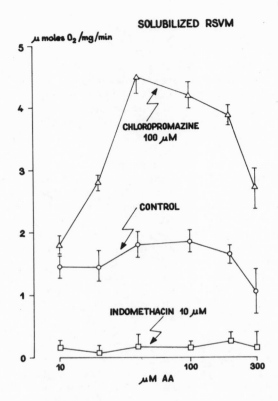

Fig. 2. Oxygen consumption (μmoles O_2/mg protein/min) by a
mixture of solubilized ram seminal vesicle microsomes
(RSVM) incubates with various concentrations of
arachidonic acid (AA) (Control). The influence of
chloropromazine (100 μM) and indomethacin (10 μM) on
oxygen consumption. No cofactors were used. The bars
represent 2 x S.E. of mean of 3 - 6 estimation.
Unpublished results of Dr. J. Robak et al.

PGH_2/PROSTAGLANDIN ISOMERASES

There are not known selective inhibitors of isomerases which
convert endoperoxides into primary prostaglandins. PGH_2 can
be non-enzymatically converted to PGE_2 and PGD_2. The conversion
into this last prostaglandin is stimulated by albumin (21).

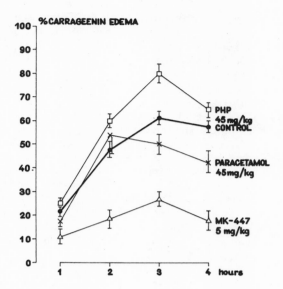

Fig. 3.   The effects on rat paw carrageenin-induced edema
          (ordinate - per cent of increase in paw volume) of three
          stimulators of prostaglandins biosynthesis MK-447 (18),
          p-acetamidophenol (paracetamol) and PHP (see tect).
          The compounds were given orally at doses of 5, 45 and
          45 mg/kg, respectively, before an intraplantar injection
          of carrageenin.

THROMBOXANE SYNTHETASE

     In contrast to primary prostaglandins, thromboxane A_2
(TXA_2) and prostacyclin (PGI_2) are generated from endoperoxides
only in the presence of corresponding synthetases. Thromboxane
synthetase is located mainly in blood platelets and prostacyclin
synthetase mainly in vascular tissue. Inhibitors of the above
enzymes may influence haemostasis.

     By definition thromboxane synthetase inhibitors invalidate
the conversion of endoperoxides to TXA_2. A selective thromboxane
synthetase inhibitor is expected not to influence the activities
of cyclo-oxygenase and prostacyclin synthetase. The superiority
of thromboxane synthetase inhibitors over cyclo-oxygenase
inhibitors is based on the fact that the former do not inhibit
the generation of prostacyclin by vascular walls. Depending on
the choice of Needleman's (22) or Gorman's (23) point of view a
search for selective thromboxane synthetase inhibitors may be
considered as a search for drugs which will alleviate acute
ischemia occuring during intravascular platelet aggregation

(24,25,26) or as a search for potential anti-thrombotic agents
that may replace heparin, K antivitamins, aspirin, sulfinpyrazone,
dipyridamole and clofibrate in prevention of myocardial re-infarction,
as well as a supplement for prostacyclin therapy in the treatment
of atherosclerosis (27).

The known thromboxane synthetase inhibitors do not constitute
a homogenous group, either chemically or pharmacologically (28,29,
30). Two non-acidic anti-inflammatory drugs, first known as
cyclo-oxygenase inhibitors benzydamine (31) and nictindole (L8027)
(32) were reported to inhibit TXA_2 synthetase at IC_{50} of 300 μM
and 1 μM, respectively. Both drugs at the above concentrations do
not influence cyclo-oxygenase activity from ram seminal vesicle
microsomes. The inhibition of thromboxane synthetase by
benzydamine was denied (28). It was confirmed for nictindole
(28), however, in vivo is practically impossible to separate
inhibition of thromboxane synthetase from inhibition of cyclo-
oxygenase by nictindole (33).

Imidazole, a compound first known as a stimulator of cAMP
phosphodiesterase has been found to inhibit thromboxane
synthetase (28,29,30,34). Imidazole is a weak (IC_{50} = 375 μM)
but selective thromboxane synthetase inhibitor (34). Therefore
imidazole derivatives (34,35), histamine and antagonists of H_2
histamine receptors such as burimamide, metiamide and cimetidine
(36) have been studied as potential thromboxane synthetase
inhibitors. Among histamine antagonists only burimamide inhibits
TXA_2 synthetase (IC_{50} = 25 μM) (36). 1-Substituted alkyl
and arylalkyl derivatives of imidazole such as 1-butyl-
imidazole or 1-(2-isopropylphenyl)imidazole (35) are much better
inhibitors of the enzyme than the parent compound. Unexpectedly,
the influence of imidazole on platelet aggregation is rather erratic.
Imidazole causes a delay in platelet aggregation in PRP but is
without any effect in washed platelet suspensions aggregated with
AA or with PGH_2 (22,29). At high concentrations, imidazole may
in fact, enhance platelet aggregability through a mechanism
independent of thromboxane synthesis (37). Perhaps a direct
stimulatory effect of imidazole on phosphodiesterase activity or
on Ca^{2+} transport through biomembranes may offer an explanation for
the pro-aggregatory action of this compound. Imidazole is
irritant to mammalian tissues. Thus for different reasons
nictindole and imidazole are both useless for the in vivo inhibition
of thromboxane synthetase.

Eakins et al (38) have demonstrated the p-benzyl-4-(1-oco-
(4-chlorobenzyl)-3-phenyl propyl) phenyl phosphate (N-0164) at
concentrations of 1 - 10 μM antagonizes the contractile action of
prostaglandins at their "receptor sites" in gastro-intestinal
smooth muscle. Later, it has been shown that N-0164 selectively
blocks "receptor sites" for PGD_2 and fails to antagonize the action

of PGE_1 and PGI_2 on platelet membranes (39).   In addition, high concentrations of N-0164 (20 - 100 μM) inhibit TXA_2 synthetase in human platelets (40).   Again, the inhibition of platelet aggregation by N-0164 cannot be considered as a result of the selective inhibition of thromboxane synthetase in platelets but it may be rather attributed of the extracellular action of N-0164.

Thromboxane synthetase was also claimed to be inhibited by nicotinic acid (41), extracts from onion (allium cepa) and garlic (allium sativum)(42) and microsomes from the bovine heart (43).

A new approach to the selective inhibition of thromboxane synthetase was initiated by the synthesis of the substrate analogs for this enzyme. The chemical group of the synthetic endoperoxide analogs and related prostanoic structures are of great biological interest. A replacement of the 9,11 oxygen-oxygen bridge in a molecule of PGH_2 by an azo (44) or an epoxymethano (45) bridges yield prostanoids which mimic biological activity of the parent structure, i.e. they induce platelet aggregation and contract aortic strips, although in platelet microsomes they may inhibit thromboxane synthetase (45). Synthetic analgos of PGH_2 cannot be converted to a TXA_2-like material by platelet microsomes and possibly therefore there still exist differences between their pro-aggregating and pro-secretory actions and those of original PGH_2 (46).

If in the azo or epoxyimino analogs of PGH_2 the 15-hydroxy group is replaced by a hydrogen atom then there arises a series of potent and markedly selective thromboxane synthetase inhibitors (37,47,48,49). The most thoroughly investigated was 9.11-azaprosta, 5,13-dienoic acid (U-81606) (23,37,48,49), which inhibits TXA_2 generation and PGH_2-induced platelet aggregation both in washed platelet suspension and in PRP. U-51605 also inhibits the activity of cyclo-oxygenase in the ram seminal vesicle microsomal preparation and prostacyclin synthetase from sheep aorta and rabbit lungs. It is, however, in this respect 10 - 40 times weaker than a thromboxane synthetase inhibitor in human platelet microsomes. Even a more interesting inhibitor of PGH_2-induced aggregation of human platelets is 9,11-epoxyiminoprosta-5,13-dienoic acid (47,50). This analog seems to antagonize directly the "receptor sites" for TXA_2 in platelets (50). It has been rightly pointed out by the authors that: "Just as experiments with dichloroisoproterenol advanced the understanding of the β-adrenergic receptor, we believe that experiments with 9.11-epoxyiminoprosta-5,13-dienoic acid will advance the understanding of TXA_2 receptors in platelets".

PROSTACYCLIN SYNTHETASE

Prostacyclin synthetase from porcine aortic microsomes is effectively inhibited by 15-hydroperoxyarachidonic acid (51) and by a number of other lipid peroxides (52). A much weaker inhibitor to the enzyme is tranylcypromine (51). Tranylcypromine (10 mg/kg i.p.) enhances platelet aggregation in murine cerebral microvessels while another monoaminoxidase inhibitor (iproniazid) which is devoid of inhibitory action on prostacyclin synthetase, inhibits platelet aggregation (53). In the same experimental model imidazole failed to influence platelet aggregation. These data support our concept (51) that prostacyclin is an important physiological inhibitor of platelet aggregation, while the in vivo role of TXA_2 for platelet aggregability is of a smaller importance.

In perfused rabbit heart nicotine inhibits the transformation of AA to 6-keto-$PGF_{1\alpha}$ and diverts AA metabolism to PGE_2 (54) in a similar way as in perfused guinea pig lungs imidazole diverts AA metabolism from TXA_2 to $PGF_{2\alpha}$ (55). Nicotine inhibits also the release of prostacyclin from pulsating rat aorta (56).

REFERENCES

1. G. J. Blackwell, W. G. Duncombe, R. J. Flower, M. F. Parsons, and J. R. Vane, The distribution and metabolism of arachidonic acid in rabbit platelets during aggregation and its modification by drugs. Br. J. Pharmacol., 59:353 (1977).
2. A. Derksen and P. Cohen, Patterns of fatty acid release from endogenous substrates by human platelet homogenates and membranes. J. Biol. Chem., 250:9342 (1975).
3. W. C. Pickett, R. L. Jesse and P. Cohen, Initiation of phospholipase A_2 activity in human platelets by the calcium ion ionophore A23187. Biochem. Biophys. Acta., 486:209 (1977).
4. J. G. White, J. M. Gerrard, Platelet morphology and the ultra-structure of regulatory mechanisms involved in platelet activation. In:"Platelets: A Multidisciplinary Approach". G. de Gaetano and S. Garattini,eds., Raven Press, New York (1978).
5. B.B.Vargaftig, Carrageenan and thrombin trigger prostaglandin synthetase-independent aggregation of rabbit platelets: inhibition by phospholipase A_2 inhibitors. J. Pharm. Pharmac. 29:222 (1977).
6. R. J. Gryglewski, B. Panczenko, R. Korbut, L. Grodzinska and A. Ocetkiewicz, Corticosteroids inhibit prostaglandin release from perfused lungs of sensitized guinea pigs. Prostaglandins, 10:343 (1975).

7. R. J. Gryglewski, Steroid hormones, anti-inflammatory steroids and prostaglandins. Pharmacol. Res. Commun., 8:337 (1976).

8. R. J. Flower, Steroidal anti-inflammatory drugs as inhibitors of phospholipase A_2. In: "Advances in Prostaglandin and Thromboxane Research". C. Galli, G. Galli and G. Porcellati, eds., Vol. 3, Raven Press, New York (1978).

9. Y. Floman, N. Floman and U. Zor, Inhibition of prostaglandin E. release by anti-inflammatory steroids. Prostaglandins, 11:591 (1976).

10. F. P. Nijkamp, R. J. Flower, S. Moncada and J. R. Vane, Partial purification of rabbit aorta contracting substance-releasing factor and inhibition of its activity by anti-inflammatory steroids. Nature (London), 263:479 (1976).

11. R. J. Flower and G. J. Blackwell, Anti-inflammatory steroids induce the biosynthesis of a phospholipase A_2 inhibitor which prevents prostaglandin generation. Nature, 278:456 (1979).

12. B. Samuelsson, P. Borgeat, S. Hammarström and R. C. Murphy, Introduction of a nomenclature: Leukotriens: In: "Abstracts of International Conference on Prostaglandins," Washington D.C. 28th May, 1979.

13. R. J. Flower, Drugs which inhibit prostaglandin biosynthesis. Pharmacol. Rev., 26:33 (1974).

14. J. R. Vane, Inhibition of prostaglandin synthesis as a mechanism of action of aspirin-like drugs. Nature New Biol. 231:232 (1971).

15. J. B. Smith and A. L. Willis, Aspirin selectively inhibits prostaglandin production in human platelets. Nature New Biol., 231:235 (1971).

16. S. H. Ferreira, S. Moncada and J. R. Vane, Indomethacin and aspirin abolish prostaglandin release from the spleen. Nature New Biol., 231:237 (1971).

17. R. J. Flower, R. J. Gryglewski, K. Herbaczynska-Cedro and J. R. Vane, The effect of anti-inflammatory drugs on prostaglandin biosynthesis. Nature New Biol, 238:104 (1972).

18. F. A. Kuehl, J. L. Humes, R. W. Egan, E. A.Ham, G. C. Beveridge and C. G. Van Arman, Role of prostaglandin endoperoxide PGG_2 in inflammatory processes. Nature, 265:170 (1977).

19. P. Krupp and M. Wesp, Inhibition of prostaglandin synthetase by psychotropic drugs. Experientia (Basel) 31:330 (1975).

20. R. E. Lee, The influence of psychotropic drugs on prostaglandin biosynthesis. Prostaglandins, 5:63 (1974).

21. M. Hamberg and B. B. Fredholm, Isomerization of prostaglandin H_2 into prostaglandin D_2 in the presence of serum albumin. Biochem. Biophys. Acta, 431:189 (1976).

22. P. Needleman, M. Minkes and A. Raz, Thromboxanes: selective biosynthesis and distinct biological properties. Science 193:163 (1976).

23. R. R. Gorman, Modulation of human platelet function by prostacyclin and thromboxane A_2. Federation Proc., 38:83 (1979).

24. J. Dyeberg, H. O. Bang, E. Stoffersen and J. R. Vane, Eicosapentanoic acid and prevention of thrombosis and atherosclerosis? Lancet, 2:117 (1978).

25. S. Morooka, M. Kobayaski and T. Shimamoto, Experimental ischemic heart disease induced by thromboxane A_2 in rabbits. Jap. Circ. J. 41:1373 (1977).

26. M. D. Schneider and B. J. Kelman, A proposed mechanism/s of transitory ischemic injury to myocardium. Am. J. Vet. Res. 40:170 (1979).

27. A. Szczeklik, R. Nizankowski, S. Skawinski, J. Szczeklik, P. Gluszko and R. J. Gryglewski, Successful therapy of advanced arteriosclerosis obliterans with prostacyclin. Lancet, 1:1111 (1979).

28. U. Diczfalusy and S. Hammarström, Inhibitors or thromboxane synthase in human platelets. Febs Letters, 82:107 (1977).

29. P. Needleman, B. Bryan, A. Wyche, S. D. Bronson, K. Eakins, J. A. Ferendelli and M. Minkes, Thromboxane synthetase inhibitors as pharmacological tools: differential biochemical and biological effects on platelet suspensions. Prostaglandins, 14:897 (1977).

30. H-H Tai and B. Yuan, Studies on the thromboxane synthetizing system in human platlet microsomes. Biochim. Biophys. Acta., 531:286 (1978).

31. S. Moncada, P. Needleman, S. Bunting and J. R. Vane, Prostaglandin endoperoxide and thromboxane generating systems and their selective inhibition. Prostaglandins, 12:323 (1976).

32. R. J. Gryglewski, A. Zmuda, R. Korbut, E. Krecioch and K. Bieron, Selective inhibition of thromboxane A_2 biosynthesis in blood platelets. Nature, 267:627 (1977).

33. R. J. Gryglewski, R. Korbut, A. Ocetkiewicz and J. Stachura, In vivo method for quantitation of antiplatelet potency of drugs. Naunyn-Schmiedeberg's Arch. Pharmacol., 302:25 (1978).

34. S. Moncada, S. Bunting, K. Mullane, P. Thorogood, and J. R. Vane, Imidazole: a selective inhibitor of thromboxane synthetase. Prostaglandins, 13:611 (1977).

35. H-H Tai and B. Yuan, On the inhibitory potency of imidazole and its derivatives on thromboxane synthetase. Biochem. Biophys. Res. Comm., 80:236 (1978).

36. G. Allan, K. Eakins, Burimamide is a selective inhibitor of thromboxane A_2 biosynthesis in human platelet microsomes. Prostaglandins, 15:659 (1978).

37. F. A. Fitzpatrick and R. R. Gorman, A comparison of imidazole and 9,11-azaprosta-5,13-dienoic acid – two selective thromboxane synthetase inhibitors,. Biochim. Biophys. Acta., 539:162 (1978).

38. K. E. Eakins, V. Rajadhyaksha and R. Schroer, Prostaglandin antagonism by sodium p-benzyl-4-(1-oxo-2-(-4-chlorobenzyl)-3-phenyl propyl) phenyl phosphonate (N-0164). Br.J. Pharmacol., 58:333 (1976).

39. B. J. R. Whittle, S. Moncada and J.R. Vane, Formation of prostacyclin by the gastric mucosa and its actions on gastric function. Prostaglandins, 15:704 (1978).

40. K. E. Eakins and P. S. Kulkarni, Selective inhibitory actions of sodium p-benzyl-4-(1-oxo-2-(4-chlorobenzyl)-3-phenyl propyl) phenyl phosphate (N-0164) and indomethacin on the biosynthesis of prostaglandins and thromboxanes from arachidonic acid. Br. J. Pharmacol., 60:135 (1977).

41. J. E. Vincent and F. J. Zijlstra, Nicotinic acid inhibits thromboxane synthesis in platelets. Prostaglandins, 15:629 (1978).

42. A. N. Makheja, J. Y. Vanderhoek and J. M. Bailey, Properties of inhibitor of platelet aggregation and thromboxane synthesis isolated from onion and garlic. Thrombosis. Haemostas., 42:74 (1979).

43. P. H. Chanch, I. Sokan, A. P. H. Chanch and P. Clavel, A comparative study of anti-thromboxane synthetase activity of the microsomes from different parts of the bovine heart. Abstracts of the IVth International Prostaglandin Conference in Washington, D.C. May 27-31 1979.

44. E. J. Corey, K. C. Nicolaou, Y. Machida, C. Malmsten and B. Samuelsson, Synthesis and biological properties of a 9,11-aza-prostanoid; highly active biochemical mimic of prostaglandin endoperoxides. Proc. Natl. Acad. Sci. USA., 72:335 (1975).

45. F. F. Sun, Biosynthesis of thromboxanes in human platelets. I. Characterization and assay of thromboxane synthetase. Biochem. Biophys. Res. Comm., 74:1432 (1977).

46. J. F. Charo, R. D. Feinman, T. C. Detwills, J. Smith, C. M. Ingerman and M. J. Silver, Prostaglandin endoperoxides and thromboxane A_2 can induce platelet aggregation in the absence of secretion. Nature, 269:66 (1977).

47. G. L. Bundy and D. C. Peterson, The synthesis of 15-deoxy-9-11-epoxyimino prostaglandins potent thromboxane synthetase inhibitors. Tetrahedron Letters, 1:41 (1978).

48. R. R. Gorman, G. L. Bundy, D. C. Peterson, F. F. Sun, O. V. Miller and F. A. Fitzpatrick, Inhibition of human platelet thromboxane synthetase by 9,11-azaprosta-5,13-dienoic acid. Proc. Natl. Acad. Sci. USA, 74:4007 (1977).

49. R. R. Gorman, F. A. Fitzpatrick and O. V. Miller, A selective thromboxane synthetase inhibitor blocks the cAMP lowering activity of PGH_2. Biochem. Biophys. Res. Commun., 79:305 (1977).

50. F. A. Fitzpatrick, G. L. Bundy, R. R. Gorman and T. Honohan, 9,11-Epoxyiminoprosta-5,13-dienoic acid is thromboxane A_2 antagonist in human platelets. Nature, in press.

51. R. J. Gryglewski, S. Bunting, S. Moncada, R. J. Flower and
     J. R. Vane, Arterial walls are protected against deposition
     of platelet thrombi by a substance (Prostaglandin X) which
     they make from prostaglandin endoperoxides. Prostaglandins
     12:685 (1976).
52. J. A. Salmon, D. R. Smith, R. J. Flower, S. Moncada and
     J. R. Vane, Further studies on the enzymatic conversion of
     prostaglandin endoperoxide into prostacyclin by porcine
     aorta microsomes. Biochim. Biophys. Acta, 523:250 (1978).
53. W. I. Rosenblum and F. El-Sabban, Enhancement of platelet
     aggregation by tranylcypromine in mouse cerebal micro-
     vessels. Circulat. Res., 43:238 (1978).
54. A. Wennmalm, Effects of nicotine on cardiac prostaglandin
     and platelet thromboxane synthesis. Br. J. Pharmac.,
     64:559 (1978).
55. F. P. Nijkamp, S. Moncada, H. L. White and J. R. Vane,
     Diversion of prostaglandin endoperoxide metabolism by
     selective inhibition of thromboxane A$_2$ biosynthesis in
     lung, spleen or platelets. Eur. J. Pharmacol., 44:179 (1977).
56. F. ten Hoor and J. F. A. Quadt, Effect of nicotine on
     prostacyclin production by the isolated pulsatingly perfused
     rat aorta. Abstracts of IVth International Prostaglandin
     Conference in Washington, D.C. May 28-31, 1979.

PROSTAGLANDIN SYSTEM AND INFLAMMATION

G. P. Velo*, M. E. Fracasso*, R. Leone* and
R. Milanino**

*Istituto di Farmacologia, Università di Padova,
Policlinico Borgo Roma, 37100 Verona, Italia

**Dipartimento di Farmacologia, Divisione Ricerche,
Laboratori Glaxo S.p.a. - Duncan Farmaceutici S.p.a.
Via A. Fleming, 2, 37100 Verona, Italia

Prostaglandins (PGs) were first described by Goldblatt and von Euler, in the early thirties, as compounds contained in the crude extract of seminal vesicles and capable of lowering blood pressure and contracting smooth muscles, especially those coming from the gastro-intestinal tract (1,2).

Since then a great deal of research has been done, and now we usually better refer to prostaglandins speaking in terms of "PG system" or "arachidonic acid cascade".

Leukotrienes A,B and C are the most recently discovered components of the PG-system archidonic acid cascade (leukotriene C probably corresponds to the slow-reacting substance of analylaxis - SRS A) (3). They are produced, by leucocytes, from archidonic acid via lipoxygenase and 5-HPETE (Figure 1). The discovery of lipoxygenase alternative pathway in the metabolism of arachidonic acid is due to the work of Hamberg and Samuelsson (4) and Nugteren (5). 12-HETE was found in the skin and it was shown that its concentration rises during psoriasis (6); this compound was also shown to possess chemotactic activity (7,8). Other components of the lipoxygenase pathway, other than 12-HETE, may have chemotactic function.

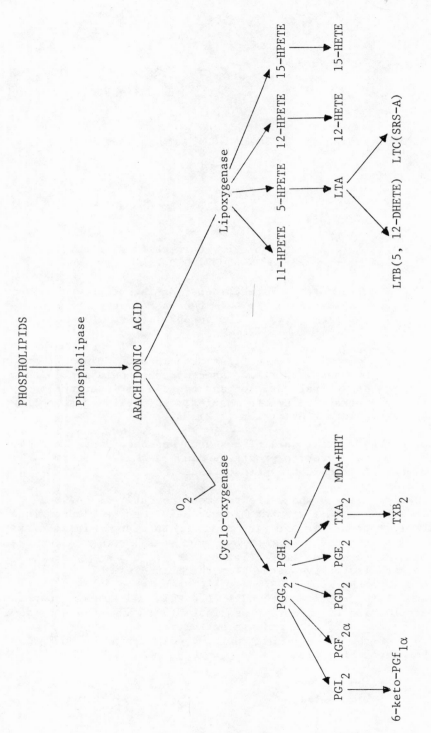

Fig. 1. Arachidonic acid cascade

INFLAMMATORY ACTIONS OF THE PG-SYSTEM

At the present time many evidences underline the involvement
of the PG-system in the inflammatory process, and the prostaglandin
contribution to a variety of inflammatory symptoms is clear
(figure 2).

The pro-inflammatory activity of some PGs was reported by
Horton (9) who was able to show an increase of vascular
permeability (guinea pig) and a rise of blood flow (cat),
following PGE_1 injections. The intradermal injection of PGE_1
causes a 10 hours lasting erythema in man (10). Crunkhorn and
Willis showed that PGE_1 and PGE_2 are capable to increase
vascular permeability in rat's skin, while PGFs have no effect
in this system (11). These Authors proposed that the effect of
PGEs could be partially mediated by the local liberation of
histamine; as a matter of fact previous administration of histamine-
antagonists or histamine-depleting agents are both able to reduce
the vascular response of PGE_2 (12). These findings were also
substantiated, in man, by Søndergaard and Greaves (13). It is
possible that PGE_1 and PGE_2 exert their effect on vascular
permeability both directly , and indirectly by liberation of
histamine. We also like to remind that PGEs potentiate the
activity of mediators like bradykinin and histamine on vascular
permeability (14,15).

Kaley and Weiner, using a modification of the Boyden chamber
technique, were able to show that PGE_1 has a strong chemotactic
activity on rabbit's polymorphonuclear leucocytes (PMN) (16).
This chemotactic activity of PGE_1 is probably present also in man,
as shown by the skin window technique (17).

Ferreira reported that PGE_1 causes hyperalgesia and
potentiates the histamine and/or bradykinin-induced pain (18).
Similar results were also obtained in man (19).

All data mentioned so far sustain the possible role of PGEs
in potentiating the inflammatory activity of different mediators.

In 1970 a prostaglandin-like substance was identified in the
cerebro-spinal fluid of a hyperpyretic cat (20). Later work
showed that PGA_1, PGE_1 and $PGF_{1\alpha}$ were able to induce hyperpyrexia
when injected into the lateral-ventricle of the cat; these results
were similar in other animal species, injecting PGE_1 (21).

Effects

PGE

VASODILATION

INCREASED VASCULAR PERMEABILITY

HISTAMINE RELEASE

PAIN

SENSITIZATION OF RECEPTOR SITES

FEVER

COLLAGEN BIOSYNTHESIS

CHEMOTAXIS

INCREASED cAMP PRODUCTION

PGE_α

VASOCONSTRICTION

DECREASED VASCULAR PERMEABILITY

INCREASED cGMP PRODUCTION

Fig. 2. PGE, PGF_α and some inflammatory actions

Recently the attention has been focused on prostaglandin D_2 (PGD_2) which is able to inhibit platelet aggregation (22,23). PGD_2 is also ausing long-lasting erythema in the human forearm, increased vascular permeability in rat's skin and potentiation of the effect of histamine on vascular permeability (24).

The cyclic endoperoxides (PGG_2 and PGH_2) have shown to potentiate both inflammatory oedema in rat (25) and cutaneous response in man (26). Lewis et al. (27) have shown, in the hamster cheek pouch preparation, that PGG_2 administration produces a transient vasoconstriction followed by a long-lasting vasodilation, this latter effect being probably due to the formation, from PGG_2, of prostacyclin (PGI_2) (28).

At the present time the role of thromboxane A_2 (TXA_2) in the development of the inflammatory process is still unclear. TXA_2 has a strong platelet aggregating action and it shows a contrictory effect on arteries (29). Thromboxane B_2 (TXB_2), the stable metabolite of TXA_2, is chemotactic for PMN in vivo and in vitro (30).

TXB_2 is also able to inhibit the increase of cutaneous vascular permeability induced by PGE_2 (30), to stimulate DNA synthesis and cellular division of carrageenan granuloma-derived fibroblasts in vitro, and it increases the syntheses of RNA and hexosamine-containing substances (31).

PGI_2 is an in vivo vasodilator (28), it induces smooth muscle relaxation in vitro (32,33) and it shows anti-aggregating properties (34). PGI_2 increases also the vascular permeability, it potentiates the bradykinin induced plasma exudation and the effect of other mediators, and, when injected into the rat paw, it is capable of increasing the reaction to carrageenan administration (35,36,37,38,39). It seems likely that the vasodilatory capacity and the effect on vascular permeability exerted by PGI_2 could both take part in the development of the inflammatory oedema and erythema. The stable metabolite of PGI_2 (6-keto-$PGF_{1\alpha}$), is approximately 500 times less potent than PGI_2 in causing oedema formation (37), and 20 to 30 times less active than PGI_2 in its vasodilatory effect (40). PGI_2 is capable of inducing hyperalgesia showing, compared to PGE_2, a 5-times greater (37), yet shorter-lasting (41), effect. Like PGEs, also PGI_2 seems to have the ability to sensitize pain receptors to different stimuli (37); on the other hand, Ferreira et al. suggest that PGI_2 could be the true mediator of pain (41).

We discussed, so far, the pro-inflammatory properties of the PG-system, yet, the role of the PG-system itself in the overall inflammatory process is far more complex.

Actually the PGs have also anti-inflammatory properties and the development of inflammation is probably dependent on the balance of the pro- and anti-inflammatory effects, whose expression could be regulated by a feedback mechanism. Interesting to this topic are the studies carried on by Hillier and Karim on human vessels (42), by Crunkhorn and Willis on vascular permeability (43), and by Velo et al. and Willoughby et al. on different models of inflammation in the rat (44,45). The latter Authors have focused their attention on the role played by the ratio PGE/PGF in the development of inflammatory exudate. They suggested for PGEs and PGFs a Yin-Yang hypothesis (Taoist concept of opposing forces modulating each other), similar to that proposed by Goldberg et al. for cAMP and cGMP (46,47,48).

Finally, PGI_2 inhibits the PMN's motility (49,50), probably stimulating the synthesis of cAMP (51); as a matter of fact it is known that cAMP itself inhibits both chemotactic response and motility of PMN s(52).

PRESENCE OF PG-COMPONENTS IN THE INFLAMMATORY PROCESS

Prostaglandins are present in many experimentally induced inflammations, in man skin inflammatory processes and in the synovial fluid of patients suffering from rheumatoid arthritis; PGs have also been studied in different cellular systems in vitro.

Following rabbit's iris irritation it is possible to isolate a substance (initially called irin) which is formed by a mixture of different components of the PG-system (53). Willis has shown the presence of PGs in the late phase of rat carrageenan oedema (54). Anderson et al. have found PGs, mainly PGE_2, in the exudate from the air bleb 3 hours after carrageenan injection; these Authors have also shown a parallel increase of PGE_2 and β-glucuronidase (55). Velo et al. have found the presence of PGE_2 and $PGF_{2\alpha}$ in the exudate from carrageenan-induced pleurisy and peritonitis, and in the synovial fluid derived from patients with rheumatoid arthritis (44). Other Authors have also measured the level of PGs in synovial fluids (56,57).

More recent studies have confirmed the importance of PGE_2 in the acute inflammatory process. This was shown, for instance, in the inflammation induced by implantation of carraggeenan-impregnated polyester sponges (58), in carrageenan-induced granuloma (59) and in the acute urate crystals arthritis of the chicken (60), also if, in this last inflammatory process, PGD_2 seems to be the most relevant component among the one's of the PG-system (60). During carrageenan-induced inflammation it is possible to show the presence of thromboxane B_2, 6 keto-$PGF_{1\alpha}$ (58) and of PGI_2, being the latter measurable in amounts greater than PGE_2 (59). The amounts of TXB_2, measured after few days, are

comparable with those obtained from the synovial fluid of
rheumatic patients (61). Yet, also in view of Chang's et al.
results (62,63), the role of these compounds remains to be
clarified.

The majority of the studies has been performed in experimentally
induced inflammations, nevertheless the presence of prostaglandins
has also been shown in perfusates of human skin affected by
allergic contact eczema, primary irritant dermatitis and after
exposure to ultraviolet radiations (64,65).

During phagocitosis PMNs release PGs(66,67) and thromboxanes
(68,69,70). Activated macrophages produce PGE_2 (71,72,73)
and TXB_2 (74), the latter being a potent chemotactic factor (75).

Also if the all picture is still rather unclear, these
data speak in favour of an important role of the latter components
of arachidonic acid cascade in the inflammatory process. We like
to stress again on the fact that the PG-components can be mediators
and modulators of the inflammatory process. They can modulate
each other directly and are self-modulating via the cyclic
nucleotides.

REFERENCES

1. M. W. Goldblatt, A depressor substance in seminal fluid,
   J. Soc. Chem. Ind., 52:1056 (1933).
2. U. S. von Euler, On the specific vasodilating and plain muscle
   stimulating substances from accessory genital glands in
   man and certain animals (prostaglandin and vesiglandin),
   J. Physiol., 88:213 (1936).
3. B. Samuelsson, P. Borgeat, S. Hammarström and R. C. Murphy,
   Introduction of a nomenclature: Leukotrienes,Abstract, Paper
   presented during the Prostaglandin Conference in Washington
   28-31 May, 1979.
4. M. Hamberg and B. Samuelsson, Prostaglandin endoperoxides.
   Novel transformations of arachidonic acid in human platelets,
   Proc. Natl. Acad. Sci. USA, 71:3400 (1974).
5. D. A. Nugteren, Arachidonate lipoxygenase in blood platelets,
   Biochim. Biophys. Acta., 380:299 (1975).
6. S. Hammarström, M. Hamberg, B. Samuelsson, E. A. Duell, M.
   Stawiski and J. J. Voorhees, Increased concentrations of
   free arachidonic acid, prostaglandins E_2 and $F_{2\alpha}$ and of 12L-
   hydroxy-5,8,10,14 - eicosatetraenoic acid (HETE) in epidermis
   of psoriasis; Evidence for perturbed regulation of arachidonic
   acid levels in psoriasis, Proc. Natl. Acad. Sci. USA, 72:
   5130 (1975).
7. S. R. Turner, J. A. Tainer and W. S. Lynn, Biogenesis of
   chemotactic molecules by the arachidonate lipoxygenase system
   of platelets, Nature, 257:680 (1975).

8. E. J. Goetzl, J. M. Woods and R. R. Gorman, Stimulation of
    human eosinophil and neutrophil polymorphonuclear leukocyte
    chemotaxis and random migration by 12-L-hydroxy-5,8,10,14-
    eicosatetraenoic acid, J. Clin. Invest., 59:179 (1977).
9. E. Horton, Action of prostaglandin E_1 on tissues which respond
    to bradykinin, Nature, 200:892 (1963).
10. L. M. Solomon, L. Juhlin and M. B. Kirschenbaum, Prostaglandin
    on cutaneous vasculature, J. Invest. Derm., 51:280 (1968).
11. P. Crunkhorn and A. L. Willis, Actions and interactions of
    prostaglandin administered intradermally in rat and in man,
    Br. J. Pharmac., 36:216P (1969).
12. P. Crunkhorn and A. L. Willis, Cutaneous reactions to intra-
    dermal prostaglandins, Br. J. Pharmac., 41:49 (1971).
13. J. S. Søndergaard and M. W. Greaves, Continuous skin perfusion
    in vitro as a method for study of pharmacological agents in
    human skin, Acta Dermatovener., 51:50 (1971).
14. S. Moncada, S. H. Ferreira and J. R. Vane, Prostaglandins,
    aspirin-like drugs and the oedema of inflammation, Nature,
    246:217 (1973).
15. G. Thomas and G. B. West, Prostaglandins, kinin and
    inflammation in the rat, Br. J. Pharmac., 50:231 (1974).
16. G. Kaley and R. Weiner, Effect of prostaglandin E on
    leucocyte migration, Nature New Biology, 234:114 (1971).
17. J. S. Søndergaard and P. Wolf-Jorgensen, The cellular exudate
    of human cutaneous inflammation induced by prostaglandins
    E_1 and $F_{1\alpha}$, Acta. Dermatovener, 52:361 (1972).
18. S. H. Ferreira, Prostaglandins, aspirin-like drugs and
    analgesia, Nature New Biology, 240:200 (1972).
19. M. W. Greaves and W. McDonald-Gibson, Itch: role of
    prostaglandins, Br. Med. J., 3:608 (1973).
20. A. S. Milton and S. Wendlandt, A possible role for
    prostaglandin E_1 as a modulator for temperature regulation
    in the central nervous system in the cat, J. Physiol. (Lond.)
    207:76P (1970).
21. W. Feldberg and P. N. Saxena, Fever produced by prostaglandin
    E_1, J. Physiol. (Lond.), 317:547 (1971).
22. J. B. Smith, M. J. Silver, C. M. Ingerman and J. J. Kocsis,
    Prostaglandin D_2 inhibits the aggregation of human platelets,
    Thrombosis Res., 5:291 (1974).
23. E. E. Nishizawa, W. L. Miller, R. R. Gorman, G. L. Bundy,
    J. Svensson and M. Hamberg, Prostaglandin D_2 as a potential
    antithrombotic agent, Prostaglandins, 9:109 (1975).
24. R. J. Flower, E. A. Harvey and W. P. Kingston, Inflammatory
    effects of prostaglandin D_2 in rat and human skin, Br. J.
    Pharmac., 56:229 (1976).
25. J. R. Vane, Prostaglandins as mediators of inflammation, in:
    Advances in Prostaglandin and Thromboxane Research, Vol.2,
    B. Samuelsson and R. Paoletti, eds., p.791 (Raven Press,
    New York, 1976).

26. O. Hagermark, K. Strandberg and M. Hamberg, Potentiating
     effects of prostaglandin E_2 and the prostaglandin
     endoperoxide PGH_2 on cutaneous responses in man, J. Invest.
     Derm., 66:266P (1976).
27. G. P. Lewis, J. Westwick and T. J. Williams, Microvascular
     responses produced by the prostaglandin endoperoxide PGG_2
     in vivo, Br. J. Pharmac., 59:442P (1977).
28. G. A. Higgs, S. Moncada and J. R. Vane, Prostacyclin as a
     potent dilator of arterioles in the hamster cheek pouch,
     J. Physiol. (Lond.), 275:30P (1978).
29. S. Samuelsson, Introduction: new trends in prostaglandin
     research, in: Advances in Prostaglandin and Thromboxane
     Research, Vol. 1, B. Samuelsson and R. Paoletti, eds.,
     p.1 (Raven Press, New York, 1976).
30. J. R. Boot, W. Dawson and E. A. Kitchen, The chemotactic
     activity of thromboxane B_2: A possible role in inflammation,
     J. Physiol., 257:47P (1976).
31. S-I. Murota, W-C. Chang, S. Tsurufuji and I. Morita, The
     possible roles of prostacyclin (PGI_2) and thromboxanes in
     chronic inflammation, in: Advances in Inflammation Research,
     Vol. 1, G. Weissmann, B. Samuelsson, R. Paoletti, eds.,
     P.439 (Raven Press, New York, 1979).
32. S. Bunting, R. Gryglewski, S. Moncada and J. R. Vane,
     Arterial walls generate from prostaglandin endoperoxides a
     substance (Prostaglandin X) which relaxes strips of
     mesenteric and coeliac arteries and inhibits platelets
     aggregation, Prostaglandins, 12:897 (1976).
33. G. J. Dusting, S. Moncada and J. R. Vane, Prostacyclin (PGX)
     is the endogenous metabolite responsible for relaxation of
     coronary arteries induced by arachidonic acid, Prostaglandins,
     13:3 (1977).
34. S. Moncada, R. J. Gryglewski, S. Bunting and J. R. Vane,
     Further studies on the enzymatic conversion of prostaglandin
     endoperoxides to an unstable substance that inhibits
     platelet aggregation, Nature, 263:663 (1976).
35. S-I. Murota, I. Morita, S. Tsurufuji, H. Sato and K. Sugio,
     Effect of prostaglandin I_2 and related compounds on vascular
     permeability response in granuloma tissues, Prostaglandins,
     15:297 (1978).
36. M. J. Peck and T. J. Williams, Prostacyclin (PGI_2)
     potentiates bradykinin-induced plasma exudation in rabbit
     skin, Br. J. Pharmac., 62:464P (1978).
37. E. A. Higgs, S. Moncada and J. R. Vane, Inflammatory effects
     of prostacyclin (PGI_2) and 6-oxo-$PGF_{1\alpha}$ in the rat paw,
     Prostaglandins, 16:153 (1978).
38. A. W. Ford-Hutchinson, J. R. Walker, E. M. Davidson and
     M. J. H. Smith, PGI_2: a potential mediator of inflammation,
     Prostaglandins, 16:253 (1978).
39. K. Komoriya, H. Ohmori, A. Azuha, S. Kurozumi, Y. Hashimoto,
     K. C. Nicolaou, W. E. Barnette and R. L. Magolda, Prostaglandin
     I_2 as a potentiator of acute inflammation in rats, Prostaglandins,
     15:557 (1978).

40. G. A. Higgs, E. A. Higgs and J. A. Salmon, Prostacyclin in
     inflammation, in: Prostacyclin, J. R. Vane and S. Bergström
     Eds., p. 187 (Raven Press, New York,1979).

41. S. H. Ferreira, M. Nakamura and M. S. Abreu Castro, The
     hyperalgesic effects of prostacyclin and PGE_2, Prostaglandins,
     16:31 (1978).

42. K.Hillier and S. M. M. Karim, Effects of prostaglandins E_1,
     E_2, $F_{1\alpha}$ and $F_{2\alpha}$ on isolated human umbilical and placental
     blood vessels, J. Obstet. Gynaec. Br. Commonwealth, 75:667
     (1968).

43. P. Crunkhorn and A. L. Willis, Interaction between prosta-
     glandins E and F given intradermally in the rat, Br. J.
     Pharmac., 41:507 (1971).

44. G. P. Velo, C. J. Dunn, J. P. Giroud, J. Timsit and D. A.
     Willoughby, Distribution of prostaglandins in inflammatory
     exudate, J. Pathol., 111:149 (1973).

45. D. A. Willoughby, J. P. Giroud, G. P. Velo, Progrès dans l'
     inflammation applicable à la polyarthrite cronique évolutive,
     Brux. Med., 54:135 (1974).

46. N. D. Goldberg, M. K. Haddox, D. K. Hartle and J. W. Hadden,
     The biological role of cyclic 3'-5'-guanosine monophosphate,
     in: Pharmacology and the Future of Man, Vol. 5, G. H. Acheson
     Ed., p.146 (Karger, Basel,1973).

47. G. P. Velo and S. E. Abdullahi, General concepts of
     inflammation, in: Inflammatory Arthropathies, E. C. Huskisson
     and G. P. Velo,Eds., p. 3 (Excerpta Medica, Amsterdam,1976).

48. J. P. Giroud, G. P. Velo and D. A. Willoughby, The role of
     prostaglandins and cyclic nucleotides in inflammation, in:
     Prostaglandins and Thromboxanes, F. Berti, B. Samuelsson and
     G. P. Velo, Eds., p.323 (Plenum Press, New York, 1977).

49. B. B. Weksler, J. M. Knapp and E. A. Jaffe, Prostacyclin
     (PGI_2) synthesized by cultured endothelial cells modulates
     polymorphonuclear leukocyte function, Blood 50(5) suppl.1:
     287 (1977).

50. G. A. Higgs, S. Moncada and J. R. Vane, Prostacyclin reduces
     the number of "slow moving" leukocytes in hamster cheek pouch
     venules, J. Physiol., 280:55P (1978).

51. J. E. Tateson, S. Moncada and J. R. Vane, Effects of
     prostacyclin (PGX) on cyclic AMP concentrations in human
     platelets, Prostaglandins, 13:389 (1977).

52. J. Rivikin, J. Rosenblatt and E. L. Becker, The role of
     cyclic AMP in the chemotactic responsiveness and spontaneous
     motility of rabbit peritoneal neutrophils, J. Immunol.,
     115:1126 (1974).

53. N. Ambache, L. Kavanagh and J. Whiting, Effect of mechanical
     stimulation on rabbit eyes: release of active substances in
     anterior chamber perfusates, J. Physiol. (Lond.), 176:
     378 (1965).

54. A. L. Willis, Parallel assay of prostaglandin-like activity
     in rat inflammatory exudate by means of cascade superfusion,
     J. Pharm. Pharmac., 21:126 (1969).
55. A. J. Anderson, W. E. Brocklehurst and A. L. Willis, Evidence
     for the role of lysosomes in the formation of prostaglandins
     during carrageenin-induced inflammation in the rat, Pharmac.
     Res. Comm., 3:13 (1971).
56. D. R. Robinson and L. Levine, Prostaglandin concentrations
     in synovial fluids in rheumatic diseases, in: 66th Annual
     Meeting of the American Society for Clinical Investigation,
     Abstr., 246 (1974).
57. D. R. Robinson, M. B. MacGuire and L. Levine, Prostaglandins
     in the rheumatic diseases, Ann. N.Y. Acad. Sci., 256:318 (1975).
58. G. A. Higgs and J. A. Salmon, Cyclo-oxygenase products in
     carrageenin-induced inflammation, Prostaglandins, 17:737
     (1979).
59. J. A. Splawinski, B. Wojtaszek, J. Swies and R. J. Gryglewski,
     Endogenous factors affecting arachidonic acid metabolism:
     I. Biosynthesis of prostacyclin and prostaglandins by
     carrageenin granulomas of rats, Prostaglandins, 16:683 (1978).
60. B. A. Peskar and K. Brune, Prostaglandin D_2: The prevailing
     prostaglandin in acute inflammation, in: Arachidonic Acid
     Metabolism in Inflammation and Thrombosis, K. Brune and
     M. Baggiolini, eds., p.260 (Birkhäuser, Basel,1979).
61. L. E. Trang, E. Granstrom and O. Lovgren, Levels of
     prostaglandins $F_{2\alpha}$ and E_2 and thromboxane B_2 in joint fluid
     in rheumatoid arthritis, Scand. J. Rheum., 6:151 (1977).
62. W-C. Chang, S-I. Murota, M. Matsuo and S. Tsurufuji, A new
     prostaglandin transformed from arachidonic acid in
     carrageenin-induced granuloma, Biochem. Res. Commun., 72:1259
     (1976).
63. W-C. Chang, S-I. Murota and S. Tsurufuji, Thromboxane B_2
     transformed from arachidonic acid in carrageenin-induced
     granuloma, Prostaglandins, 13:17 (1977).
64. J. Søndergaard and M. W. Greaves, Release of prostaglandins
     in human cutaneous sustained inflammatory reactions, in:
     Future Trends in Inflammation, G. P. Velo, D. A. Willoughby,
     J. P. Giroud, eds., p.45 (Piccin, Padova 1974).
65. M. W. Greaves and J. S. Søndergaard, Pharmacological agents
     released in ultraviolet inflammation studied by cutaneous
     skin perfusion, J. Invest. Derm., 54:365 (1970).
66. R. B. Zurier and D. M. Sayadoff, Release of prostaglandins
     from human polymorphonuclear leukocytes, Inflammation,
     1:93 (1975).
67. G. A. Higgs, M. E. McCall and L. J. F. Youlten, A chemotactic
     role for prostaglandins released from polymorphonuclear
     leukocytes during phagocytosis, Br. J. Pharmac., 53:539
     (1975).
68. G. A. Higgs, S. Bunting, S. Moncada and J. R. Vane,
     Polymorphonuclear leukocytes produce thromboxane A_2-like

activity during phagocytosis, Prostaglandins, 12:749 (1976).

69. I. M. Goldstein, C. L. Malmsten, H. B. Kaplan, H. Jindahl,
     B. Samuelsson and G. Weissmann, Thromboxane generation by
     stimulated human granulocytes. Inhibition by gluco-
     corticoids and superoxide dismutase, Clin. Res., 25:518A
     (1977).

70. E. M. Davison, A. W. Ford-Hutchinson, M. J. H. Smith and J.
     R. Walker, The release of thromboxane B2 by rabbit peritoneal
     polymorphonuclear leukocytes, Br. J. Pharmac., 63:407P
     (1978).

71. D. Gordon, M. A. Bray and J. Morley, Control of lymphokine
     secretion by prostaglandins, Nature, 262:401 (1976).

72. J. L. Humes, R. J. Bonney, L. Pelus, M. E. Dahlgran, S. J.
     Sadowski, F. A. Kuehl Jr. and P. Davies, Macrophages
     synthesise and release prostaglandins in response to
     inflammatory stimuli, Nature, 269:149 (1977).

73. M. Glatt, H. Kälin, K. Wagner and K. Brune, Prostaglandins
     release from macrophages: An assay system for anti-inflammatory
     drugs in vitro, Agents and Actions, 7:321 (1977).

74. J. Morley, M. A. Bray R. W. Jones, D. H. Nugteren and D. A.
     van Dorp, Prostaglandin and thromboxane production by human
     and guinea-pig macrophages and leucocytes, Prostaglandins,
     17:730 (1979).

75. J. R. Boot, W. Dawson and E. A. Kitchen, The chemotactic
     activity of thromboxane B2: A possible role in inflammation,
     J. Physiol, 257:47P (1976).

FREE RADICAL REACTIONS IN RELATION TO LIPID PEROXIDATION

INFLAMMATION AND PROSTAGLANDIN METABOLISM

T. F. Slater*and Chiara Benedetto**

*Department of Biochemistry, Brunel University,
 Uxbridge, Middlesex, U.K.
 and
**Institute of General Pathology,
 University of Turin, Italy

Chemical bonds in organic structures normally involve the
sharing of pairs of electrons; the two electrons in each pair
have opposite spins that create opposing small magnetic dipoles.
When a single unpaired electron is present, the resultant
compound has a number of novel chemical and biological properties:
such compounds are called free radicals. The presence of the
unpaired electron is conventionally represented by a heavy dot :
R·. Reviews that may be consulted for general background
references on free radicals are by Isenberg (1), Pryor (2),
Slater (3), Pryor (4), Slater (5).

Free radicals can be electrically neutral species, or may
have a net positive or negative charge; examples to illustrate
this point are shown in Figure 1.

The single unpaired electron in general gives the free
radical a rather high chemical reactivity. However, free radicals
are known that range in reactivity from examples that are
exceptionally reactive through to those being stable at room
temperature. The hydroxyl radical (OH·) is a very powerful
oxidising agent and its half-life in aqueous biological
environments is only a few micro-seconds (for discussion of its
rates of reaction with biomolecules see 6); the superoxide
radical ($O_2^-·$) is much less reactive than OH· under normal
conditions in biological systems (6), whereas diphenyl
picrylhydrazyl is a stable radical that may be stored almost
indefinitely (see 2).

$$Pr + OH^{\cdot} \longrightarrow Pr^{+\cdot} + OH^{-}$$

$$O_2 + e^{-} \longrightarrow O_2^{-\cdot}$$

$$CCl_4 + e^{-} \longrightarrow CCl_3^{\cdot} + Cl$$

Fig. 1.   This illustrates three free radical reactions in which a
         cationic ($Pr^{+\cdot}$), an anionic ($O_2^{-\cdot}$) and a neutral free
         radical ($CCl_3^{\cdot}$) are formed. In the first case, the
         phenothiazine drug promethazine is oxidised by $OH^{\cdot}$; in
         the second, oxygen is reduced to form the superoxide
         free radical; in the third, CCl_4 undergoes dissociative
         electron capture to yield the
         radical.

     When free radicals of high chemical reactivity are produced
inside cells, the variety of neighbouring chemical substances
ensures that the reactive free radical cannot diffuse very far
before undergoing chemical modification. In fact, chemical
reactivity and the radius of diffusion in biological systems are
inversely related as shown in Figure 2. Free radicals that can
diffuse long distances (in cellular terms) are not very reactive
chemically; highly reactive free radicals, on the other hand, are
essentially trapped in their micro-environment at their locus of
formation (5). Somewhat paradoxically, therefore, we can
expect the free radicals of intermediate reactivity to be the
most active in producing cellular damage distant to their site of
formation. Another factor that affects diffusion of the primary
radical species is their lipophilicity: free radicals such as
the arachidonate radical (see later), if formed in the membranes
of the endoplasmic reticulum, will generally only be 'free' to
diffuse within the plane of the membrane due to their high
lipophilicity (for discussion of membrane fluidity and diffusion
of membrane components see 7).

     Chemically reactive free radicals generally occur only in
very low concentrations in biological systems as a consequence of
normally low metabolic rates of formation and rapid rates of
utilisation :

$$A \xrightarrow{\text{slow}} A^{\cdot} \xrightarrow{\text{fast}} \text{non-radical products}$$

In consequence, direct study of free radicals in tissues or
subcellular fractions is often difficult due to the low steady
state or transient radical concentrations that occur.

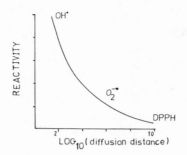

Fig. 2.   This represents in a diagrammatic fashion the relation-
          ship between chemical reactivity of free radicals (in
          arbitrary units) and the average diffusion radius from
          the site of formation. To illustrate this point, the
          approximate positions for a highly reactive radical
          (OH$^{\cdot}$), a moderately reactive radical (O$_2^{-\cdot}$) and a stable
          radical (DPPH) are shown.

        The most direct method for studying free radicals is
electron spin resonance spectroscopy (ESR), which depends on the
small magnetic dipole of the unpaired electron. When the free
radical is placed in a high magnetic field (H) the magnetic
dipole can either line-up parallel to (low energy) or anti-parallel
to (high energy) the applied magnetic field. If micro-wave
radiation (E) is now directed onto the sample an absorption of
energy can 'flip' the magnetic dipole of the free radical from
the low energy to the high energy state. This will occur at a
particular frequency ($\bar{v}$) of the microwave radiation such that

$$h\,\bar{v} = E$$

where h is Planck's constant and E is the energy for producing
the dipole transition. Moreover, E = gβH, where 'g' is a
spectroscopic factor related to the radical under study, β is a
constant (the Bohr magneton) and H is the magnetic field.

Thus: $$h\,\bar{v} = g\,\beta\,H$$

If the frequency is held constant (h and β are also general
constants, and g is constant for a particular free radical) and
H is varied there will be an absorption of microwave radiation
when H satisfies the above equation. A spectrum of energy
absorption against H not only indicates the presence of a free
radical but the position (g-value) and height of the absorption
line(s) give information about the type of radical under study.

For technical reasons the derivative of the energy absorption is usually plotted against H.

Biological samples usually give many absorption lines due to radical species such as semiquinones, flavine radicals, metal complexes, superoxide, etc. An example of a particularly strong ESR signal in a human tissue is illustrated for normal human cervix in Figure 3.

Reviews that may be consulted for further details of ESR are by Swartz et al. (9), and by Symons (10).

ESR is the most direct method available for studying free radical reactions in biological systems but unfortunately the method is not very sensitive. If very reactive radicals are under study their concentration may be far below the limits of ESR spectroscopy due to very rapid annihilation reactions. Under these conditions a less direct technique known as spin trapping (11) may be used. In this procedure, the reactive radical interacts with a stable nitroso or nitrone-compound to yield a stable nitroxy-radical that progressively accumulates (Figure 4). The nitroxy-radicals have characteristic ESR triplet spectra and can be rather easily detected. This technique is being increasingly applied to studies on lipid peroxidation in microsomal membranes (12,13) and in vivo (14).

Free radicals can be formed in biological situations by a variety of reactions. Firstly, they can be formed by the direct impact of high energy radiation on to biological material (see 6). Generally this results in the formation of the highly reactive hydroxyl radical (OH$^{\cdot}$). Low energy radiation (e.g. visible light) can also generate free radicals when appropriate photosensitisers (e.g. porphyrins) are present (15). Under these latter conditions the primary activated species is singlet oxygen (for discussion see 16); singlet oxygen may also be involved under particular conditions in the process of lipid peroxidation (17).

Free radicals can also be formed by enzyme redox reactions where single electrons are transferred to or from the substrate resulting in a free radical product. Examples here are NAD(P)H-linked flavo enzymes that can donate electrons to a variety of acceptors (e.g. O_2 (18), nitro-compounds and quinones (19)) and the reduction of ferric-lipoxygenase I by linoleic acid to yield the linoleic acid radicals (20). Such enzyme reactions can be highly localised within the cell due to precise localisation of the relevant enzyme carrying out the redox reaction, and/or to the local bio-availability of the substrate.

A third main pathway to free radical formation in vivo and in vitro involves transitional metal ions (see refs. 2,3) that

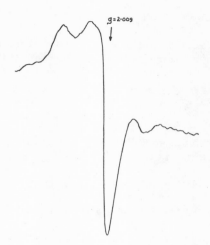

Fig. 3. Electron spin resonance spectrum of a sample of frozen
         powdered human cervix. The spectrum was obtained using
         a Varian E-4 spectrophotometer with cavity temperature
         at -140°C.

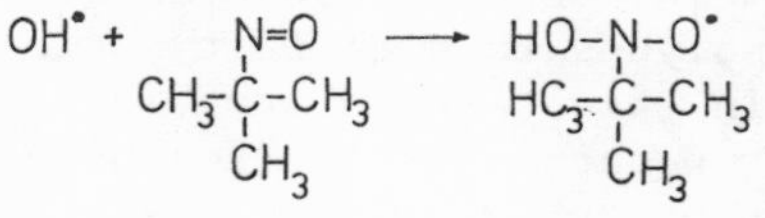

Fig. 4. The trapping of a reactive free radical (OH·) by a
         spin trap (2-methyl-2-nitroso-propane) to yield a
         'stable' nitroxy-radical.

readily undergo one-electron oxidation or reduction; the major
example here involves Fe^{2+}/Fe^{3+}. In the presence of ascorbate,
or H_2O_2, or free-SH then free radicals can be generated in
considerable concentrations and variety. This type of free
radical generation can be affected by changes in the intracellular
distribution of the Fe^{2+}/Fe^{3+} as well as by localised availability
of the relevant oxidant or reductant. In brief, Fe/vit.c or
H_2O_2 can produce the highly oxidising radical OH·; Fe/-SH
produces mainly the weakly reactive O_2^{-}·. Experiments with ESR
and spin traps have shown (21) that O_2^{-}· and H_2O_2 can produce OH·
through the Haber-Weiss reaction:

$$O_2^{-\cdot} + H_2O_2 \longrightarrow O_2 + OH^- + OH^\cdot$$

In this way a rather unreactive radical ($O_2^\cdot$) can participate in the production of a much more reactive species ($OH^\cdot$) that can produce a variety of important biological disturbances.

Free radicals can cause damage to cells and tissues in a variety of ways.

i) by direct attack on -SH groups including those essential for enzymic activities:

$$\text{Protein -SH} + R^\cdot \longrightarrow \text{Protein-S}^\cdot + RH$$

$$\text{Protein -S}^\cdot + R^\cdot \longrightarrow \text{Protein-S-R}$$

$$\text{Protein-S}^\cdot + X\text{-S}^\cdot \longrightarrow \text{Protein-S-S-X}$$

ii) by substitution into aromatic or heterocylic rings of amino acids and coenzymes. This often results in loss of relevant biological activity. The $OH^\cdot$ radical, for example, reacts rapidly with thymine to give an adduct (22,23).

iii) many reactive radicals can also produce damage by abstracting a hydrogen-atom ($H^\cdot$), and this is particularly relevant for methylene hydrogens associated with allylic-sequences in polyunsaturated fatty acids (e.g. arachidonic acid, AAH). In this case an arachidonyl radical ($AA^\cdot$) is formed that reacts quickly (24) with oxygen to give the peroxy-derivative.

$$\text{AAH} + R^\cdot \longrightarrow AA^\cdot + RH$$
$$\downarrow O_2$$
$$AAO_2^\cdot$$

The formation of $AA^\cdot$ is the initiation reaction in the peroxidation of arachidonic acid, and which results in a breakdown of AAH to a complex variety of products, many of high pharmacological activity.

Lipid peroxidation is now known to be a major mechanism of cell injury in a variety of pathological conditions. For example, free radical initiated lipid peroxidation has been shown to be involved in inflammatory processes (25); in liver injury by many agents such as halogenoalkanes (such as CCl_4 (26)) or paracetamol (27);in iron overload conditions (28); in ozone toxicity (29); in cytotoxicity due to adriamycin or bleomycin (30); in radiation injury (6) etc. Some aspects of lipid peroxidation

relevant to the theme of this meeting on Prostaglandins will be
discussed below; more general reviews on lipid peroxidation that
may be consulted are by Slater (31), Mead (32), Witschi and Plaa
(33), Dianzani and Ugazio (34).

Reactive free radicals like OH· react with alkyl hydrogens
in polyunsaturated fatty acids as well as with the more susceptible
methylene hydrogens between two double bonds. Some hydrogen
abstraction from the numerous alkyl hydrogens can be expected (24)
in addition to the several allytic positions available (e.g.
in arachidonate). In consequence a variety of peroxy radicals
may be formed that lead to complex different pathways of
degradation. In fact, it seems likely that, depending on the
nature of the initiating radical (in particular, its chemical
reactivity, its precise locus of formation, and its ability to
penetrate into membranes, etc.) or of the particular enzyme
involved, the chemical structure of the arachidonyl radical
produced will vary and thus result in different groups of
products.

Initial reactions of O_2 with fatty acid radicals have been
studied in model systems by Hasegawa and Patterson (24).
Enzymic studies on mechanisms of peroxidation have largely
concerned the plant lipoxygenase (see, for example, 35, 36).
In studies on the latter enzyme Hamberg and Samuelsson (35)
showed that oxygen is rather specifically introduced at w-6 in a
wide range of natural and synthetic unsaturated fatty acids. A
requirement for peroxidation was the presence of a cis-cis-1,4-
pentadiene group with a methylene group at w-8. Moreover, as
shown by Holman et al (37) a free, sterically unhindered carboxyl
group is necessary for activity of the enzyme.

The soya-bean plant lipoxygenase is therefore rather specific
in its action on unsaturated fatty acids and generally results in
a w-6 hydroperoxide. A mammalian enzyme, sheep vesicular gland
lipoxygenase, however, produced a different product from linoleic
acid to that formed by soya-bean lipoxygenase (36) and recent
studies by Borgeat and Samuelsson (38) have provided evidence
for an additional type of arachidonate hydroperoxide in rabbit
polymorphonuclear leucocytes.

In rat liver microsomes, a number of peroxidising systems
have been studied (39) that differ in their variation with
changes in temperature, with ageing of the microsomal membranes,
and with respect to the action of free radical scavengers. The
microsomal systems that have been studies involve NADPH,
$NADPH/ADP/Fe^{2+}$, $NADPH/CCl_4$, and ascorbate/ADP/Fe. Presumably,
these systems involve different initiating radicals (e.g. OH·,
CCl_3^- , O_2^{-}·) and different mixtures of products. In these rat
liver systems the nature of the immediate products of peroxidation

(i.e. the fatty acid peroxy radicals, and hydroperoxides) have not yet been studied in the same way as for plant lipoxygenase.

The pathobiological consequences of lipid peroxidation have been extensively studied for the hepatotoxic agent carbon tetrachloride. This agent produces centrilobular necrosis and fatty degeneration of the liver, and lipid peroxidation is a major feature of the overall liver injury. In fact, the early damage involves the endoplasmic reticulum (where CCl_4 is activated to CCl_3^- , and specifically requires NADPH (see 40). Moreover, the peroxidation process stimulated by CCl_4 mainly involves arachidonic acid that is present in phosphatidyl ethanolamine (41).

From these and earlier comments concerning soya-bean lipoxygenase we can speculate that the nature and distribution of the initiating enzyme-catalysed event in physiological peroxidative reactions within the phospholipid environment of a biomembrane (plasma membrane, endoplasmic reticulum, etc.) together with local distribution of free radical scavenging materials can result in controlled types of peroxidation with the subsequent controlled production of desirable products. Disturbance of these carefully balanced reactions pushes lipid peroxidation into pathological events that may be profoundly damaging to the cell.

Lipid peroxidation has long been known to yield a complex variety of products; two important reviews that may be consulted are by Schauenstein (42,43). Among the products are mixtures of peroxides and hydroperoxides, and a considerable number of aldehydes, unsaturated aldehydes and hydroxy-alkenals. A number of studies have associated these products of free radical initiated lipid peroxidation with components of the inflammatory response.

The role of free radicals in early stages of the acute inflammatory response has been stressed by several groups of investigators. McCord (44) for example has shown the importance of $O_2^-\cdot$; these studies have been reviewed and extended recently in a Ciba Symposium (45). Krishna-Murti (25)et al, showed some years ago that experimental inflammation induced by carrageenin resulted in an increased lipid peroxidation in liver homogenates; the increase was prevented by prior administration of phenyl-butazone. Although Robak (46) also found a small increase in liver peroxidation during carrageenin inflammation it was necessary to include ascorbate/Fe. In contrast, adjuvant induced arthritis. was associated with a considerable decrease in lower peroxidation. Puig-Parellada and Planas (47) studied the degradation of synovial fluid by free radicals and found that some anti-inflammatory drugs strongly inhibited this process. Torrielli (48) has recently demonstrated the direct inflammatory effects

of various aldehydes after injection into rats and has demonstrated
the partial protection afforded by a number of free radical
scavengers.

In our view, the experimental situations studied are rather
difficult to interpret clearly and we believe the systems studied
involve complex inter-relationships between free radical reactions,
lipid peroxidation, peroxidative product activity, prostaglandin
synthesis and cyclic nucleotide metabolism. A simplified summary
of important interactions is shown in Figure 5.

Brief comments on individual steps shown in Figure 5 are as
follows: Reactions (1) and (2): as already outlined, it is
probable that the chemical structure of the lipid hydroperoxide
(LOOH) produced can be different according to the particular
enzymic or radical initiatory step involved. In consequence,
LOOH may be a family of related lipid hydroperoxides where the
individual chemical species in the family have different
activities with respect to subsequent reactions and biological
properties. Reaction (3): generally speaking, lipid peroxidation
is considerably reduced in tumour tissues(49,50) compared to the
corresponding normal tissue. This results from any or all of the
following known parameters: an increased antioxidant level in
tumours (51), a decreased poly-unsaturated fatty acid content of
tumour microsomal membranes, or a change in distribution of polyunsaturated fatty acids relative to the initiation site. Reactions
(4) and (5): lipid peroxides are known to be toxic especially
when administered parenterally. The LD_{50} of methyl linoleate
peroxide when given i.p. to rats was 12 mg/kg (see 52). It is
not surprising therefore that quite efficient metabolising
systems occur in mammalian tissues and which result in the
formation of much less toxic products; Christopherson (53), for
example, has demonstrated clearly the metabolism of lipid
hydroperoxides to hydroxy fatty acids by a GSH-dependent
peroxidase. Reaction (6): intraperitoneal injection of methyl
linoleate peroxide to rats produced massive ascites (see 52)
which most probably relates to a strong action of lipid peroxides
in increasing capillary permeability (54). It is not known whether
this is a direct action of lipid peroxides or whether some
secondary effect (e.g. on prostaglandin/cyclic nucleotide systems,
reactions 17, 19, 20) is involved. Reaction (7): lipid peroxidation in liver microsomes is accompanied by a rapid destruction
(55) of cytochrome P-450, a hemoprotein enzyme that is effective
in metabolising many xenobiotic substances. Lipid peroxides,
in vitro, destroy cytochrome P-450 so that any significant
peroxidation in tissues active in drug metabolism may well be
associated with a significantly reduced metabolism of clinically
administered drugs. This may be clinically important in some
types of acute inflammation. Reaction (8): this results in the
production of a variety of aldehydes and aldehyde-derivatives

that often have considerable biological activity. Peroxidising
liver microsomes, for example, produce 4-hydroxy-alkenals that
strongly inhibit many enzyme activities. An important recent
finding in this respect is the identification of 4-hydroxy-
nonenal in peroxidising rat liver microsomes (56). In this way
a localised peroxidation can cause biological damage at a distance.

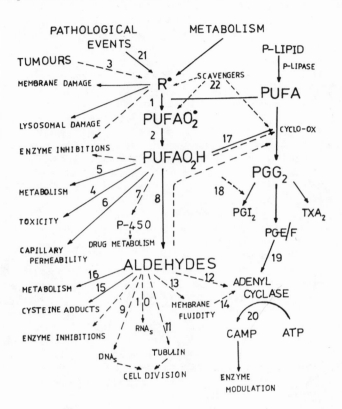

Fig. 5.   Interactions of lipid peroxidation and prostaglandin
          metabolism. A poly-unsaturated fatty acid (PUFA) is
          shown entering the sequence leading to peroxides and
          aldehydes or to prostaglandins. Explanatory notes on
          reactions shown are given in the text; dashed lines
          indicate inhibitory effect; DNA$_s$, DNA-synthesis.

Reactions (9) - (16): aldehydes, keto-aldehydes and hydroxy-
alkenals have been shown to inhibit nucleic acid and protein
synthesis in a number of experimental systems. Detailed studies
have been conducted with methyl glyoxal and with 4-hydroxypentenal
in particular. In general, it seems that 4-hydroxy alkenals have
a much stronger action (see 43) on DNA-synthesis than on RNA or

protein synthesis; this is one reason why they have been tested
for anti-tumour activity (see 57, 58). Some aldehydes have been
shown to cause disturbance in micro-tubule function (59); this is
of relevance to the anti-tumour activity previously mentioned.
Recently, Dianzani's group in Turin have shown that μ-molar
concentrations of some aldehydes (e.g. methyl glyoxal) strongly
inhibit adenyl cyclase in rat liver plasma membrane suspensions
(59). In our opinion, this is an important finding for it
demonstrates that aldehydes of the type produced by peroxidation
can have specific effects at micro-molar levels as opposed to
unspecific denaturation effects that require concentrations of
10^4 - 10^6 greater. In reaction (13), it has been shown that
lipid peroxidation in rat liver microsomes is associated with a
decreased membrane fluidity (60), probably as a result of protein
cross-linking through aldehydic products. Such effects of
fluidity can be expected to have general biological consequences
for many protein-protein interactions in membranes are probably
governed at least in part by local fluidity factors. Changes in
fluidity, for example, have been shown to affect adenyl cyclase
activity (61) (reaction 14). Aldehydes (and especially hydroxy-
alkenals) undergo interesting reactions with thiol-groups and
this modified the biological activity of the aldehydes considerably.
Recently, the reaction of lipid peroxides with cysteine has been
demonstrated (62) and this type of product needs to be considered
pharmacologically in view of the relationship to the cysteine
adducts of the leucotriene group (63). In reaction 16 are
indicated metabolic pathways of aldehydes, in which the aldehyde
dehydrogenases are a major feature. There are various aldehyde
dehydrogenases in mammalian tissues and they differ especially
with respect to the K_m (substrate). Changes have been reported
to occur in the aldehyde dehydrogenase activity in some animal
tumours (64). Reactions (17) - (20): an important inter-relationship of lipid peroxidation and prostaglandin metabolism was
reported by Land's group (65). Low concentrations of lipid
peroxide were found to stimulate cyclo-oxygenase in sheep
visicular glands whereas higher concentrations inhibited.
Moreover, lipid peroxides are known to strongly depress
prostaglandin synthetase (66). The result of these effects can be
to increase prostacyclin and thromboxane synthesis at the expense
of prostaglandin; this would have significant path - physiological
consequences. Moreover, the increased synthesis of prostaglandins
can be coupled to a stimulation of adenyl cyclase with subsequent
production of c-AMP. Reactions (21)- (22): the reactions
described above all depend on an initial free radical initiation
step leading to a lipid peroxy-radical and then to a lipid hydroperoxide. As described previously in this article there is some
evidence that inflammatory processes are associated with the local
production of free radicals ($O_2^{\cdot -}$, $OH^{\cdot}$) that can subsequently
initiate peroxidation. An important area of future study, in our
opinion, is to clarify the protective role of free radical

scavengers in acute and chronic inflammation since it may prove possible in this way to profoundly attenuate the associated pathological events in a clinically acceptable manner. In controlling the free radical reactions that initiate lipid peroxidation, it is of significance that recent evidence has shown that chains of free radical scavengers may function more efficiently that individual scavengers (67).

The overall impression of Figure 5 and the accompanying remarks in the text may be one of considerable complexity. There is no doubt that lipid peroxidation can result in a bewildering spectrum of events both physiological and pathological. The detailed scheme of Figure 5 can be greatly simplified by the use of a set diagram to give the scheme of Figure 6. Here, lipid peroxides can be visualised to produce either a set of toxic reactions (set 2), profound direct actions on prostaglandin and cyclic nucleotide metabolism (set 3), with interactions between the sets shown by the overlap.

At present we are only just beginning to appreciate the varied nature of the interactions between the lipid peroxidation pathways and the prostaglandin in cyclic nucleotide cascades. The possibilities available for affecting which pathway is followed at any particular instant of time are numerous : variations in localised concentrations of the polyunsaturated fatty acids; in membrane asymmetry and fluidity; in oxygen, radical initiator and scavenger concentrations; in modulations of enzyme catalysed steps for supplying or removing substrate, as well as initiating the important first radical step - these are all identifiable and possible ways for directing the peroxidative sequences.

Perhaps in such shifting dynamic equilibria of lipid phases in biomembranes, with allosteric control of membrane enzyme specificities and with variable lipophilic gradients of selective scavengers and pro-oxidants, we are beginning to see the dim outlines of a new and complex hierarchy of metabolic control mechanisms impinging closely on our appreciation of pharmacological and pathological phenomena.

ACKNOWLEDGMENT

The preparation of this paper was facilitated by financial support from the National Foundation for Cancer Research.

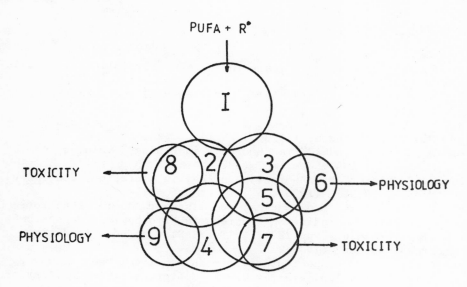

Fig. 6. Set-representation of the inter-relating reactions
         shown in Figure 5.

Poly-unsaturated fatty acids and a free radical initiator
(or initiating reaction) are shown entering set I where
a variety of PUFA$^\bullet$ and PUFAO$_2^-$ free radicals are formed.
These either enter the degradative lipid peroxidation
pathway (set 2) or, via cyclo-oxygenase, the prostaglandin
pathway (set 3). Inter-actions between lipid
peroxidation and prostaglandin synthesis are shown in the
overlap of sets 2 and 3. Lipid peroxidation results in
the formation of aldehydes (set 4) that can have a
variety of physiological properties (set 9) when sets 1,
2 and 4 are under metabolic control, or can result in
toxic manifestations (set 8) when peroxidation overwhelms
normal protective mechanisms. The prostaglandin pathway
interacts with cyclic nucleotides (set 5) and can likewise
be directed into physiological (set 6) or pathological
(set 7) consequences.

It is envisaged that the arrangement shown is a dynamic
one, where the relative importance of the sets and
the corresponding overlaps are determined by features
in the local environment.

REFERENCES

1. I. Isenberg, Free radicals in tissues, Physiol. Revs., 44:487,
    (1964).
2. W. A. Pryor, "Free Radicals", McGraw-Hill Inc., New York,
    (1966).
3. T. F. Slater, "Free Radical Mechanisms in Tissue Injury",
    Pion Ltd., London, (1972).
4. W. A. Pryor (ed.) "Free Radicals in Biology" volumes 1-3,
    Academic Press, New York, (1977).
5. T. F. Slater, Biochemical pathology in microtime, Panminerva
    Medica, 18:381, (1976).
6. R. L. Willson, Free radical and tissue damage: mechanistic
    evidence from radiation studies, in "Biochemical Mechanisms
    of Liver Injury" pp.123-224, T. F. Slater, ed., Academic
    Press, London, (1978).
7. A. Stier, Membrane fluidity, in "Biochemical Mechanisms of
    Liver Injury" pp. 219-364, T. F. Slater, ed., Academic Press,
    London, (1978).
8. C. Benedetto and T.F. Slater, Electron spin resonance studies
    on human endometrium and cervix, in "Recent Studies on lipid
    Peroxidation in Health and Disease", T. F. Slater, ed., in
    press, (1980).
9. H. Swartz, J. Bolton and D. Borg, (eds.) "Biological
    Applications of Electron Spin Resonance", Wiley-Interscience,
    New York, (1972).
10. M. Symons, "Chemical and Biochemical Aspects of Electron Spin
    Resonance Spectroscopy", Van Nostrand-Rheinhold Co. Ltd.,
    (1978).
11. C. A. Evans, Spin trapping, Aldrichimica Acta, 12:23,
    (1979).
12. C-S. Lai, T. A. Grover and L. M. Piette, Hydroxyl-radical
    production in a purified NADPH-cytochrome C (P450) reductase
    system, Archs. Biochem. Biophys., 193:373, (1979).
13. A. Ingall, K. A. K. Lott, T. F. Slater, S. Finch and A. Stier,
    Metabolic activation of CCl_4 to a free-radical product:
    studies using a spin trap, Biochem. Soc. Trans., 6:962,(1978).
14. E. K. Lai, P. B. McCay, T. Noguchi and K-L. Fong, In vivo
    spin trapping of trichloromethyl radicals formed from CCl_4,
    Biochem. Pharmac., 28:2231, (1979).
15. T. F. Slater and P. A. Riley, Photosensitisation and
    lysosomal damage, Nature,Lond., 209:151, (1966).
16. R. K. Clayton, "Light and Living Matter" vol.2, pp.203-213,
    McGraw-Hill Inc., New York, (1971).
17. C. Auclair and M-C. Lecomte, Singlet oxygen production associated
    with hydroperoxide induced lipid peroxidation in liver micro-
    somes, Biochem. Biophys. Res. Commun., 85:946, (1978).

18. S. D. Aust, D. L. Roerig and T. C. Pederson, Evidence for superoxide generation by NADPH-cytochrome c reductase of rat liver microsomes, Biochem. Biophys. Res. Commun., 47:1133, (1972).

19. N. R. Bachur, S. L. Gordon, M. V. Gee and M. Kon, NADPH-cytochrome P-450 reductase activation of quinone anticancer agents to free radicals, Proc. Natl. Acad. Sci. U.S.A., 76:954, (1979).

20. J. J. M. C. De Groot, G. J. Garssen, J. F. G. Vliegenthart and J. Boldingh, The detection of linoleic acid radicals in the anaerobic reaction of lipoxygenase, Biochim. Biophys. Acta., 326:279, (1973).

21. T. Ozawa and A. Hanaki, Hydroxyl radical produced by the reaction of superoxide ion with hydrogen peroxide: electron spin resonance detection by spin trapping, Chem. Pharm. Bull., 26:2572, (1978).

22. R. Latarjet, B. Ekert and P. Demerseman, Peroxidation of nucleic acids by radiation: biological implications, Rad. Res. Suppl., 3:247, (1963).

23. R. L. Willson, P. Wardman and K-D. Asmus, Interaction of dGMP radical with cysteamine and promethazine as possible model of DNA-repair, Nature, Lond., 252:323, (1974).

24. K. Hasegawa and L. K. Patterson, Pulse radiolysis studies in model lipid systems: formation and behaviour of peroxy-radicals in fatty acids, Photochem. Photobiol., 28:817, (1978).

25. S. C. Sharma, H. Mukhtar, S. K. Sharma and C. R. Krishna Murti, Lipid peroxide formation in experimental inflammation, Biochem. Pharmac., 21:1210, (1972).

26. G. Ugazio, Halogenoalkanes and liver injury, in "Biochemical Mechanisms of Liver Injury", pp.709-744, T. F. Slater, Ed., Academic Press, London, (1978).

27. A. Wendel, S. Feuerstein and K-H. Konz, Acute paracetamol intoxication of starved mice leads to lipid peroxidation in vivo, Biochem. Pharmac., 28:2051, (1979).

28. D. S. P. Patterson, W. M. Allen, S. Berrett, D. Sweasey and J. T. Dore, The toxicity of parenteral iron preparations in the rabbit and the pig with a comparison of the clinical and biochemical responses to iron-dextran in 2-day old and 8-day old piglets, Vet. Med. A., 18:453, (1971).

29. D. B. Menzel, The role of free radicals in the toxicity of air pollutants (nitrogen oxides and ozone), in "Free Radicals in Biology" vol.2., pp.181-202, W. A. Pryor, ed., Academic Press Inc., New York, (1976).

30. J. Goodman and P. Hochstein, Generation of free radicals and lipid peroxidation by redox cycling of adriamycin and daunomycin, Biochem. Biophys. Res. Commun., 77:797, (1977)

31. T. F. Slater, The role of lipid peroxidation in liver injury, in "Pathogenesis and Mechanisms of Liver Cell Necrosis", D. Keppler, ed., MTP Press, Lancaster, U.K., (1975).

32.   J. F. Mead, Free radical mechamisms of lipid damage and
      consequences for cellular membranes, in "Free Radicals in
      Biology" vol.1., pp.51-68, W. A. Pryor, ed., Academic Press,
      New York, (1976).
33.   G. L. Plaa and H. Witschi, Chemicals, drugs and lipid
      peroxidation, Ann. Rev. Pharmacol., 16:125, (1976).
34.   M. U. Dianzani and G. Ugazio, Lipid peroxidation, in
      "Biochemical Mechanisms of Liver Injury" pp.669-708,
      T. F. Slater, ed., Academic Press, London, (1978).
35.   M. Hamberg and B. Samuelsson, On the specificity of the
      oxygenation of unsaturated fatty acids catalysed by
      soybean lipoxidase, J. Biol. Chem., 242:5329, (1967).
36.   M. Hambers, B. Samuelsson, I. Björkhem and H. Danielsson,
      Oxygenases in fatty acid and steroid metabolism,in "Molecular
      Mechanisms of Oxygen Activation" pp.30-85, O. Hayaishi, ed.,
      Academic Press Inc., New York, (1974).
37.   R. T. Holman, P. O. Egwim and W. W. Christie, Substrate
      specificity of soybean lipoxidase, J. Biol. Chem., 244:1149,
      (1969).
38.   P. Borgeat and B. Samuelsson, Arachidonic acid metabolism
      in polymorphonuclear leukocytes: unstable imtermediate in
      formation of dihydroxy acids, Proc. Natl. Acad. Sci., U.S.A.
      76:3213, (1979).
39.   T. F. Slater, Mecha isms of protection against the damage
      produced in biological systems by oxygen-derived radicals,
      in "Oxygen Free Radicals and Tissue Damage" Ciba Foundation
      Symposium 65 (new series), D. W. Fitzsimons, ed., Excerpta
      Medica, Amsterdam, (1979).
40.   T. F. Slater and B. C. Sawyer, The stimulatory effects of
      carbon tetrachloride and other halogenoalkanes on peroxidative
      reactions in rat liver systems in vitro, Biochem. J., 123:805,
      (1971).
41.   A. Benedetti, A. F. Casini, M. Ferrali and M. Comporti, Early
      alterations induced by carbon tetrachloride in the lipids of
      the membranes of the endoplasmic reticulum of the liver cell,
      Chem. Biol. Interactions, 17:167, (1977).
42.   E. Schauenstein, Autoxidation of polyunsaturated esters in
      water: chemical structure and biological activity of the
      products, J. Lipid. Res., 8:417, (1967).
43.   E. Schauenstein, H. Esterbauer and N. Zollner, "Aldehydes in
      Biological Systems Pion Ltd., London, (1977).
44.   J. M. McCord, Free radicals and inflammation : protection of
      synovial fluid by superoxide dismutase, Science, 185:529,
      (1974).
45.   D. W. Fitzsimons (ed.), "Oxygen Free Radicals and Tissue
      Damage", Ciba Foundation Symposium 65 (new series) ,Excerpta
      Medica, Amsterdam, (1979).
46.   J. Robak, Adjuvant-induced and carrageenin-induced inflammation
      and lipid peroxidation in rat liver, spleen and lungs,
      Biochem. Pharmac., 27:531, (1978).

47. P. Puig-Parellada and J. M. Planas, Synovial fluid
    degradation induced by free radicals : in vitro action of
    several free radical scavengers and anti-inflammatory drugs,
    Biochem. Pharmac., 27:535, (1978).
48. M. V. Torrielli, Lipid peroxidation in experimental
    inflammation models, in "Recent Studies in Lipid Peroxidation
    in Health and Disease", T. F. Slater, ed., in press, (1980).
49. E. D. Lash, The antioxidant and pro-oxidant activity in
    ascites tumours, Archs. Biochem. Biophys., 115:332, (1966).
50. K. Utsumi, G. Yamamoto and K. Inaba, Failure of Fe^{2+} - induced
    lipid peroxidation and swelling in the mitochondria from
    ascites tumour cells, Biochim. Biophys. Acta., 105:368, (1965).
51. R. M. Arneson, V. J. Aloyo, G. S. Germain and J. E. Chenevey,
    Antioxidants in neoplastic cells : changes in the antioxidative
    capacity of mouse neuroblastoma cells measured by a single-
    phase assay, Lipids, 13:383, (1978).
52. A. A. Barber and F. Bernheim, Lipid Peroxidation : its
    measurement, occurrence and significance in animal tissues,
    Adv. Gerontol Res., 2:355, (1967).
53. B. O. Christopherson, Reduction of linolenic acid hydroperoxide
    by a glutathione peroxidase, Biochim. Biophys. Acta., 176:463,
    (1969).
54. G. Ugazio, M. V. Torrielli, E. Burdino, B. C. Sawyer and
    T. F. Slater, Long-range effects of products of carbon
    tetrachloride-stimulated lipid peroxidation, Biochem. Trans.,
    4:353, (1976).
55. P. J. O'Brien, Hydroperoxides and superoxides in microsomal
    oxidations, Pharmacol. Therapeut., 2:517, (1978).
56. H. Esterbauer, A. Benedetti and M. Comporti, in press, (1980).
57. E. Schauenstein, M. Ernet, H. Esterbauer and H. Zollner,
    Experiments on the therapeutic effect of 4-hydroxypentenal:
    II, inhibition of the growth of Sarcoma 180, Z. Krebs Forsch.,
    75:90, (1971).
58. P. J. Conroy, J. T. Nodes, T. F. Slater and G. W. White,
    Carcinostatic activity of 4-hydroxy-2-pent-en-1-al against
    transplantable murine tumour lines, Eur. J. Cancer, 11:231,
    (1975).
59. M. U. Dianzani, Mechanisms of liver cell damage in carbon
    tetrachloride poisoning : a general reconsideration, in
    "Recent Studies on Lipid Peroxidation in Health and Disease",
    T. F. Slater, ed., in press, (1980).
60. A. Ingall, K. A. K. Lott, T. F. Slater and A. Stier, Effects
    of lipid peroxidation on fluidity of rat liver endoplasmic
    reticulum membranes as shown by spin label techniques, in
    press (1980).
61. I. Dipple and M. D. Houslay, The activity of glucagon-
    stimulated adenylate cyclase from rat liver plasma membranes
    is modulated by the fluidity of its lipid environment,
    Biochem. J., 174:179, (1978).

62. H. W. Gardner, R. Kleiman, D. Weisleder and G. E. Inglett,
     Cysteine adds to lipid hydroperoxide, Lipids, 12:655, (1977).
63. E. Granstrom, Biosynthesis, in "Advances in Endoperoxide
     Prostacyclin and Thromboxane Research", F. Berti and G. P.
     Velo, eds., Plenum Press, (1980).
64. R. N. Feinstein, R. J. M. Fry, E. C. Cameron, C. Peraino, and
     H. P. Morris, New aldehyde dehydrogenase isozymes in
     chemically-induced liver tumours in the rat, Proc. Soc. Exp.
     Biol. Med., 152:463, (1976).
65. M. E. Hemler, H. W. Cook and W. E. M. Lands, Prostaglandin
     biosynthesis can be triggered by lipid peroxides, Archs.
     Biochem. Biophys., 193:340, (1979).
66. S. Moncada, R. J. Gryglewski, S. Bunting and J. R. Vane, A
     lipid peroxide inhibits the enzyme in blood vessel micro-
     somes that generates from prostaglandin endoperoxides the
     substance (Prostaglandin x) which prevents platelet
     aggregation, Prostaglandins, 12:715, (1976).
67. J. E. Packer, T. F. Slater and R. L. Willson, Direct
     observation of a free radical interaction between vitamin E
     and vitamin C, Nature, Lond., 278:737, (1979).

PROSTAGLANDINS AND INFLAMMATORY HYPERALGESIA

S. H. Ferreira

Department of Pharmacology,
Faculty of Medicine of Ribeirão Preto
University of São Paulo, Ribeirão Preto
S.P., Brazil

In our "Discussion on the mode of action of anti-inflammatory drugs" (in this book) it is pointed out that the therapeutic effects of aspirin-like drugs are symptomatic.   These drugs do not interfere with the evolution of the chronic processes but act on the expression of some inflammatory signs and symptoms. Possibly, most of the therapeutic use of aspirin-like drugs in many diseases is due to their antialgic effect rather than to their anti-oedematogenic properties. If one day, we have drugs which really interfere with the progression of chronic diseases, aspirin-like drugs, i.e. cyclo-oxygenase inhibitors, will be classified as pseudo-anti-inflammatory drugs.

Opiates is thought to cause analgesia by a central mechanism while aspirin-like drugs act peripherally (24). Our suggestion (10) that the antialgic effect of non-steroid drugs resulted from the prevention of the development of hyperalgesia due to the inhibition of prostaglandins generation at the inflammatory site, has been supported by findings from several independent laboratories. It is clear now that prostaglandins (E_1, E_2 and I_2) contribution to inflammatory pain is associated with the sensitization of pain receptors (hyperalgesia) to other chemical mediators or mechanical stimuli (10, 13-16, 19, 20, 21, 26, 27, 32). The hyperalgesia induced by prostaglandins probably results from the lowering of the threshold of C fiber polymodal nociceptors (27). Agents which by systemic administration display a _direct_ analgesic effect on inflammatory hyperalgesia have not yet been described so far. Such a development would constitute a major therapeutic advance. It is our belief that the understanding of the physiopathological

events associated with prostaglandin induced hyperalgesia will
lead to such class of analgesic agents.

We shall review here recent observations made in our
laboratory which stress the importance of prostaglandins in
inflammatory pain and enlarge the understanding of the mechanism
of the analgesic action of aspirin-like drugs and possibly of
opioids. We shall discuss a) the "immediate" hyperalgesic effect
of prostacyclin (PGI_2); b) the central antialgic effect of
aspirin-like drugs on carrageenin rat paw hyperalgesia; c)
prostaglandin hyperalgesia as a mechanism related to $cAMP/Ca^{2+}$,
and d) the peripheral analgesic effect of morphin, enkephalins
and opioids antagonists on the "delayed" hyperalgesic effect of
prostaglandins E_2.

The Hyperalgesic Effect of Prostaglandin and Prostacyclins (PGI_2)

It is a common clinical observation, in various pathological
conditions such as rheumatoid arthritis or special types of
headaches that the antialgic effect of aspirin-like drugs take a
few hours to establish. This can be explained by the long lasting
hyperalgesic effect of prostaglandins (10). However, it is of
general knowledge that for some type of pain aspirin-like drugs
have a relatively quick effect. The hyperalgesic effect of
prostaglandins in the rat paw is long lasting (13, 32) but
aspirin-like drugs are capable of reducing already established
carrageenin hyperalgesia within an hour (33). An explanation
for this discrepancy has been recently obtained in our laboratories.
Using two experimental models, a modification of the Randall-
Selitto method (38) and the dog incapacitation test (8), it was
shown that prostacyclin was a more potent hyperalgesic agent than
PGE_2 (16). Furthermore, the hyperalgesia induced by prostacyclin
was immediate and of a much shorter duration. Prostacyclin
(PGI_2) like PGE_1 and PGE_2 is a product of the oxidation of
arachidonic acid by cyclo-oxygenase, therefore its release is
also blocked by aspirin-like drugs. The presence of prostacyclin
stable metabolite 6-keto prostaglandin $F_{1\alpha}$, has been demonstrated
in the exudate of carrageenin granuloma (3). An alternative
explanation might be that aspirin-like drugs are blocking the
release of substances sharing the pain producing activity of
fatty acid hydroperoxides. Intradermal injections of hydroperoxides
of arachidonic, linoleic and linolenic acids induced a much more
intense immediate overt pain that the original fatty acids or
acetyl-choline, bradykinin, histamine or PGE_1 (10). Thus, it is
conceivable that the endoperoxides, intermediate in prostaglandins
synthesis, can also be responsible for the type of pain which is
quickly blocked by aspirin-like drugs.

The Central Effect of Aspirin-Like Drugs

Flower and Vane (17) explained the antialgic or anti-pyretic effect of paracetamol or phenacetin by a selective effect on the prostaglandin synthetase enzymes of the CNS. This can explain why these agents (as well as dypirone, 6) display an anti-algic effect without conspicuous local anti-inflammmatory (anti-oedematogenic) action. Such interpretation presuppose that the prostaglandins responsible for causing hyperalgesia are generated at the sensory nerves by the same group of cyclo-oxygenase found in the CNS in contrast to that responsible for the oedema and vasodilatation, which would be of vascular origin. Recently we have proposed an additional interpretation (13).

Using carrageenin hyperalgesia tests in rats, we have observed that hyperalgesia developed much faster when the con-tralateral paw had been previously treated with carrageenin. This was taken as an indication that the local inflammation evoked a central mechanism, which facilitated local hyperalgesia. We have also studied the effects of aspirin, indomethacin, paracetamol and phenacetin injected into the paw and into the cerebral ventricles. There was a synergic antialgic effect between central and peripheral administration of these agents. Administration of a specific prostaglandin antagonist (SC-19220), either into the cerebral ventricles or into the paw, significantly inhibited carrageenin-evoked hyperalgesia. This hyperalgesia in the rat paw could be mimicked only by a combined central and peripheral administration of prostaglandins. These results suggest that, in the rat, inflammatory hyperalgesia has two components resulting from prostaglandin release: a peripheral one and a central one, due to the participation of central pain circuits. The anti-algic effect of paracetamol or phenacetin may be partially related to an action on this central component. We do not know yet, if this concept can be extended to other models of inflammation, but it is plausible that it will be applicable to those models in which fever due to prostaglandin release in CNS occurs during the development of inflammation.

Prostaglandin Hyperalgesia as a Mechanism Related to cAMP/Ca^{2+}

In the experiments described here the hyperalgesia was measured by our modification of the Randall-Selitto method (13, 28). In this modification, instead of increasing pressure a constant pressure of 20 mm Hg is applied to the rat paw and the time of appearance of a characteristic response is measured. The rats were treated with indomethacin (2 mg/kg, IP, 30 min before starting the experimental session) in order to avoid the release of PGs by the injection trauma or by injectedd test substances.

The time course of hyperalgesia induced by intraplantar injection of PGE_2, Db-cAMP, isoprenaline, $BaCl_2$ and Ca^{2+} ionophore (A 23187) was similar. The plateau effect was attained within 2-3 hours and remained up to the 4th or 5th hour. PGE_2 induced hyperalgesia at doses in the ng range while 500-1000 fold quantities of other agents were necessary to cause an equivalent effect. All agents caused a dose-dependent effect and were potentiated by local administration of methyl-xanthines. Caffeine (10 µg) and theophylline (20 µg) had no analgesic effect on normal paws. Potentiation of the hyperalgesic effect of PGE_2 by methyl-xanthines could only be demonstrable in rats not pretreated with indomethacin, since this treatment inverted the effect of the methyl-xanthines, causing analgesia instead of enhancing the hyperalgesia. Indomethacin treatment had no effect on the other hyperalgesic stimuli. Adrenaline (100 µg) was equipotent to isoprenaline and twice as potent as noradrenaline. The hyperalgesia induced by isoprenaline was abolished by propranolol which, in contrast, had no effect on PGE_2 induced hyperalgesia. Thus indicating that effect of simpathomimetic is mediated through a β receptor.

These results support the hypothesis that rat paw hyper-algesia induced by prostaglandin is related to a $cAMP/Ca^{2+}$ dependent process. We suggest that the interaction of prostaglandin or catecholamines with the receptor at the peripheral nociceptive terminations activate an adenylate-cyclase (cAMP-ase) associated with pharmacological receptors, causing an increase in the intracellular concentration of cAMP. This assumption is based on the fact that local administration of Db-cAMP or of adenylate-cyclase activators such as catecholamines and prosta-glandins induced hyperalgesia. This local hyperalgesic effect of Db-cAMP may explain the observation that a single intravenous injection of this cAMP derivate in man causes headaches, abdominal pain, myalgias and other types of pain. In several biological systems increased levels of cAMP are associated with an increased Ca^{2+} concentration (30). In our system substances which increase intracellular Ca^{2+} concentration ($BaCl_2$ and Ca^{2+} ionophore) induced hyperalgesia while those known to block Ca^{2+} influx were analgesics. A Ca^{2+} related mechanism may also be involved in CNS activity since intraventricular administration of lanthanum causes antinociception. On the base of the present results it is difficult to know whether intracellular Ca^{2+} concentration regulates adenylate-cyclase activity or vice versa. It seems that in our system methyl-xanthines potentiate hyper-algesia by a mechanism other than inhibition of phosphodiesterase since Db-cAMP, a resistant cAMP derivative (30), similarly to PGE_2, isoprenaline, $BaCl_2$ and Ca^{2+} ionophore was also potentiated. In our working hypothesis, intracellular concentration of Ca^{2+} at nociceptive termination plays a major role in controlling its threshold sensitivity, possibly through a modulation of adenylate-cyclase which activity may control the induction of generator potentials at the nociceptors.

cGMP, in several biological systems, had the opposite effect of cAMP (18). In our system, direct administration of cGMP or substances which stimulate the synthesis of cGMP (Ach and carbachol) caused peripheral analgesia. The effects of Ach or carbachol were associated with a muscarinic receptor since atropine abolished the analgesia. It is interesting to point out that the analgesic effect of cholinergic substances could only be demonstrable after treatment of the rats with indomethacin. This may be due to a local release of PGs, as it is described to occur in isolated lungs by Ach administration (1). The peripheral analgesic effect of cGMP seems to occur at various levels of the CNS, since its central administration also caused antinociception (4). We have shown that substances which lower intracellular Ca^{2+} concentration were analgesics but there is no experimental evidence indicating that this effect is related to an increased activity of cGMP. The importance of the analgesic effect of cGMP for development of a new class of peripheral analgesic agents is discussed later in this paper.

Prostaglandin Metabotropic Effect

One intriguing characteristic of prostaglandin hyperalgesia is its long duration. Prostaglandins of the E series administered intradermally in man, in the rat paw or in dog knee joints induce a hyperalgesia which lasts more than four hours (10,16, 29,32). Another characteristic, which has called our attention, is its delayed onset and the long time needed to reach the plateau after a single dose of PGE_2. In the rat paw the maximum effect of small doses of prostaglandin E_2 is attained two to three hours after its administration. This delayed and long lasting hyperalgesic effect of prostaglandins of E series is suggestive of a basic change in the normal metabolism of nociceptors. Recently, Eccles and McGeer (7) called attention to two different features of neurotransmission. In the ionotropic transmission the mediator acts to open ionic gates while in the metabotropic transmission the mediator acts indirectly, by triggering a biochemical change at the post-synaptic membrane. Ionotropic differs from metabotropic transmission because of its short latency and by its increased conductance at the postsynaptic membrane. This concept may well be valid for the nociceptors related to inflammatory hyper-algesia. Considering the differences in their mode of action (26) bradykinin and prostaglandins effects could be considered as ionotropic and metabotropic respectively.

In order to support the idea that prostaglandin hyperalgesia
is a metabotropic effect we have treated rats with cyclo-
hexemide known to inhibit the synthesis of proteins and
peptides. Cyclohexmide strongly inhibit the hyperalgesia
induced by prostaglandin E_2 without affecting the hyperalgesia
caused in the contralateral paw by Db cAMP. This result is
suggestive of a protein or a peptide triggered by prostaglandin
E_2.

The Peripheral Action of Morphine and its Antagonists

Recently we presented evidence that morphine and enkephalins
have a peripheral analgesic effect (11). At this site the
"pure" opioid antagonist, naloxone, does not antagonize
morphine but is an algesic agonist. Hyperalgesia due to intra-
plantar injection of PGE_2 is fully developed by about three hours
and remains constant for up to six hours. Intraplantar injection
of 10 µg of morphine given when hyperalgesia was already fully
developed greatly reduced its intensity for two and half hours.
Met-enkephalin had a similar effect but of shorter duration at
the dose used (50 µg). Both substances cause hypoalgesia
when injected in control saline treated paws. Morphine treatment
of the contralateral paw did not affect the intensity of hyperalgesia induced by prostaglandin or the threshold of saline
treated paws. This result excludes a possible central
component in the analgesia observed.

To characterize further this peripheral site of action of
morphine, we investigated the effects of naloxone, a "pure"
morphine antagonist. The results showed unexpectedly that
naloxone by itself had an agonist morphine like effect in
reducing hyperalgesia. Furthermore, naloxone given at the same
time as morphine did not show any antagonism in analgesic
effect but caused an effect greater than that attained by each
substance given separately. Although naloxone is generally
accepted as a "pure" antagonist it might have at this peripheral
site partial agonist activity. One of the characteristics of
a partial agonist is that antagonistic activity last longer than
its agonist effect. However, morphine still displayed an
analgesic effect when given two hours after naloxone, thus
excluding this possible interpretation.

We estimated the potency of opioids and enkephalins at
this peripheral site, relative to a standard locally acting
analgesic agent lidocaine. From our results, two important
points emerge. First, lidocaine is about one hundred times
less potent than the opioids agonists and antagonists. Therefore,
the effects observed cannot be explained by a local anaesthetic
effect. Second, although enkephalins are rapidly inactivated
by plasma, met-enkephalin was only four less potent than morphine.

The comparative low potency of leu-enkephalin is in accord with its potency in other systems. From these results, we calculated from linear regression the ID_{50} values for each substance, to be: morphine 14.3 nmoles; nalorphine 17.8 nmoles; naloxone 20.4 nmoles; pentazocine 22.4 nmoles; met-enkephalin 74.5 nmoles, leu-enkephalin 126.6 nmoles and lidocaine 1774 nmoles.

Our experiments so far had established the analgesic agonist effect of opiates and of morphine-antagonist injected intraplanatarly.

Morphine and met-enkephalin have a clear peripheral analgesic effect on prostaglandin hyperalgesia. Morphine also reduced the hyperalgesic effect of isoprenaline and $BaCl_2$ but no effect on Db-cAMP hyperalgesia. This last observation is in accord with our idea that these analgesics are acting on a step preceding cAMP generation in some step in the process by which prostaglandins activate adenylate-cyclase.

Relevance of the Peripheral Analgesic Effect of Morphine and of Morphine Antagonists

In order to compare the central with the peripheral effect of these agents we have investigated their effect by administration in the cerebral ventricles (13). The doses given intraventricularly were the ED_{50} calculated from the peripheral analgesic effect. The tests were performed on groups of 5 rats and the results are expressed as the mean values obtained four and a half hours after the induction of hyperalgesia by prostaglandins and two hours after the intraventricular injection of the test drug. Control intraventricular injection of saline (10 µl) had no effect on the threshold response of normal (46 ± 0.15 sec) as well as of hyperalgesic paws (19.7 ± 0.4 sec). Morphine caused an intense analgesia in both control (18.8 ± 4.3 sec) and hyperalgesic (6.3 ± 1.8 sec) paws (compared with the former group). For naloxone the intensity of hyperalgesia was: 7.2 ± 0.5 sec for the control and 25.4 ± 0.4 sec for hyperalgesic paws. The values for nalorphine-treated rats were 8.7 ± 0.6 sec and 26.0 ± 0.7 sec for control and hyperalgesic paws, respectively. Intraventricular administration of pentazocine did not change the response of normal (0.3 ± 0.1 sec) or hyperalgesic paws (19.8 ± 0.3 sec). These results clearly indicate that, morphine antagonists in contrast to morphine are devoid of central analgesic effects. In fact they cause hyperalgesia. Analgesia by pentazocine could be mainly due to a peripheral action. In the next series of experiments we looked for such an activity after systemic (intraperitoneal) injection of morphine antagonists in an attempt to evaluate the contribution of peripheral analgesia to the total analgesic effect. In the same series of experiments, we included morphine and pentazocine for comparison. The doses

used have been shown to be effective in the original Randall-
Selitto test but are generally ineffective in tests based upon
reaction to thermal stimuli (31-33). All agents cause analgesia
thirty minutes after systemic administration. However, with
nalorphine and naloxone the analgesic activity was short-lasting
and after half an hour was replaced by a hyperalgesic effect,
manifest in prostaglandin and saline-treated paws, which was
further increased at the second hour. This hyperalgesia is
most probably due to a central effect since these agents have
only analgesic activity when given intraplantarly. At thirty
minutes, the analgesic activity of pentazocine and of a lower
dose of morphine (0.1 - 0.5 mg/kg/IP) is probably due to a
peripheral action since these drugs have little influence on
saline-treated paws.

Looking for New Mild Analgesics

It may well be that the understanding of the mechanism of
antialgic action of aspirin-like drugs will not allow us to
improve this group of agents. This is because the mechanism
of analgesia induced by such drugs as well as their side effects
are probably linked with the inhibition of cyclo-oxygenase (12).
One would also expect that a general prostaglandin antagonist
would have similar side effects. However, since cyclo-oxygenase
from different tissues shows different sensitivity to aspirin-
like drugs, the possibility to develop a tissue specific
analgesic remains open to investigation.

On the other hand our results clearly indicate a new approach
to the problem. The observed peripheral analgesic activity of
morphine antagonists suggests the presence of a receptor different
from that already postulated in the CNS and in the periphery (22,
25). At the peripheral pain terminations naloxone and nalorphine
are agonists as potent as morphine, pentazocine or met-enkephalin
(N receptor) in contrast to their antagonist effect on central
analgesic morphine (M) receptors. It would be desirable to
develop drugs which act exclusively at the N receptors. We
postulated that the N receptors are associated with inhibition
of an adenylate-ciclase capable of being stimulated by prostaglandins
and β sympathomimetics. The results of Ferri et al. (9) and
Collier and Roy (5) support the idea that central morphine
analgesia may result from an inhibition of prostaglandin activation
of adenylate-cyclase.

The ideal peripheral analgesic should be unable to cross the
blood brain barrier,(BBB),thus avoiding any central side effects,
but should have a strong peripheral action on inflammatory hyperalgesia. Such substance should be inactive in the tail flick test.

We recently described a prototype of such an agent (11).
BW 180c is an enkephalin analog displaying increased resistante
to hydrolysis, and which does not cross the BBB (2)·BW 180c
had a strong local analgesic effect and, when given intraperitoneally,it antagonized both prostaglandin E_2 and carrageenin
induced hyperalgesia. We expect a similar effect of morphine
antagonists or opiate-analogs which do not cross the BBB.
Another lead for such agents may be a long-lasting cGMP derivative.
This substance is thought not to cross the BBB and to have an
analgesic effect when administered systemically.

In summary, prostaglandins are inflammatory mediators:
a) they have been detected in several types of inflammation;
b) drugs which inhibit their synthesis in vivo diminish the
intensity of inflammatory signs and symptoms; c) prostaglandins
cause vasodilation, fever and act sinergistically with other
mediators to cause inflammatory oedema. Prostaglandins E_1 and
E_2 cause a long lasting hyperalgesia, in several models.
Prostacyclin (PGI_2)causes an intense but short lasting hyperalgesia. Aspirin-like drugs, at therapeutic doses, block the
synthesis of prostaglandins in vivo.

The term antialgic (antialgesic) rather than analgesic
should be used for the effect of aspirin-like drugs. These agents
do not directly block the hyperalgesic effect of prostaglandins
or the direct action of nociceptive stimuli. By inhibiting
cyclo-oxygenase they prevent the development of hyperalgesia
induced by PGE_2 release by inflammatory stimuli. If prostaglandins are released at the CNS, parallel to their release at the
inflammatory site, it shall enhance the local hyperalgesia. In
such instance, a central effect of aspirin-like drugs, in
addition to their local effect, would also be expected.

The direct peripheral hyperalgesic effect of prostaglandins
is blocked by opioids and their antagonists. It is possible that
an endogenous opioid (endorphins or enkephalins) regulated the
threshold sensitivity at several levels of the nociceptive
system. Prostaglandins may cause hyperalgesia by off setting
this mechanism. An important practical consequence of the
peripheral analgesic action of the opioids and their antagonists
is the possibility of development of a new class of morphine
like analgesics with selective peripheral action. Many of the
presently used assays measure mainly analgesia at a central
site, selecting for pain relieving properties, as well as for
addition liability (23,31). However, the ideal analgesic
should have high activity in the peripheral assays and no effect
in the central assays. Such a compound might be one excluded
from the CNS by its physicochemical characteristics. This
analgesic, would constitute a major therapeutic advance, lacking
both the unwanted central effects of opioids and the peripheral

side effects of aspirin-like drugs. The described interrelationship between prostaglandins, aspirin-like drugs and opioids
provide an unifying hypothesis to interpret the mechanism of
action of different types of "pain killers".

Acknowledgements

We thank FAPESP (Brazil) and The Wellcome Foundation for
research grants.

REFERENCES

1. V. A. Alabaster and Y. S. Bakhle. Release of smooth muscle-
    contracting substances from isolated perfused lungs. Europ.
    J. Pharmac., 35:349-360 (1976).
2. C. R. Beddell, R. L. Follenfant, L. A. Lowe, F. B. Ubatuba,
    S. Wilkinson and R. J. Miller. Analogues of the enkephalins
    - Structural requirements for opioid activity. In:
    "Biological Activity and Chemical Structure". J. A. Keverling
    Buisman, ed., Elvesier Scientific Publishing Company, New
    York, pp.177-193 (1977).
3. W. C. Chang, S. Murota and S. Tsurufugi. A new prostaglandin
    transformed from arachidonic acid in carrageenin-induced
    granuloma. Biochem. Biophys. Res. Comm., 72:1259-1264
    (1976).
4. M. L. Cohn, M. Cohn and F. H. Taylor. Guanosine 3', 5'
    -monophosphate: A central nervous system regulator of
    analgesia. Science, 199:319-322 (1978).
5. H. O. Collier and A. C. Roy. Inhibition of E- rostaglandins
    sensitive adenyl cyclase as the mechanism of morphine
    analgesia. Prostaglandins, 7:361-376 (1974).
6. A. Dembiska-Kiec, A. Zmuda and J. Krupinska. Inhibition
    of prostaglandin synthetase by aspirin-like drugs in
    different microsomal preparations. In: "Advances in
    Prostaglandins and Thromboxane Research", vol. 1. B.
    Samuelsson and R. Paoletti, eds., Raven Press, New York, pp.99-
    103 (1976).
7. J. C. Eccles and P. L. Mcgeer. Ionotropic and metabotropic
    transmission. Trends in Neurosciences, 2:39-40 (1979).
8. J. Faires and D. J. McCarty. Acute arthritis in man and
    dog after intrasynovial injection of sodium urate
    crystals. Lancet, 11:682-685 (1962).
9. S. Ferri, A. Santagostino, P. C. Braga and I. Galatelas.
    Decrease antinociceptive effect of morphine in rats treated
    intraventricularly with prostaglandin E_1. Psychopharmacologia
    (Berl.), 39:231-235 (1974).
10. S. H. Ferreira. Prostaglandins, aspirin-like drugs and
    analgesia. Nature, New Biol., 240:200-203 (1972).

11. S. H. Ferreira and M. Nakamura. Prostaglandin hiperalgesia: I, A cAMP/Ca^2 dependent process; II, The peripheral analgesic activity of morphine, enkephalins and opioid antagonists; III, Relevance of the peripheral effect for the analgesic action of opioid antagonists. Prostaglandins, in press (1979).

12. S. H. Ferreira and J. R. Vane. Mode of action of anti-inflammatory agents which are prostaglandin synthetase inhibitors. In: "Anti-Inflammatory Drugs", J. R. Vane and S. H. Ferreira, eds., Handbook of Experimental Pharmacology, vol. 50/II - Springer Verlag, Berlin, Heidelberg, pp.348-398 (1978).

13. S. H. Ferriera, B. B. Lorenzetti and F. M. A. Correa. Central and peripheral antialgesic action of aspirin-like drugs. European J. Pharmacol., 53:39-48 (1978).

14. S. H. Ferreira, S. Moncada and J. R. Vane. Some effects of inhibiting endogenous prostaglandin formation on the responses of the cat spleen. Br. J. Pharmac., 47:48-58 (1973).

15. S. H. Ferreira, S. Moncada and J.R. Vane. Prostaglandins and the mechanism of analgesia produced by aspirin-like drugs. Br. J. Pharmac., 49:86-97 (1973).

16. S. H. Ferreira, M. Nakamura and M. S. A. Castro. The hyperalgesic effects of prostacyclin and prostaglandin E_2. Prostaglandins, 16:31-37 (1978).

17. R. J. Flower and J. R. Vane. Inhibition of prostaglandin synthetase in brain explains the anti-pyretic activity of paracetamol (4-acetamido - phenol). Nature, 240:410-411 (1972).

18. N. D. Goldberg, M. K. Haddox, S. E. Nicol, D. B. Glass, C. H. Sanford, F. A. Kuehl Jr. and R. Estensen. Biologic regulation through opposing influences of cyclic GMP and cyclic AMP: The yin yang hypothesis. In: "Advances in Cyclic Nucleotides Research", G. I. Drummond, P. Greengard and G. A. Robinson, eds. Raven Press, New York, vol. 5 pp. 307-330 (1975).

19. A. G. Herman and S. Moncada. Release of prostaglandins and incapacitation after injection of endotoxin in the knee joint of the dog. Br. J. Pharmac., 53:465p (1975).

20. H. Juan and F. Lembeck. Action of peptides and other algesic agents on paravascular pain receptors on the isolated perfused rabbit ear. Naunym-Schmiedeberg's Arch. Pharmac., 283:151-164 (1974).

21. H. Juan and F. Lembeck. Inhibition of action of E-prostaglandins (PGs) on paravascular pain receptors. Naunym-Schmiedebergs Arch. Pharmac.,285: R36 (1974).

22. J. Knoll, S. Fürst and S. Makleits. The pharmacology of N-substituted azido-morphines. Arch. Int. Pharmacodyn., 228:268-292 (1977).

23. L. Lasagna. The clinical pharmacology of analgesics and analgesic antagonists. In: "Proc. of the 3rd International Pharmacol. Meeting", R. K. S. Lim, ed. Pergamon Press,Oxford, vol. 9: 113-120 (1968).

24. R. K. S. Lim, F. Guzman, D. W. Rodgers, K. Goto, G. Braun, G. D. Dickerson and R. J. Engle. Site of action of narcotic and non-narcotic analgesics determined by blocking bradykinin-evoked visceral pain. Arch. Int. Pharmacodyn., 152:25-59 (1964).

25. W. R. Martin. Opioids antagonists. Pharmacol. Reviews, 4:463-521 (1967).

26. S. Moncada, S. H. Ferreira and J. R. Vane. Inhibition of prostaglandin biosynthesis as the mechanism of analgesia of aspirin-like drugs in the dog knee joint. Europ. J. Pharmacol., 31:250-260 (1975).

27. E. R. Perl. Sensitization of nociceptors and its relation to sensation. In: "Advances in Pain Research and Therapy", J. J. Bonica and D. Albe-Fessard, eds., Raven Press, New York, vol. I, pp.17-34 (1976).

28. L. O. Randall and J. J. Selitto. A method for measurement of analgesic activity on inflammed tissue. Arch. Int. Pharmacodyn., 111:409-419 (1957).

29. M. E. Rosenthale, A. Dervinis, J. Kassarich and S. Singer. Prostaglandins and anti-inflammatory drugs in the dog knee joint. J. Pharm.Pharmac., 24:149-152 (1972).

30. E. W. Sutherland, G. A. Robison and R. W. Butcher. Some aspects of the biological role of adenosine 3', 5'-monophosphate (Cyclic AMP). Circulation, 37:279-306 (1968).

31. J. W. Ward, M. Foxwell and W. H. Funderburk. The detection of analgesia produced by morphine antagonists in laboratory animals. Pharmacologist, 7:163 (1965).

32. A. L. Willis and M. Cornelsen. Repeated injection of prostaglandin E_2 in rat paw induced chronic swelling and marked decrease in pain threshold. Prostaglandins, 3: 353-357 (1973).

33. C. A. Winter and L. Flataker. Reaction thresholds to pressure in edematous hindpaws of rats and responses to analgesic drugs. J. Pharmacol. Exp. Therapeutics, 150:165-171 (1965).

A DISCUSSION ON THE MODE OF ACTION OF NON-STEROID ANTI-INFLAMMATORY

DRUGS: INHIBITION OF PROSTAGLANDIN SYNTHESIS

S. H. Ferreira

Faculty of Medicine of Ribeirão Preto,
Department of Pharmacology, 14100 - Ribeirão Preto
São Paulo, Brazil

At present there are two lines of thought regarding the mode
of action of non-steroid anti-inflammatory drugs: a) the
multiple effect theory which explains their mechanism through
interference with various molecular or cellular events (102,103)
and b) the PG theory which considers the inhibition of the synthesis
of prostaglandins as the common denominator of the mechanism of
action of aspirin-like drugs (116).

Non-steroid anti-inflammatory drugs (NSAID) have a high
chemical reactivity towards proteins. Thus, it is not surprising
that they inhibit a great number of enzymic systems in vitro.
However, inhibition of an in vitro system has a pharmacological
meaning only when it is shown to be reproducible in vivo at a
therapeutic dosage. Furthermore, the in vivo effect of a NSAID
needs to be causally related to the attenuation of one or
several inflammatory signs or symptoms. For example, in order
to accept an effect on leucocytes as a mode of action of NSAID,
it is mandatory to demonstrate that such effect can be induced
in vivo by several agents of the group and also to explain how
those cells are related to the development of erythema, oedema
or hyperalgesia, or any other inflammatory event.

Presently, for many students to profess either the multiple
effect or the prostaglandin theory tends to be a dogmatic matter.
Maybe an agreement could be reached if a basic scientific dogma
is accepted for sake of discussion, i.e., the best theory is the
simplest theory which encompasses the greatest number of observations. In fact, to accept inhibition of cyclo-oxygenases as
the common denominator of the mechanism of action of NSAID, does
not preclude that the drug has other actions, which may be important

as explanations of differences in therapeutic usefulness, specific toxicity and other effects not related to inflammation.

A general acceptance of a mode of action of a drug implies at least a common understanding of the basic chain of events, responsible for the development of the physiopathological state in which this drug interferes. Thus, it is impossible to conduct a logical discussion on the mode of action of aspirin like drugs, without a previous agreement on the main events involved in the establishment of the inflammatory signs and symptoms. We proposed elsewhere (35) a simple but comprehensive model of the inflammatory events in order to facilitate the discussion on possible sites of action of anti-inflammatory agents. A slightly modified version will be used in this discussion (Fig. 1).

The four basic components of inflammatory reactions are: i) the trauma; ii) the injury of local or migrating cells; iii) generation of inflammatory mediators and iv) tissue responses. In several instances the primary trauma is not directly responsible for the tissue injury. In infections for example, the effective trauma are substances generated by the microorganisms which are responsible for the tissue injury. In many chronic inflammatory diseases the primary event is not known but immunocomplexes may actually be the effective trauma. The trauma may affect local or migrating cells. Presence of migrating cells can be either a pro or an anti-inflammatory event. Phagocytes together with humoral factors, are primarilly associated with the inactivation and/or removal of the effective trauma. Those cells also play an important role in the removal of the debris resulting from cell destruction. However, if PMN or macrophages (for any reason) are unable to remove the injuring stimuli, they may become an amplifying factor of the lesion, due to the release of enzymes (neutral proteases or lysosomal enzymes (140).

Trauma of local or migrating cells leads to the release of inflammatory mediators (Fig. 1, site 4). However, inflammatory mediators may be generated without intervention of cells by the action of an effective trauma on plasma systems (e.g. endotoxin can directly activate kinin or complement systems). But injured cells are bound to release factors which activate plasma mediatorgenases. A mediatorgenase is an enzyme or a cascade of enzymes which activated, generate one or several inflammatory mediators. There are three important plasma systems which are interconnected and, depending on the type of trauma, may play a relevant role in the development of the inflammatory signs and symptoms: kinin, complement and coagulation systems (42,84,113).

Any endogenous substance the level of which increases at the site of inflammation in association with a tissue response (or structural change), can be considered as an inflammatory mediator.

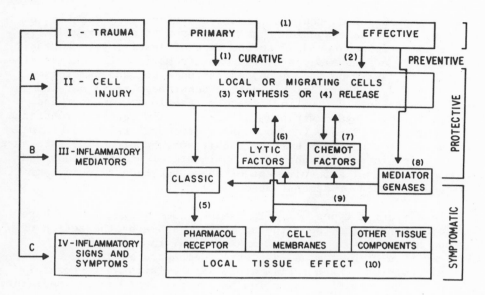

Fig. 1.   Pathways leading to inflammation. Four components of
          inflammation can usually be recognized. Trauma (I)
          causes injury (II) to local or migrating cells. This
          leads to appearance of local inflammatory mediators
          (III) which induce tissue respons (IV) that are the
          basis of inflammatory signs or symptoms (arrow A).
          In some instances, a trauma can induce formation of
          inflammatory mediators, acting directly on plasma systems
          (arrow B). A trauma can produce a sign or a symptom
          directly (arrow C; burning, for example) but in such
          instances anti-inflammatory drugs are of little or no use.

Since several structures present in tissue respond to the appearance
of these mediators, the inflammatory signs and symptoms develop:
erythema, oedema, tissue destruction, hyperalgesia, overt pain,
etc.

     According to their mode of action, three main groups of
inflammatory mediators can be envisaged. 1) classical mediators,
such as histamine, which act via a pharmacological receptor at
the membrane of the effector cells; 2) lytic factors, which
are responsible for the damage of the tissue components (they
can be lytic enzymes or endogenous detergent-like substances);
3) chemotactic factors which stimulate migration of any type of
cell to the inflammatory site. There is another group of mediators
which will not be discussed here, because it is related mainly
to the systemic effect of inflammation (for example, the
endogenous pyrogen).

It is recognised that inflammation differs from species to species, in the same species from one tissue to another and also in the same tissue according to the type of trauma; yet the early inflammatory events induced by various trauma in different species and tissues have much in common, as far as signs and symptoms are concerned. Several highly active substances are liberated locally in tissues during inflammatory reactions. Among these are histamine, 5-hydroxytryptamine (5-HT), slow reacting substance of anaphylaxis (SRS-A), various chemotactic factors, bradykinin (Bk), a PGs of the E or F series, rabbit aorta contracting substance (RCS), which is now thought to be a mixture of endoperoxides and thromboxane A_2. The involvement of these substances in inflammation has been proposed or demonstrated (137).

In different types of inflammation, some mediators may have more prominent roles than others; this is shown by the action of various antagonists. In some immunological reactions the participation of histamine is clearly demonstrated by the use of anti-histaminics. Each inflammatory sign or symptom is possibly caused by the co-ordinated action of several inflammatory mediators and this must also depend on the sensitivity of the responding cells. This interplay is very important and the absence of any one factor can substantially change the final response. Generally speaking, even though the inflammatory response has an abundance of mediators each one is important in itself; otherwise it would be difficult to reduce preferentially some of the signs or symptoms.

Although we cannot prevent the outcome of most chronic inflammatory diseases, because we do not know how to prevent the ongoing tissue injury, we can at least ameliorate the situation and sometimes even recover impaired functions. Chronic inflammation, broadly speaking, differs from the acute by the increased activity or by proliferation of cellular components (e.g. macrophages and fibroblasts and by the presence of tissue lesions). We believe, however, that some inflammatory signs and symptoms observed in chronic inflammation are caused by the same set of mediators which participate in acute inflammation. This is the reason why drugs which development was based on models of acute experimental inflammation such as carrageenin oedema, are effective in some forms of chronic arthropathies. While discussing the mode of action of aspirin like drugs one should always have in mind which is the type of therapy provided by the non-steroid anti-inflammatory agents.

Four main types of therapy for the inflammatory process are suggested in our diagram: curative, preventive, protective and symptomatic. In the curative therapy the drugs are directed towards the primary trauma and success is achieved with the termination of injuriousing stimuli. A curative therapy (Fig. 1,

site 1, e.g. antibiotics) avoids both the direct tissue injury and
the generation of any other effective trauma. The term preventive
therapy (or suppressive therapy)is used in our context to
describe drugs which avert the generation of an effective trauma,
(site 2) but when their administration is discontinued, the
injuringing stimulus may reccur. This would be the case of
drugs such as allopurinol, which blocks the synthesis of uric
acid, or immunosuppressants, that interfere with the generation
of immunocomplexes. Both curative and preventive therapics are
expected to hinder the progression of pathological lesions.

It is interesting that substances belonging to those two
categories (with exception of allopurinol) are not classified as
anti-inflammatory drugs. To illustrate further the problems of
in vitro against in vivo effect, NSAID are able to inhibit
bacterial growth (98, 122) but have no effect on animal infections
(94).

Antigen-antibody reactions in vitro were inhibited by
non-steroid anti-inflammatory drugs but only at toxic concentrations
(62). Cytostatic effects could affect antibody formation but
this response is not significantly impaired by non-steroid
anti-inflammatory drugs (71,87). In contrast to immunosuppressants,
these drugs are effective in the immunopathological events
subsequent to the interation antigen-antibody.

Immunocomplexes have been implicated in the pathogenesis
of several human diseases. Although the primary cause of the
diseases is frequently difficult to establish, the effective
trauma has been related to an autoimmune disease. There are
several immunological reactions in which aspirin-like drugs do
have effects, such as systemic anaphylaxis induced by egg-white
challenge in rabbits, Shwartzman reaction, reverse passive
Arthus reaction, allergic encephalomyelitis in guinea-pig,
serum sickness in man and adjuvant arthritis in rats (62,64,79,
95, 99,115).

In rheumatoid diseases there are reduced sulphydryl levels,
which led Lorber et al. (68) to suggest that this change may
contribute to the formation of autoantigen. Similarly,
inhibition of autoantigen production due to inhibition of protein
denaturation was proposed as a possible mode of action of
aspirin-like drugs (74). Hichens (50) remarks that "to speak of
inhibiting in vivo production of an autoantigen is to over-
estimate the value of aspirin-like drugs, especially because it
overlooks the fact that they exhibit most dramatic effects in
experimental conditions not related to autoimmune phenomena".

In conclusion, the experimental evidence supports the
ideas that therapy NSAID is neither curative or suppressive,

because they do not act at the level of the trauma (sites 1 and 2).

Protective Therapy

A protective therapy would act by minimizing the ongoing
tissue destruction. This type of therapy may affect several
different events of the inflammatory process, and would be
expected eventually to slow down the progression of the tissue
destruction. Thus by interfering for example with the generation
or release of lytic factors originated by plasma systems
(activation of mediatorgenases) or by injured cells.

One of the most important plasma systems related with tissue
injury is the complement. Inhibition of the complement cascade
would have an effect on inflammatory vascular events by blocking
the generation of C3a, C5a, etc. (84,113). In fact complement-
reactive proteins decrease after salicylate therapy (54) but
this effect has not been causably related to the rheumatic
process (92). There are also reports showing aspirin-like drugs
to possess anti-complementary action. Cobra venom and zymosan
deplete C3 and diminish inflammatory responses. Fichel et al. (36)
found that salicylate and cortisone had an anti-complement effect
through an anti-esterase activity. Recently, Di Perri and Auteri
(26) showed that aspirin, flufenamic acid, indomethacin and
phenylbutazone inhibited in vitro the activation of several
components of complement. However, the relevance of this
observation to an anti-inflammatory effect is not clear for
in vivo the drugs were shown to be effective on the complement
system only in very high doses (100 mg/kg, i.v. for indomethacin).

An effect on migrating cells either by diminishing their
number at the inflammatory site or by bloking the release of
neutral proteases or lysosomal enzymes certainly would minimize
inflammatory tissue destruction. Lysosomal enzymes and related
hydrolytic enzymes can break down many tissue components and
degradation of tissue is one of the basic features of chronic
inflammation. Repeated intra-articular injection of lysosomal
enzymes can induce several signs and symptoms of chronic
inflammation (123). Inflammatory exudates contain a large
variety of enzymic activities, originating from various sources.
Collagenase, for instance, is present in polymorphonuclear
leucocytes (63), in skin (41) and rheumatoid synovium (29).
A specific inhibitor of any lysosomal enzyme certainly would be
of value on controlling inflammation. Flufenamic acid and aspirin,
but not phenylbutazone and ibufenac, inhibit collagenase activity
of a lysosomal preparation in vitro (1). To our knowledge,
there is no lysosomal enzyme that is selectively inhibited in
vivo by aspirin-like drugs.

Unspecific binding of aspirin-like drugs to cell membrane

proteins could help to stabilize lysosomal membranes and inhibit
platelet aggregation or red cell lysis. Some of these effects
could be relevant to the amelioration of inflammatory signs and
symptoms because they would ultimately block the release either
of inflammatory mediators or of lytic enzymes. But, how relevant
are the actions of aspirin-like drugs on lysosomal membranes
to their anti-inflammatory action? The effect of aspirin like
drugs on lysosome membranes in vitro have been inconsistent.
Some investigators report labilization and others stabilization.
These discrepancies possibly reflect differences in methodology
(50,55). Gluco-corticoids, as shown by Weissmann and Thomas (124),
have a direct stabilizing action on lysosome membranes against
disrupting trauma such as hypoxia, bacterial and chemical toxins
or UV light. Although very much depending on the preparation of
the lysosomes, buffer conditions and disrupting stimuli, several
aspirin-like drugs stabilize lysosomes in vitro (11,58,73,108).
Recently, Ignarro renewed interest in lysosomal membrane
stabilization as a possible mechanism of action of aspirin-like
drugs (58,59). However, the rank order or potency of the drugs
tested was inverted when inhibition of oedema was compared with
inhibition of extrusion of lysosome enzymes, i.e. aspirin>
phenylbutazone>indomethacin regarding the latter (see 33).

   The experiments of Chayen are possibly relevant to the
discussion because they show that in a more complex system (a
very thin fragment of human skin), aspirin-like drugs are
effective stabilizing agents (15-17). Anderson (1) found that
phenylbutazone reduced the increased lysosomal enzyme activity in
the paws of rats with adjuvant arthritis. Hichens (50) interpreted
these effects, as well as those described by Coppi and Bonardi
(22) and Ignarro and Slywka (60), as secondary to the reduction
of cellular infiltration. However the interference of aspirin-
like drugs in the migration of cells into tissues is still a
matter of controversy and in many experimental models they have
little or no effect on the cell content of acute inflammatory
exudates 9 2,52,114).

   Most of the lysosomal enzymes in inflammatory exudates are
thought to be derived from leucocytes, especially from PMN cells,
released during phagocytosis. Inhibition of phagocytosis,
lysosomal degranulation or fusion of lysosomes with vacu
may ameliorate the inflammatory reaction by avoiding extrusion of
the enzymes (site 6). Colchicine affects PMN cell function by
disrupting microtubules and consequently blocking the fusion of
phagocytic vacuoles with lysosomes. In vivo, it does not seem
that aspiring-like drugs interfere with the phagocytic function
of PMN cells, for there is no change in the content of lysosome
enzymes in inflammatory exudates (131).

Even disregarding the fact that aspirin-like drugs may have a labilizing effect on lysosomal membranes (47), it is difficult to accept that the stabilization of the membrane is important for the mechanism of anti-inflammatory and analgesic effect of aspirin-like drugs. This conclusion had already been reached by Winter in 1966 (135).

Inhibition of migration of PMN cells (39), or monocytes (28) has been suggested as a mode of action of non-steroid anti-inflammatory agents.

Since leucocytes play an important role in the development of acute and chronic inflammation, inhibition of their migration might account for part of the anti-inflammatory effect of some drugs, such as corticoids and immunossuppressants. Non-steroid anti-inflammatory drugs in doses which block increased permeability, seem: a) to interfere with migration of cells in some models, such as pleurisy induced by carrageenin (7); b) not to interfere in others such as the inflammation in the dog knee joint (114, 115); c) to have different effects depending on the type and intensity of the stimulus, such as in the migration of leucocytes into subcutaneous implanted sponges (52,103).

As we already pointed out, migrating cells may be involved in the amplification of an inflammatory reaction possibly by "regurgitation during feeding" of lysosomal enzymes and neutral proteases (25-125-126). Certainly T lymphocytes, through the secretion of lymphokinins and cooperation with the macrophages, are key cells in the development of delayed hypersensitivity (80,113). Blockade of cell migration would certainly reduce tissue destruction. But do aspirin-like drugs have such an effect?

Recently we have shown that aspirin, indomethacin and dexamethasone had a marked effect in leucopenic rats (treated with methotrexate) where the oedematogenic response was partially (60%) restored by administration of folinic acid (Fig.2). This experiment clearly indicates that NSAID and corticoids have a marked antioedematogenic effect independent of an action of leucocytes. This experimental evidence certainly is in disagreement with the views of Smith et al., (102,103).

In fact, it is a dayly clinical observation that NSAID have none or little effect on the number of cells of inflammatory exudates. Probably it is because of the absence of effect on cell migration and on the release of lytic enzymes that NSAID do not reduce the progression of the destructive lesions in chronic inflammation and as we shall discuss below their administration constitutes just a symptomatic therapy.

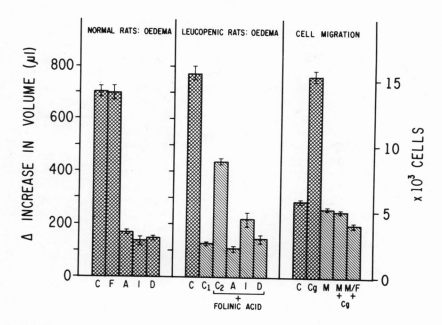

Fig. 2.   Effect of aspirin, indomethacin and dexamethasone on
carrageenin oedema induced in normal and methotrexate/
folinic acid treated animals.

Left panel: effect of Aspirin (300 mg/kg,A),
indomethacin (2 mg/kg,I) and dexamethasone (0.2 mg/kg,D)
in normal rats.   The oedema was measured 4 hours after
carrageenin challenge.   Control carrageenin oedema (C)
was not modified by treatment of (n=5) the animals with
folinic acid (F = 1 mg/kg).

Central panel: effect of aspirin, indomethacin and
dexamethasone in methotrexate-folinic acid treated animals.
C, control normal rats; C_1, methotrexate treated rats;
C_2 methotrexate-folinic acid treated animals.   (n=7).

Right panel: migration of cells induced by carrageenin
into the abdominal cavity.   The data represent the number
of white cells/mm^3 of the wash out of abdominal cavity
(10 ml). C, normal rats without carrageenin stimulation;
Cg, normal rats after carrageenin stimulation;   M,
methotrexate treated animals without carrageenin
stimulation;   M+Cg, methotrexate rats stimulated with
carrageenin;   MF+Cg, methotrexate/folinic acid treated
rats challenged with carrageenin, (n=5).

Symptomatic Therapy

The statement that NSAID represents just a symptomatic
therapy does not come as a surprise. As shown in our model,
such anti-inflammatory therapy should interfere either with some
classical mediator (site 5) or with the reactivity of the effector
cells (site 10). Diminished response of tissue structures could
be achieved by a drug acting directly on any basic metabolic
process. Salicylates uncouple oxidative phosphorylation (10)
and this has led to the suggestion that the reduction in ATP
synthesis would interfere with glycogen and protein synthesis
or with cell membrane permeability (for a review, see 128). Such
an action during therapy with aspirin-like drugs would cause a
general reduction in responsiveness of the vessels to all stimuli
causing permeability increases. This does not happen, as we shall
discuss later. Furthermore, a substance well known as an
uncoupler of oxidative phosphorylation such as 2,4-dinitrophenol,
does not exhibit anti-inflammatory activity (see Winter, 134).
Corticosteroids on the other hand may have this type of action.
Corticosterone reduces vasodilatation (resulting in decreased
blood flow) and vascular exudation (4,77,78,104,136). Recently,
Garcia Leme and Wilhelm (43) re-stated the importance of
corticosteroids as regulators of direct vascular responsiveness to
mediators such as histamine and 5-HT. In this context, Munck
(82) suggested that corticosteroids decrease the utilization of
glucose by peripheral tissues by blocking its transport into the
cell, possibly by preventing phosphorylation. Schayer (96)
proposed that the anti-inflammatory action of corticosteroids
was caused by the passive attachment of the steroid to the microvascular smooth muscle cells, thus interfering with dilatation.

All experimental evidences point to the conclusion that
aspirin-like drugs do not affect the threshold sensitivity of
the effector cells. This is exemplified by the persistence
of the effect of prostaglandins (E_2, E_1, I_2) on production of
erythema, oedema, hyperthermia and hyperalgesia in animals treated
with aspirin-like drugs (34,35).

We may then conclude, from the above discussion, that the
basic mechanism of action of NSAID must involve one or more
classical mediators. Theoretically, a drug can interfere with the
participation of a classical mediator in the inflammatory
reaction by inhibiting its synthesis (site 3), release (site 4)
or antagonizing its association with a pharmacological receptor
(site 5).

Collier and Shorley in 1960 (21) showed that NSAID inhibited
bradykinin induced bronchoconstriction in guinea pigs. They also
have shown that in rabbits and guinea pigs (20) aspirin-like
drugs decrease the extent of hypotension induced by bradykinin.

However, it was soon shown that this effect was not specific since
bronchoconstriction induced by other substances such as ATP, slow
reacting substances C and A, arachidonic acid, collagen etc. was
also inhibited (91-118).

Some of the putative inflammatory mediators, specially Bk,
cause a contraction of isolated strips of vascular tissue, an
effect which in antagonized by aspirin-like drugs. However, there
is doubt whether this effect is selective (20). We suggested
that it reflects an inhibition of a background or stimulated
production of prostaglandins which sensitizes the isolated
smooth muscle preparations to the agonists (35,117). For example,
addition of Bk to slices of bovine mesenteric vessels stimulated
PG synthesis (110). When the direct vascular effects of several
inflammatory mediators have been studied in vivo, no general
pattern of action of aspirin-like drugs has emerged. Phenylbutazone
or aspirin were not effective in reducing the oedema produced by
intra-plantar injections of mediators such as histamine or 5-HT
or phlogogenic stimuli chicken egg white, 48/80, polyvinyl-
pyrrolidone or dextran (8,44). Furthermore, the increased
vascular permeability induced by Bk or peptides prepared from
fibrin, was unaffected by local administration of salicylate
in rats (105). However, calcium aspirin and antipyretics
inhibited the wealing induced by intradermal injection of Bk,
histamine or 5-HT in the rat (107). Arrigoni-Martelli (3) also
found that aspirin, flufenamic acid, phenylbutazone, or sodium
salicylate (in decreasing order of potency) inhibited the increased
vascular permeability induced by Bk. In the guinea pig, aspirin
or sodium salicylate did not reduce the increase of permeability
induced by Bk (21,65). In the rabbit, (67) aspirin-like drugs
diminished the permeability increase caused by Bk (but not that
induced by histamine), but Northover and Subramanian (85) found
no effect on the Bk response. When an injected substance causes
mediator release, it is difficult ot assess in vivo whether an
anti-inflammatory agent is directly inhibiting the activity of
the injected substance or blocking the formation or release of
an endogenous substance(s). Certainly, many unspecific trauma
and specific stimuli induce a quick local formation and release
of PGs. An example comes from Messina et al. (72) who studied
the vasodilator effect of Bk in the cremaster muscle. They
concluded that the effect of Bk was at least in part mediated
by a local release of PGs, since they found that vascular effects
of Bk, but not of PGs, were reduced by PG synthetase inhibitors.
It is possible that all these discrepancies between species or
investigators depend on whether or not there is a release of PGs
caused by the trauma of injection in that particular species or
experiment (117).

Aspirin-like drugs in vitro at high concentrations, inhibit
the synthesis of histamine and this has been suggested as one of

the multiple ways by which these agents could block inflammation
(100). In contrast to aspirin-like drugs, anti-histamine drugs
are anti-inflammatory only in some special types of inflammation
such as urticaria, hay fever and certain manifestations of
anaphylaxis. Passive cutaneous anaphylaxis in the rat, for example,
is inhibited by anti-histaminics, but not consistently by
aspirin-like drugs. Moreover, there is no indication that aspirin-
like drugs are effective in several inflammatory reactions in
which histamine release plays a relevant role.

Prostaglandins

The first clear demonstration of an inhibitory action of
aspirin-like drugs at low concentrations on the release of a
substance by a traumatic stimulus was made by Piper and Vane
(88-90) who showed that a previously unidentified biologically
active material, which they named rabbit aorta contracting
substance (RCS), was released from guinea pig lung during
anaphylaxis, along with histamine, SRS-A and PGs. The RCS release
was blocked by aspirin. Owing to methodological problems, they
failed to notice that there was also inhibition of PG synthesis.
Evidence to link RCS to th biosynthetic pathway came from Vargaftig
and Dao Hai (119,120) who showed that the PG precursor, arachidonic
acid, also generated RCS when infused into guinea pig lungs.
The main component of RCS activity has been re-named thromboxane
A_2 (48).

It was shown in 1971, that the generation or release of
prostaglandins could be inhibited by aspirin-like drugs in three
different systems and species. These systems were a cell-free
preparation of PG synthetase (116), a suspension of human
platelets(101) and the dog autoperfused spleen stimulated by
catecholamines (31). At that time, release of PGs was already
equated with synthesis (90), because it was known that cells do
not store PGs. These findings have been confirmed in a large
number of species using a wide range of analytical techniques,
including thin-layer and gas chromatography, radiometric, and
polarographic assays, as well as radioimmunoassays.

Vane's (116) suggestion that inhibition of PG synthesis
explained the anti-inflammatory activity of aspirin-like drugs,
enormously stimulated research in the field of inflammation. In
contrast to all other hypotheses about the mechanism of anti-
inflammatory, analgesic, and antipyretic activity of aspirin-like
drugs, inhibition of PG synthesis encompasses observations made
by biochemists, physiologists, pharmacologists and pathologists,
and forms the only unified view until now presented. Many
points that we shall briefly review in the next section have
already been discussed and subject to several reviews(32,35,37,38,
45,97).

Observations which Support a Pro-Inflammatory Role of Prostaglandins

1. All cells are capable of generating prostaglandins. There
    is no experimental demonstration that normal tissues
    expontaneously generate prostaglandins (this also applies for
    prostacyclin). Generation of prostaglandins reflects an
    injury of the cell membranes or a state of hyperactivity
    of the cell. Loss of cell compartimentalization may also be
    necessary for PG generation. Prostaglandins have been
    demonstrated in inflammatory exudates, in the venous or
    lymphatic effluent from tissues under mechanical or chemical
    stimulation or after injury. Phagocytosis by PMNs or
    macrophages is accompanied by prostaglandin release (51,80,
    81). Homogenates of phagocytosing PMNs generate more
    prostaglandins than homogenates obtained from resting PMN
    (51). This may indicate that cyclo-oxygenase is activated
    during phagocytosis. The concentration of prostaglandins
    in the inflammatory exudates does not parallel leucocyte
    number (86). This concentration probably reflects the
    degree of secretory or phagocytic activity of the migrating
    cells and/or the intensity of local cell damage rather
    than the PMN number. The contribution of the local cells
    to the prostaglandin content of the inflammatory exudates is
    illustrated by the treatment of animals with colchicine which
    abolishes cell migration without interfering or even
    increasing PGE_2 concentration (52). We believe that in
    chronic inflammmation the "functional prostaglandin" is
    generated by the effector cells themselves (local cells).
    In acute processes, with intense cell migration and damage
    "phagocytic prostaglandins" may contribute to the
    development of inflammatory signs and symptoms.

2. Each type of cell has a tendency to produce a major type of
    prostaglandins. Homogenates of phagocytosing PMNs synthetise
    prostaglandin E_2 and thromboxane A_2 when incubated with
    the endoperoxide PGH_2. In contrast, endothelial cells
    generate mainly PGI_2 (76). Prostacyclin seems to be the
    major route of endoperoxide metabolism in the other tissues
    like rat stomach, lung or uterus when cofactors are not
    added. Addition of different cofactors to partially purified
    cyclo-oxygenase preparations directed the biosynthesis
    either towards E_2 or $F_{2\alpha}$ (37,38). Variation of the content of
    cofactors during the evolution of an inflammatory reaction
    may explain why in some models of experimental inflammation
    there is an initial release of PGE_2 later followed by $F_{2\alpha}$.
    It is not yet established if conversion of endoperoxides to
    PGE_2 or $F_{2\alpha}$ is enzymatic. Certainly conversion to prostacyclin
    or thromboxane is enzyme mediated, for inhibitors have
    been described. Conversion of PGG_2 to thromboxane is inhibited
    by benzydamine while the 15-hydroperoxy-arachidonic acid

inhibits prostacyclin synthesis. Thus the type of
prostaglandin which participates in each type of inflammation
depends on the cells involved. Endothelial lesions may
contribute mainly with prostacyclin. If the vascular lesions
extend to more internal layers, prostaglandin of E type
probably predominate. Prostaglandin E_s and I_2 are described
to be generated in acute and in chronic inflammatory processes
(14,52,83,106).

3. Cyclo-oxygenase prepared from various tissues and animal
    species are inhibited by NSAID. The duration of the
    effect of NSAID in vivo is regulated by a) the access of
    the enzyme in the cell membrane; b) by the turnover of
    cyclo-oxygenase and c) by the type of inhibition. A single
    administration of aspirin inhibits cyclo-oxygenase of
    platelets for 2-3 days, possibly because it acetylated
    the enzyme and the novo synthesis of cyclo-oxygenase in this
    cell is very restricted (see 37,38). There are drugs which
    inhibit cyclo-oxygenase in vitro but have no anti-
    oedematogenic effect. However there are no drugs capable
    of inhibiting cyclo-oxygenase in vivo and which show anti-
    oedematogenic or antialgic effect (52). The body fluid
    concentration of NSAID during therapy is of the same order
    of magnitude as that necessary for inhibition of cyclo-
    oxygenase preparations. NSAID enantiomers without
    anti-inflammatory activity have no inhibitory effect upon
    cyclo-oxygenase. The PG synthetase is readily inhibited by
    a number of methyl aryl acetic acids with the S(+) absolute
    configuration, but not by their R(-) enantiomers. It is
    noteworthy that this very high degree of stereospecificity
    is the same as observed in in vivo anti-inflammatory assays
    but not shared by any other in vitro systems. For example,
    the uncoupling of oxidative phosphorylation and the
    stabilization of erythrocyte membrane are equally responsive
    to both S and R isomers. NSAID at higher concentrations
    also affect lipoxygenase activity which may explain their
    inhibitory effect on PMN migration in vivo (97).

4. Corticosteroids have no direct effect on cyclo-oxygenase
    but have been shown to inhibit prostaglandin release in
    several systems, in vitro and in vivo. The effect of
    corticosteroids in the prostaglandin synthesis depends upon
    protein synthesis (see 27). It is thought that the
    mechanism of action of corticosteroids depends on the
    generation of a peptide which by inhibiting phospholipase
    A_2 activity, diminishes prostaglandin generation (see
    Flower, this book). Corticotherapy of several chronic
    arthropathies is just symptomatic and its clinical benefit
    similar to NSAID therapy may result from action at a
    different sites of arachidonic acid metabolism.

5.   PG synthetase prepared from different tissues shows
     differential sensitivities to aspirin-like drugs. This
     property may reflect a series of isoenzymes and can
     explain the variations in activity within the compounds
     capable of inhibiting PG synthesis in vivo. Paracetamol
     and dipyrone, which is analgesic and antipyretic and
     thought to have little anti-oedematogenic effect, has a
     greater or equivalent activity than aspirin upon brain
     enzymes but is much less active on enzymes prepared from
     other tissues (37,38). A more pronounced effect of
     phenylbutazone on prostaglandin synthetase from nervous
     tissue may also explain its superior analgesic action on
     processes such as spondylitis in which pain may arise mainly
     as a consequence of the generation of PGs by the injured
     nerves themselves. One condition that may govern in vivo
     the potency of a cyclo-oxygenase inhibitor is its access
     to the enzyme within the cells. Cyclo-oxygenase from
     endothelial cells is less vulnerable to NSAID than the
     platelet enzyme. For this reason low doses of aspirin can
     affect platelet aggregation without great interference with
     the prostacyclin generation. At a high therapeutic anti-
     inflammatory dosage, prostaglandin E_2, I_2 and TXA_2 generation
     by most of tissues is inhibited.

6.   Prostaglandins administered locally mimic some inflammatory
     events and when given into the cerebral ventricles cause
     fever. We have reviewed in detail the ability of
     prostaglandins to reproduce inflammatory signs and symptoms
     (32-35) and selected for discussion only a few points
     which differentiate prostaglandins from the other classical
     inflammatory mediators, such as histamine, bradykinin, etc.

     a) While the other classical inflammatory mediators produce
         a short lasting erythema, prostaglandins of the E_2
         and E_1 series cause a long lasting effect. Prostaglandin
         I_2 considered as one of the most potent vasodilators
         but its effect is short lived (see Moncada in this
         book).

     b) Prostaglandins (E_1, E_2 and I_2) cause little exudation
         or oedema. However when associated with other mediators
         they cause an intense potentiation of exudation or
         oedema (40,53). This potentiation probably is the
         result of the vasodilatation induced by prostaglandins
         (130). However vasodilatation may not be the only factor.
         In the rat paw, prostaglandins cause a long lasting
         vasodilator effect, but the ability to potentiate
         carrageenin oedema lasts less than 30 mins. It is
         possible that endoperoxides play a role in inflammation .
         However, PGG_2 and PGH_2 also potentiate to the same extent

rat paw oedema induced by carrageenin. This is
indicative that the free radical formed in the metabolism
of PGG_2 is not very important for this potentiating
effect.

c) Cell migration. Prostaglandins of the E series cause
    chemotaxis in vitro but other products of arachidonic
    acid metabolism might play a more important role in vivo.
    HETE generated by lipoxygenase may be one of these
    substances. High doses of NSAID may effect lipoxygenase
    activity. Low doses, in fact, seem to potentiate
    migration probably by inhibiting cyclo-oxygenase and
    increase the availability of AA for HETE formation.

d) Prostaglandins hyperalgesia. The importance of this
    event is fully discussed in (75) and in another paper
    in this book (see Ferreira).

e) Prostaglandins of the E series cause fever. If
    inhibition of prostaglandins explains the anti-
    pyretic effect of NSAID is still a matter of controversy.
    Antipyretics do not antagonise the direct hyperthermic
    effect of prostaglandins. NSAID abolish CNS generation
    of prostaglandins induced by systemic administration
    of pyrogens parallel to a return to normal body
    temperature. However prostaglandins E_2 antagonists did
    not reduce the fever induced by leucocyte pyrogen and
    only partially reduced the response to centrally
    administered arachidonate. These observations may
    suggest that there are other matabolites of arachidonic
    acid not related to cyclo-oxygenase involved in the
    pyrogenic effect of some substances. There is also
    the possibility that the endoperoxides are matabolized
    in CNS to other pyrogenic prostaglandins different from
    the E series. This would explain the failure of
    prostaglandin antagonists. The problem is discussed in
    length in recent reviews (18,30).

f) Finally I shall call attention to one point which has
    caused misinterpretations in the literature. Because
    the concentration of prostaglandins found in some
    inflammatory exudates is below the threshold to induce
    an inflammatory event, it has been concluded that
    prostaglandins play, at the best, a minor role (14).
    This interpretation does not take into consideration that
    some of the inflammatory effects of prostaglandins are
    long lasting. Thus the effect of the continous release
    of minute amounts during a long period of time is
    cumulative, eventually leading to the establishment of
    an inflammatory sing or symtpom like erythema or
    hyperalgesia.

The Anti-Inflammatory Effect of Prostaglandins

There is an apparent anomaly in the prostaglandin theory, for prostaglandins can be anti-inflammatory in acute and chronic models (5,46,139,141). However these effects have only been shown with very high amounts of prostaglandins, which make it improbable that endogenously released prostaglandins would play an important role as anti-inflammatory substances. Two mechanisms could account for these pharmacological effects of prostaglandins, especially of prostaglandin E_1. They could act through a release of an endogenous anti-inflammatory factor and/or by inhibiting the release of inflammatory mediators. Prostaglandins given in such high doses (up to 1 mg a day) undoubtedly cause an increased vascular permeability and could be acting as an irritant (9). Vasoactive drugs such as isoprenaline, histamine, 5-hydroxytryptamine, saponin, digitonin and ethyl alcohol also have a similar effect. It has been shown, however, that concentrations of prostaglandins E_1 or E_2 higher than those found in inflammatory exudates block the release in vitro: a) of histamine and SRS-A from lung fragments and basophiles (66,109); b) of lysosomal enzymes from human leucocytes (9,13,127,140); c) of lymphokines from macrophages (80), and d) prevent lymphocyte-mediated cytotoxicity (49). These effects in vitro correlate with an increase in intra-cellular cAMP and may explain why administration of cAMP suppresses acute and chronic inflammation in several experimental models (56,57). The inhibitory effect of pharmacological doses of prostaglandins has also been shown in vivo for cartilage destruction and lysosomal enzyme release (5,138). But if endogenous prostaglandins were depressing cartilage destruction or lysosomal enzyme release in any type of chronic inflammation, treatment with a prostaglandin synthetase inhibitor should accelerate the evolution of the physiopathological lesions; this does not happen. Alternatively it could be that the cyclo-oxygenase of the cells involved in the bone erosi. sensitive to NSAID.

Thus, it is likely that endogenous prostaglandins play a pro-inflammatory rather than an anti-inflammatory role and the anti-inflammatory effect of exogenous prostaglandins is either by releasing endogenous anti-inflammatory substances or by blocking the release of inflammatory mediators.

Much has been said about the modulating role of prostaglandins in inflammation: PGEs are regarded as pro-inflammatory and PGFs as anti-inflammatory. PGE_2 together with PMNs predominate at the peak of plasma exudation, but $PGF_{2\alpha}$ rises at the time when exudation decreases (13,45,121,133). These authors demonstrated the occurrence of a similar pattern of responses for several types of inflammatory reaction in the pleural cavity of the rat (induced

by carrageenin, calcium pyrophosphate, reverse passive Arthus
reaction, delayed hypersensitivity). The basic assumption
underlying this theory is that $PGF_{2\alpha}$ is "anti-inflammatory".
This idea started with the observation that in the rat the
permeability increase induced by bradykinin was partially
curtailed by $PGF_{2\alpha}$ (111,112,132); Crunkhorn and Willis (23,24)
observed that $PGF_{2\alpha}$ reduced the effect of PGE_1 and PGE_2.
Recently, Juan and Lembeck (61) showed that $PGF_{2\alpha}$ reduced the
algesic effect of bradykinin on isolated perfused ear of the
rabbit. They concluded that $PGF_{2\alpha}$ did not directly reduce the
effect of bradykinin but inhibited the enhancement of its algesic
effect produced by prostaglandin E that is released endogenously
by bradykinin. First it should be pointed out that these effects
of $PGF_{2\alpha}$ are species dependent because in man $PGF_{2\alpha}$ is a
vasodilator and causes hyperalgesia (34). $PGF_{2\alpha}$ has no antagonistic
effect upon the potentiating effect of PGE_2 on carrageenin or
on oedema in rats or on the effect of Bk in rabbits (130).

We believe that experiments made with bolus injections
bear little similarity to what occurs in inflammation. In
inflammation mediators are released in small quantities during
a relative long period of time. This is the situation when
prostaglandins due to their long lasting effect on vessels and
sensory terminations, enhance oedema and cause hyperalgesia.
Moreover the $PGF_{2\alpha}$ feed back theory implies also an effect on the
release of lysosomal enzymes. The rise of prostaglandin levels
(E_2 or $F_{2\alpha}$) in the exudate would induce a rise of cyclic AMP in
PMNs with consequent reduction of the extrusion of acid hydrolases.
There is no experimental observation <u>in vivo</u> to support this
hypothesis. On the contrary there was no change of lysosomal
enzymes in inflammatory exudates when the generation of
prostaglandins was inhibited by aspirin like drugs (131).
Furthermore the amount of lysosomal enzymes increased parallel
to the concentration of prostaglandins in the inflammatory
exudate (2).

Several prostaglandins of the E and A series were found to
affect gastrointestinal functions and to exert therapeutic effects
on a variety of lesions of the stomach and small intestine in
animals (6,19,69,93). It is well known that non-steroid anti-
inflammatory drugs cause gastric lesions and it has been suggested
that this side effect could result from an abolition of the
release of prostaglandins (116). Anti-secretory prostaglandins
inhibit gastric secretion and prevent gastric mucosal erosion
in rats (129). Although the inhibition of gastric secretion is
likely to be the primary mechanism, these prostaglandins block
gastric mucosal erosion even in the presence of perfused acid,
thus indicating that other protective mechanisms must be
operative, as suggested by Robert (93). It is possible that in
the gastrointestinal tract endogenous prostaglandins (PGI_2?) play

an important role in maintaining the integrity of a tissue which is constantly threatened by a variety of traumatic stimuli. Prostaglandins causing local vasodilatation (one component of the inflammatory reaction!) possibly increase the interstitial wash-out, thus protecting mucosa integrity (from the back diffusion of acid, for example). The fact that a therapeutic dose of a prostaglandin analogue displays antiulcerogenic activity does not necessarily indicate that endogenous prostaglandins are anti-inflammatory.

Conclusions

NSAID therapy is simply symptomatic implying that in chronic inflammation it does not affect those mechanisms involved in the progression of tissue destruction, such as inhibition of phagocyte migration or the release of lysosomal enzymes.

There is no drug which inhibits in vivo generation of prostaglandins and which does not have anti-oedematogenic or antialgic effect. Prostaglandins of E_1, E_2, I_2, D_2 series when administered in animals pretreated with NSAID reproduce some of the basic inflammatory events such a hyperalgesia, erythema and potentiate exudation induced by other inflammatory mediators. The site of generation of prostaglandins is suggested to be the structure which they affect. "Exudate prostaglandins" probably are relevant when the trauma is intense with consequent tissue and migrating cell destruction. Cyclo-oxygenases from various tissues show a differential sensitivity towards NSAID. This explains why a particular NSAID (dypirone or paracetamol) at a therapeutic dosage may have a more intense antialgic than an anti-oedematogenic effect, or why low doses of aspirin inhibit the synthesis of thromboxane A_2 by platelet or of PGE_2 by PMN while that of prostacyclin by endothelial cells is still preserved.

Acknowledgements

We thank FAPESP (Brazil) and the Wellcome Foundation for research grants.

REFERENCES

1. A. J. Anderson, Lysosomal enzyme activity in rats with adjuvant-induced arthritis. Ann. Rheum. Dis., 29:307-313 (1970).
2. A. J. Anderson, W. E. Brocklehurst and A. L. Willis, Evidence for the role of lysosomes in the formation of prostaglandins during carrageenin induced inflammation in the rat. Pharmacol. Res. Commun., 3:13-19 (1971).

3. E. Arrigoni-Martelli, Antagonism of anti-inflammatory drugs on bradykinin-induced increase of capillary permeability. J.Pharm. (Lond.), 19:617-620 (1967).

4. N. Ashton, C. Cook, In vivo observations of the effects of cortisone upon the blood vessels in rabbit ear chambers. Brit. J. Exp. Path., 33:445-450 (1952).

5. R. L. Aspinall and P. S. Cammarata, Effect of prostaglandin E$_2$ on adjuvant arthritis. Nature, 224:1320-1321 (1969).

6. A. Bennett, Effects of prostaglandins on the gastrointestinal tract. In: "The Prostaglandins: Progress in Research", S. M. M. Karim, ed., MTP Med. and Tec. Publ. Co., Oxford, pp.205-221 (1972).

7. A. Blackham and R. T. Owen, Prostaglandin synthetase inhibitors and leucocytic emigration. J. Pharm. (Lond.), 27:201-203 (1975).

8. I. L. Bonta, Time-effect course and drug antagonism pattern of various kinds of rat paw oedemas. In: "Non-Steroidal Anti-Inflammatory Drugs", International Symposium, Milan, S. Garattini, M. N. G. Dukes, eds., p.236. Amsterdam-London: Excerpta Medica Foundation (1965).

9. I. L. Bonta, Endogenous modulators of the inflammatory response. In: "Inflammation", J. R. Vane and S. H. Ferreira, eds. Handbook of Experimental Pharmacology vol.50/I, Springer-Verlag, Berlin, Heidelberg, p.523-560 (1978).

10. T. M. Brody, Action of sodium salicylate and related compounds on tissue metabolism in vitro. J. Pharmacol. Exp. Ther., 117:39-51 (1956).

11. J. H. Brown, N. L. Schwartz, Interaction of lysosomes and anti-inflammatory drugs. Proc. Soc. Exp. Biol. (N.Y.), 131:614-620 (1969).

12. K. Brune, B. Minder, M. Glatt and L. Schmid: Do polymorphonuclear leucocytes function as mediators in acute inflammation? In: "Future Trends in Inflammation", G. P. Velo, D. A. Willoughby, J. P. Giroud, eds., pp.289-300. Padua-London: Piccin Medical Books (1974).

13. F. Capasso, C. J. Dunn, S. Yamamoto, D. A. Willoughby and J. P. Giroud, Further studies on carrageenin induced pleurisy in rats. J. Pathol., 116:117-124 (1975).

14. W. C. Chang, S. Murota and S. Tsurufuji Role of prostaglandin E in carrageenin induced inflammation in rats. Bioch. Pharmac., 25:2045-2050 (1976).

15. J. Chayen and L. Bitensky, Lysosomal enzymes and inflammation with particular reference to rheumatoid diseases. Ann.Rheum. Dis., 30:522-536 (1971).

16. J. Chayen, L. Bitensky, R. G. Butcher and B. Gashman, Evidence for altered lysosomal membrane in synovial lining cells from human rheumatoid joints. Beitr. Path. Anat., 142:137-149 (1971).

17. J. Chayen, L. Bitensky, R. G. Butcher, L. W. Poulter and
    G. S. Ubhi, Methods for direct measurement of anti-
    inflammatory action on human maintained in vitro. Brit. J.
    Derm., 82:Suppl. 6, 62 (1970).
18. W. G. Clark, Mechanisms of antipyretic action. Gen.
    Pharmacol., 10:71-77 (1979).
19. M. M. Cohen and B. C. Vancouver, Mucosal cytoprotection by
    prostaglandin E$_2$. Lancet, 8102 (II):1253-1254 (1978).
20. H. O. J. Collier, A pharmacological analysis of aspirin.
    Advanc. Pharmacol. Chemother.,7:333-405 (1969).
21. H. O. J. Collier and P. G. Shorley, Analgesic antipyretic
    drugs as antagonists of bradykinin.Brit. J. Pharmacol.,
    15:601-610 (1960).
22. G. Coppi and G. Bonardi, Effect of two non-steroidal anti-
    inflammatory agents on alkaline and acid phosphatases of
    inflamed tissues. J. Pharm. (Lond.), 20:661-662 (1968).
23. P. Crunkhorn and A. L. Willis, Actions and interactions
    of prostaglandins administered intradermally in rat and
    man. Br. J. Pharmac., 36:216-217 (1969).
24. P. Crunkhorn and A. L. Willis, Cutaneous reactions to
    intradermal prostaglandins. Br. J. Pharmac., 41:47-49
    (1971).
25. P. Davies and A. S. Allison, The release of hydrolitic
    enzymes from phagocytic and other cells participating in
    acute and chronic inflammation. In: "Inflammation",J. R.
    Vane and S. H. Ferreira, eds., Handbook of Experimental
    Pharmacology vol. 50/I, Springer-Verlag, Berlin, Heidelberg
    p.267-294 (1978).
26. T. Di Perri and A. Auteri, On the anticomplementary action
    of some non-steroidal anti-inflammatory drugs. In:
    "Future Trends in Inflammation", G. P. Velo, D. A. Willoughby,
    J. P. Giroud, eds., p.215-225. Padua-London:
    Piccin Medical Books (1974).
27. M. Di Rosa and P. Persico, Mechanism of inhibition of
    prostaglandin biosynthesis by hydrocortisone in rat
    leucocytes. Br. J. Pharmac., 66:161-163 (1979).
28. M. Di Rosa, J. M. Papadimitriou and D. A. Willoughby,
    A histopathological and pharmacological analysis of the
    mode of action of non-steroidal anti-inflammatory drugs.
    J. Path., 105:239-256 (1971).
29. J. M. Evanson, J. J. Jeffrey and S. M. Krane, Human
    collagenase: identification and characterization of an
    enzyme from rheumatoid synovium in culture. Science, 158:
    499-502 (1967).
30. W. S. Feldberg and A. S. Milton, Prostaglandins and body
    temperature. In: "Inflammation", J. R. Vane and S. H.
    Ferreira, eds., Handbook of Experimental Pharmacology
    vol. 50/I, Springer-Verlag, Berlin, Heidelberg
    p.617-649 (1978).

31. S. H. Ferreira, S. Moncada and J. R. Vane: Indomethacin and aspirin abolish porstaglandin release from the spleen. Nature (New Biol.),231:237-239 (1971).

32. S. H. Ferreira, S. Moncada and J. R. Vane, Prostaglandins and signs and symptoms of inflammation. In: "Prostaglandin Synthetase Inhibitors", H. J. Robinson and J. R. Vane, eds., Raven Press, New York, p.157-187 (1974).

33. S. H. Ferreira and J. R. Vane, Aspirin and prostaglandins. In: "The Prostaglandins II", P. W. Ramwell, ed., Plenum Press, New York, London, p.1-39 (1974).

34. S. H. Ferreira and J. R. Vane, New aspects of the mode of action of non-steroid anti-inflammatory drugs. Ann. Rev. Pharmacol., 14:57-73 (1974).

35. S. H. Ferreira and J. R. Vane, Mode of action of anti-inflammatory agents which are prostaglandin synthetase inhibitors. In: "Anti-Inflammatory Drugs", J. R. Vane and S. H. Ferreira, eds. Handbood of Experimental Pharmacology vol. 50/II, Springer-Verlag, Berlin, Heidelberg p.348-398 (1978).

36. E. E. Fichel, C. W. Frank, A. J. Boltax and M. Arcasoy, Observations on the treatment of rheumatic fever with salicylate, ACTH and cortisone. II. Combined salicylate corticoid therapy and attempts at rebound-suppression. Arthr. Rheum., 1:351-366 (1958).

37. R. J. Flower, Drugs which inhibit prostaglandin biosynthesis. Pharm. Revs., 26:33-67 (1974).

38. R. J. Flower, Prostaglandin and related compounds. In: "Inflammatory drugs" J. R. Vane and S. H. Ferreira, eds. Handbook of Experimental Pharmacology vol. 50/II, Springer-Verlag, Berlin, Heidelberg p.374-422 (1978).

39. A. W. Ford-Hutchinson, M. J. M. Smith, P. N. Elliott, J. G. Bolam, J. R. Walker, A. A. Lobo, J. K. Badcock, A. J. Colledge and F. J. Billimoria, Effects of a human plasma fraction on leucocyte migration into inflammatory exudates. J. Pharm. (Lond.), 27:106-112 (1975).

40. A. W. Ford-Hutchinson, J. R. Walker, E. M. Davidson and M. J. H. Smith, PGI_2: A potential mediator of inflammation. Prostaglandins, 16, (2): 253-258 (1978).

41. H. M. Fullmer, W. A. Gibson, G. Lazarus and A. C. Stamm, Collagenolytic activity of the skin associated with neuromuscular diseases including ammyotrophic lateral sclerosis. Lancet,I: 1007-1009 (1966).

42. J. Garcia Leme, Bradykinin System. In: "Inflammation", J. R. Vane and S. H. Ferreira, eds. Handbook of Experimental Pharmacology vol. 50/I, Springer-Verlag, Berlin, Heidelberg, p.464-487 (1978).

43. J. Garcia Leme and D. L. Wilhelm, The effects of adrenalectomy and corticosterone on vascular permeability responses in the skin of the rat. Brit. J. Exp. Path., 56:402-407 (1975).

44. J. Garcia Leme, L. Hamamura, M. P. Leite and M. Rocha
E Silva, Pharmacological analysis of the acute inflammatory
process induced in the rat's paw by local injection of
carrageenin and by heating. Brit. J. Pharmacol., 48:
88-96 (1973).

45. J. P. Giroud, G. P. Velo and D. A. Willoughby, The role of
prostaglandins and cyclic nucleotides in inflammation.
In: "Prostaglandins and Thromboxanes", F. Berti, B.
Samuelsson and G. P. Velo, eds., Plenum Press, pp.323-344
(1977).

46. E. M. Glenn and N. Rohloff, Anti-arthritic and anti-
inflammatory effects of certain prostaglandins. Proc. Soc.
Exp. Biol. Med., 139:290-294 (1972).

47. N. H. Grant, M. E. Rosenthale, H. E. Alburn and A. C. Singer,
Slowed lysosomal enzyme release and its normalization by
drugs in adjuvant-induced polyarthritis. Biochem.
Pharmacol., 20:2821-2824 (1971).

48. M. Hamberg, J. Svensson and B. Samuelsson, Novel transformations of prostaglandin endoperoxides: formation of
thromboxanes. In: "Advances in Prostaglandin and
Thromboxane Research",vol. I, B. Samuelsson and R. Paoletti,
eds., pp.p9-27. New York: Raven Press (1976).

49. C. S. Henney, H. R. Bourne and L. M. Lichtenstein, The role
of cyclic 3'5' - adenosine monophosphate in the specific
cytolytic activity of lymphocytes. J. Immunol., 108:
1526-1534 (1972).

50. M. Hichens, Molecular and cellular pharmacology of the
anti-inflammatory drugs: some in vitro properties to their
possible modes of action. In: "Anti-Inflammatory Agents,
Chemistry and Pharmacology", vol. 2, R. A. Scherrer and M. W.
Whitehouse, eds., pp.264-297. New York-San Francisco-London:
Academic Press (1974).

51. G. A. Higgs, S. Buting, S. Moncada and J. R. Vane,
Polymorphonuclear leukocytes produce thromboxane A_2-like
activity during phagocytosis. Prostaglandins, 12 (5):
749-757 (1976).

52. G. A. Higgs, E. A. Harvey, S. H. Ferreira and J. R. Vane,
The effect of anti-inflammatory drugs on the production of
prostaglandins in vivo. In: "Advances in Prostaglandin and
Thromboxane Research", vol. I, B. Samuelsson and R. Paoletti,
eds., pp.105-110. New York: Raven Press (1976).

53. E.A. Higgs, S. Moncada and J. R. Vane, Inflammatory effects
of prostacyclin (PGI_2) and 6-oxo-$PGF_{1\alpha}$ in the rat paw.
Prostaglandins, 16(2):153-160 (1978).

54. A. G. S. Hill, C-reactive protein in rheumatic fever.
Lancet, II:558-560 (1952).

55. J. Hyteel and A. Jorgensen, Studies on lysosome stabilization
by antirheumatic drugs. Europ. J. Pharmacol.,11:383-387
(1970).

56. A. Ichikawa, H. Hayas i, M. Minami and K. Tomita, An acute
     inflammation induced by inorganic pyrophosphate and adenosine
     triphosphate, and its inhibition by cyclic 3'5'-adenosine
     monophosphate. Biochem. Pharmacol., 21:317-331 (1972).

57. A. Ichikawa, M. Nagasaki, K. Umezu, H. Hayashi and K. Tomita,
     Effect of cyclic 3'5' monophosphate on oedema and granuloma
     induced by carrageenin. Biochem. Pharmacol., 21:2615-2626
     (1972).

58. L. J. Ignarro, Effects of anti-inflammatory drugs on the
     stability of rat liver lysosomes in vitro. Biochem.
     Pharmacol., 20:2847-2860 (1971).

59. L. J. Ignarro and C. Colombo, Enzyme release from guinea
     pig polymorphonuclear leucocyte lysosomes inhibited in
     vitro by anti-inflammatory drugs. Nature (New Biol.)
     239:155-157 (1972).

60. L. J. Ignarro and J. Slywka, Changes in liver lysosomes
     fragility, erythrocyte membrane stability, and local and
     systematic lysosomal enzyme levels in adjuvant-induced
     polyarthritis. Biochem. Pharmacol.,21:875-886 (1972).

61. H. Juan and F. Lembeck, Prostaglandin $F_{2\alpha}$ reduces the
     algesic effect of bradykinin by antagonizing the pain
     enhancing action of endogenously released prostaglandin E.
     Br. J. Pharmac., 59:385-391 (1977).

62. T. G. Kantor, Anti-inflammatory drugs. In: "Text Book of
     Immunopathology", P. A. Miescher and H.J. Müller-Eberhard,
     eds., pp.217-226, Grune, London, (1968).

63. G. S. Lazarus, R. S. Brown, J. R. Daniels and H. M. Füllmer,
     Human granulocyte collagenase. Science, 159:1483-1485
     (1968).

64. M. H. Lepper, E. R. Candwell, P. K. Smith, Jr., and B. F.
     Miller, Effects of anaphylactic shock of salicylates,
     aminopyrine, and other chemically and pharmacologically
     related compounds. Proc. Soc. Exp. Biol. (N.Y.)
     74:254-258 (1950).

65. G. P. Lewis, Pharmacological actions of bradykinin and its
     role in physiological and pathological reactions.
     Ann. N.Y. Acad. Sci., 104:236-249 (1963).

66. L. M. Lichtenstein and R. De Bernado, The immediate allergic
     response in vitro action evelie AMP-active and other drugs
     on the two stages of histamine release. J. Immunol.,
     107:1131-1136 (1971).

67. P. M. Lish and G. R. McKinney, Pharmacology of methdilazine.
     II. Some determinants and limits of action on vascular
     permeability and inflammation in model systems. J. Lab.
     Clin. Med., 61:1015-1028 (1963).

68. A. Lorber, C. M. Pearson, W. L. Meredith and L. E. Gantz-
     Mandell, Serum sulfhydryl determinations and significance
     in connective tissue diseases. Ann. Intern. Med., 61:423-
     434 (1964).

69. I. H. M. Main, Prostaglandins and the gastrointestinal tract.
    In: "The prostaglandins. Pharmacological and Therapeutic
    Advances", M. F. Cuthbert, ed., Heinemann, London, pp.284-
    323 (1973).

70. S. E. Malawista and P. T. Bodel, The dissociation by
    colchicine of phagocytosis from increased oxygen consumption
    in human leukocytes. J. Clin. Invest., 46:786-789
    (1967).

71. A. M. Marmont, F. Rossi and E. Damasio,Indomethacin in the
    treatment of rheumatic and non-rheumatic diseases, with
    special reference to systemic lupus erythematosus. In:
    "International Symposium on Non-Steroid Anti-Inflammatory
    Drugs", S. Garattini and M. M. G. Dukes, eds. International
    Congress Series 82, pp.363-372, New York, Excerpta Medica
    Foundation (1965).

72. E. J. Messina, R. Weiner and G. Kaley, Inhibition of
    bradykinin vasodilation and potentiation of norepinephrine
    and angiotensin vasoconstriction by inhibitors of
    prostaglandin synthesis in skeletal muscle of the rat.
    Circulat. Res., 37:430-437 (1975).

73. W. S. Miller and J. G. Smith, Effect of acetylsalicytic
    acid on lysosomes. Proc. Soc. Exp. Biol. (N.Y.),
    122:634-636 (1966).

74. Y. Mizushima and H. Suzuki, Interaction between plasma
    proteins and antirheumatic or new anti-phlogistic drugs.
    Arch. Int. Pharmac.,157:115-124 (1965).

75. S. Moncada, S. H. Ferreira and J. R. Vane, Pain and
    inflammatory mediators. In: "Anti-Inflammatory Drugs",
    J. R. Vane and S. H. Ferreira, eds. Handbook of Experimental
    Pharmacology vol. 50/II, Springer-Verlag, Berlin,
    Heidelberg, p.588-608 (1978).

76. S. Moncada, E. A. Higgs and J. R. Vane, Human arterial and
    venous tissue generate prostacyclin (prostaglandin X),
    a potent inhibitor of platelet aggregation. Lancet,
    I: 18-20 (1977).

77. V. H. Moon and G. A. Tershakovec, Influence of cortisone
    upon acute inflammation. Proc. Soc. Exp. Biol., (N.Y.),
    79:63-65 (1952).

78. V. H. Moon and G. A. Tershakovec, Effect of cortisone upon
    local capillary permeability. Proc. Soc. Exp. Biol. (N.Y.),
    85:600-603 (1954).

79. D. F. Moore, J. Lowenthal, M. Fuller and L. B. Jacques,
    Inhibition of experimental arthritis by cortisone, salicylate,
    and related compounds. Amer. J. Clin. Path., 22:936-943
    (1952).

80. J. Morley, Prostaglandins and lymphokines in arthritis.
    Prostaglandins, 8:315-326 (1974).

81. J. Morley, Lymphokines. In: "Inflammation",J. R. Vane and
    S. H. Ferreira, eds. Handbook of Experimental Pharmacology
    vol. 50/I, Springer-Verlag, Berlin, Heidelberg, p.314-344 (1978).

82. A. Munck, Glucocorticoid inhibition of glucose uptake by
     peripheral tissues: old and new evidence, molecular mechanisms,
     and physiological significance. Perspect. Bio. Med., 14:
     265-269 (1971).

83. S. Murota and I. Morita, Effect of prostaglandin I_2 and
     related compounds on vascular permeability response in
     granuloma tissues. Prostaglandins, 15 (2): 297-301 (1978).

84. A. Nicholson, P. T. Fearon and K. F. Austen, Complement.
     In: "Inflammation"?J. R. Vane and S. H. Ferreira, eds.
     Handbook of Experimental Pharmacology vol. 50/I, Springer-
     Verlag, Berlin, Heidelberg, p.424-450, (1978).

85. B. J. Northover and G. Subramanian, Analgesic-antipyretic
     drugs as antagonists of endotoxin shock in dogs. J. Path.
     Bact., 83: 463-468 (1962).

86. C. Patrono, S. Bombardieri, O. Dimunno, G. P. Pasero, F.
     Greco, D. Grossi-Belloni and G. Ciabattoni, Radioimmuno-
     assay measurement of prostaglandins $F_{1\alpha}$ and $F_{2\alpha}$ in human
     synovial fluids and in perfusates of human synovial tissue.
     In: "The Role of Prostaglandins in Inflammation",
     G. P. Lewis, ed., Hans Huber,Bern,Stuttgart,Vienna, pp.122-
     132 (1976).

87. C. E. Perry, The action of salicylates on the development
     of antibodies following anti-typhoid inoculation. J. Path.
     Bact., 53:291-297 (1941).

88. P. J. Piper and J. R. Vane, The release of prostaglandins
     during anaphylaxis in guinea-pig isolated lungs. In:
     prostaglandins, Peptides and Amines", P. Mantegazza and
     E. W. Horton, eds., Academic Press,London, pp.15-19 (1969).

89. P. J. Piper and J. R. Vane, Release of additional factors
     in anaphylaxis and its antagonism by anti-inflammatory
     drugs. Nature, 223:29-35 (1969).

90. P. J. Piper and J. R. Vane, The release of prostaglandin
     from lung and other tissue. Ann. New York Acad. Sci.,
     180:363-385 (1971).

91. P. J. Piper and J. R. Vane, Antagonism of bradykinin
     Bronchoconstriction by Anti-Inflammatory Drugs. In: "Anti-
     Inflammatory Drugs", J. R. Vane and S. H. Ferreira, eds.,
     Handbook of Experimental Pharmacology vol. 50/II, Springer-
     Verlag, Berlin, Heidelberg, p.146-163 (1978).

92. L. O. Randall, Non narcotic. In: "Physiological Pharmacology:
     a Comprehensive Treatise", W. S. Rodt and F. G. Hoffmann,
     eds., pp.214-416. New York-London: Academic Press (1963).

93. A. Robert, Effect of prostaglandins on gastrointestinal
     functions. In: "Prostaglandins and Thromboxanes", F. Berti,
     B. Samuelsson and G. P. Velo, eds., Plenum Press, New York
     and London, pp.287-313 (1977).

94. H. J. Robinson, H. F. Phares and O. E. Graessle, Prostaglandin
     synthetase inhibitors and infection. In: "Prostaglandin
     Synthetase Inhibitors", H. J. Robinson and J. R. Vane,
     eds., Raven Press, New York, p.327-342 (1974).

95. M. E. Rosenthale, Evaluation for immunosuppressive and
     anti-allergic activity. In: "Anti-Inflammatory Agents,
     Chemistry and Pharmacology", vol.2, R. A. Scherrer and M. W.
     Whitehouse, eds., p.123-192. New York-San Francisco-
     London: Academic Press (1974).
96. R. W. Schayer, A unified theory of glucocorticoid action.
     Perspect. Biol. Med., 8:71-84 (1964).
97. T. Y. Shen, Prostaglandin synthetase inhibitors. In:
     "Anti-Inflammatory Drugs", J. R. Vane and S. H. Ferreira,
     eds. Handbook of Experimental Pharmacology vol. 50/II,
     Springer-Verlag, Berlin, Heidelberg, p.305-347 (1978).
98. C. S. Schwartz, H. G. Mandel, The selective inhibition of
     microbial RNA synthesis by salicylate. Biochem. Pharmacol.,
     21:771-785 (1972).
99. G. Shwartzman and S. S. Schneierson, Inhibition of the
     phenomenon of local tissue reactivity by corticosteroids,
     salicylates and compounds related to salicylate. Ann. N.Y.
     Acad. Sci., 56:733-743 (1953).
100. I. F. Skidmore and M. W. Whitehouse, Biochemical properties
     of anti-inflammatory drugs. VIII. Inhibition of histamine
     formation catalysed by substrate specific mammalian
     histidine decarboxylases. Drug antagonism of aldehyde
     binding to protein amino groups. Biochem. Pharmacol., 15:
     1965-1983 (1966).
101. J. B. Smith and A. L. Willis, Aspirin selectively inhibits
     prostaglandin production in human platelets. Nature (New
     Biol.), 231:235-237 (1971).
102. M. J. H. Smith, Prostaglandins and aspirin: an alternative
     view. Agents and Actions, 5:315-317 (1975).
103. M. J. H. Smith, A. W. Ford-Hutchinson and P. N. C. Elliott,
     Prostaglandins and the anti-inflammatory activities of
     aspirin and sodium salicylate. J. Pharm. (Lond.), 27:
     473-478 (1975).
104. D. M. Spain, N. Molomut and A. Harber, Studies of cortisone
     effects on the inflammatory response: alterations of
     histopathology of chemically induced inflammation.
     J. Lab. Clin. Med., 39:383-389 (1952).
105. W. G. Spector and D. A. Willoughby, Anti-inflammatory
     effects of salicylate in the rat. In: "Salicylates" an
     International Symposium, London, J. A. St. Dixon, B. K.
     Martin, M. J. H. Smith and P. H. N. Wood, eds., pp.141-
     147. London: J. and A. Churchill Ltd. (1963).
106. J. A. Splawinski, B. Wojtaszek, J. Swies and R. J.
     Gryglewski, Endogenous factors affecting arachidonic
     acid metabolism: I. Biosynthesis of prostacyclin and
     prostaglandins by carrageenin granulomas of rats.
     Prostaglandins, 16 (5): 683-697 (1978).

107. M. S. Starr and G. B. West, Bradykinin and oedema formation in heated paws of rats. Brit. J. Pharmacol., 31:178-187 (1967).

108. K. Tanaka, Y. Iizuka, Suppression of enzyme release from isolated rat liver lysosomes by non-steroidal anti-inflammatory drugs. Biochem. Pharmacol., 17:2023-2032 (1968).

109. A. L. Tauber, M. Kaliner, D. J. Stechschulte and K. F. Austen, Immunologic release of histamine and slow reacting substances and anaphylaxis from human lungs V. Effects of prostaglandins on release of histamine. J. Immunol. (1973).

110. D. A. Terragno, K. Crowshaw, N. A. Terragno and J. C. McGiff, Prostaglandin synthesis by bovine mesenteric arteries and veins. Circulat. Res., 36:176-180 (1975).

111. G. Thomas and G. B. West, Prostaglandins, kinin and inflammation in the rat. Br. J. Pharmac., 50:231-235 (1974).

112. G. Thomas and G. B. West, Prostaglandins as regulators of bradykinin responses, J. Pharm. Pharmac., 25:747-748 (1973).

113. J. L. Turk and D. A. Willoughby, Immunological and para-immunological aspects of inflammation. In: "Inflammation", J. R. Vane and S. H. Ferreira, eds. Handbook of Experimental Pharmacology vol. 50/I, Springer-Verlag, Berlin, Heidelberg, p.231-260 (1978).

114. C. G. Van Arman and R. P. Carlson, Anti-inflammatory drugs and the behaviour of leucocytes. In: "Future Trends in Inflammation", G. P. Velo, D. A. Willoughby and J. P. Giroud, eds., pp.159-169. Padua-London: Piccin Medical Books (1974).

115. C. G. Van Arman, R. P. Carlson, E. A. Risley, R. H. Thomas and G. W. Nuss, Inhibitory effects of indomethacin, aspirin and certain drugs on inflammation induced in rat and dog by carrageenin, sodium urate and ellagic acid. J. Pharmacol. Exp. Ther., 175:459-468 (1970).

116. J. R. Vane, Inhibition of prostaglandin synthesis as a mechanism of action for aspirin-like drugs. Nature (New Biol.), 231:232-235 (1971).

117. J. R. Vane and S. H. Ferreira, Interactions between bradykinin and prostaglandins. International Symposium on the Chemistry and Biology of the Kallikrein-Kinin System in Health and Disease. Fogarty International Center Proceedings, 27, Life-Sci.,16:804-805 (1975).

118. B. B. Vargaftig, Interference of anti-inflammatory drugs with hypotension. In: "Anti-Inflammatory Drugs", J. R. Vane and S. H. Ferreira, eds. Handbook of Experimental Pharmacology vol. 50/II, Springer-Verlag, Berlin, Heidelberg, p.164-208 (1978).

119. B. B. Vargaftig and N. Dao Hai, Release of vaso-active substance from guinea-pig lungs by slow reacting substance C and arachidonic acid. Pharmacology (Basel), 6:99-108 (1971).

120. B. B. Vargaftig and N. Dao Hai, Selective inhibition by mepacrine of the release of rabbit aorta contracting substance evoked by the administration of bradykinin. J. Pharm. (Lond.), 24:159-161 (1972).

121. G. P. Velo, C. J. Dunn, J. P. Giroud, J. Timsit and D. A. Willoughby, Distribution of prostaglandins in inflammatory exudates. J. Pathol., 111:149-156 (1973).

122. T. Wagner-Jauregg and J. Fisher, Uber die Hemmung des Wachstums von Lactobacillus casei durch einige Antiphlogistica. Experientia (Basel), 24:1029-1031 (1968).

123. G. Weissmann, Lysosomal mechanisms of tissue injury in arthritis. New Engl. J. Med., 286:141-147 (1972).

124. G. Weissmann and L. Thomas, The effects of corticosteroids upon connective tissue and lysosomes. Recent Progr. Hormone Res., 20:215-245 (1964).

125. G. Weissmann, I. M. Goldstein, S. Hoffsteins, G. Chauvet and R. Robineaux, Yin/yang modulation of lysosomal enzyme release from polymorphonuclear leukocytes by cyclic nucleotides. IV. Role of inflammatory cells in the destruction of synovial tissues. Ann. N.Y. Acad. Sci., 256:222 (1975).

126. G. Weissmann, R. B. Zurier and S. Hoffsteins, Leukocytes proteases and the immunologic release of lysosomal enzymes. Am. J. Pathol., 68:539 (1972).

127. G. Weissmann, R. B. Zurier, P. J. Speler and I. M. Goldstein, Mechanism of lysosomal enzyme release from leukocites exposed to immune complexes and other particles. J. Exp. Med., 134:149-166 (1971).

128. M. W. Whitehouse, Some biochemical and pharmacological properties of anti-inflammatory drugs. Fortschr. Arzneimittel-Forsch, 8:321-429 (1965).

129. B. J. R. Whittle, Antisecretory prostaglandins and gastric mucosal erosions. In: "Prostaglandins and Thromboxanes", F. Berti, B. Samuelsson and G. P. Velo, eds., Plenum Press, New York and London, pp.315-322 (1977).

130. T. J. Williams, Prostaglandins E_2, prostaglandin I_2 and vascular changes of inflammation. Br. J. Pharmac., 65:517-524 (1979).

131. A. L. Willis, P. Davidson, P. W. Ramwell, W. E. Brocklehurst and B. Smith, Release and actions of prostaglandins in inflammation and fever: inhibition by anti-inflammatory and anti-pyretic drugs. In: "Prostaglandins and Cellular biology", P. W. Ramwell and B. P. Pharris, eds., Plenum Press, N.Y.-London, pp.227-259 (1972).

132. D. A. Willoughby, Effects of prostaglandins $PGF_{2\alpha}$ and
      PGE_1 on vascular permeability. J. Path. and Bacteriol.,
      96:381-387 (1968).

133. D. A. Willoughby and P. Dieppe, Prostaglandins in the
      inflammatory response-pro or anti? In: "The Role of
      Prostaglandins in Inflammation", G. P. Lewis, ed., Hans
      Uber Publishers, Vienna, pp.14-25 (1976).

134. C. A. Winter, Anti-inflammatory testing methods:
      comparative evaluation of indomethacin and other agents.
      In: "Nonsteroidal Anti-Inflammatory Drugs", S. Garattini
      and M. N. G. Dukes, eds., pp.190-202. Amsterdam:
      Excerpta Medica Foundation (1965).

135. C. A. Winter, Non-steroid anti-inflammatory agents. Ann.
      Rev. Pharmacol., 6:157-174 (1966).

136. L. C. Wyman, G. P. Fulton, M. H. Schulman and L. L. Smith,
      Vasoconstriction in the cheek pouch of the hamster
      following treatment with cortisone. Amer. J. Physiol.,
      176:335-340 (1954).

137. L. J. F. Youlten, Inflammatory mediators and vascular
      events. In: "Inflammation", J. R. Vane and S. H. Ferreira,
      eds. Handbook of Experimental Pharmacology vol. 50/I,
      Springer-Verlag, Berlin, Heidelberg, p.571-587 (1978).

138. R. B. Zurier and M. Ballas, Prostaglandin E_2 suppression
      of adjuvant arthritis histopathology. Arthritis Rheum.,
      16:251-258 (1973).

139. R. B. Zurier, S. Hoffstein and G. Weissmann, Cytochalasin
      B: effect on lysosomal enzyme release from human leucocytes.
      Proc. Nat. Acad. Sci. USA., 70:844-848 (1973).

140. R. B. Zurier and K. Krakauer, Lysosomal enzymes. In:
      "Inflammation", J. R. Vane and S. H. Ferreira, eds.
      Handbook of Experimental Pharmacology vol. 50/I, Springer-
      Verlag, Berlin, Heidelberg, p.295-313 (1978).

141. R. B. Zurier and F. Quagliata, Effect of prostaglandin E_1
      on adjuvant arthritis. Nature, 234:304-305 (1971).

STEROIDAL ANTI-INFLAMMATORY DRUGS

Roderick J. Flower

Dept. Prostaglandin Research,
Wellcome Research Laboratories, Langley Court
Beckenham, Kent BR3 3BS, U.K.

INTRODUCTION

In this chapter I will discuss the effect of the anti-
inflammatory steroids on the generation of prostaglandins and
other arachidonate oxidation products.

It was really the discovery by Vane and his colleagues in
1971 (25,6,22) that non-steroidal drugs blocked the biosynthesis
of PGs which stimulated research workers around the world to
investigate the effect of other types of anti-inflammatory drugs
on PG production. The question most often formulated was quite
simple - if the aspirin-like drugs owed their pharmacological
activity to their ability to block PG biosynthesis, do other
types of anti-inflammatory drugs have the same mode of action?
In this respect many investigators were interested in the steroids.
At the time of the original discovery, it was found that the
steroidal anti-inflammatory drugs were without effect on the
microsomal cyclo-oxygenase, even in quite high concentrations
(6,10,22,25). However, the steroids apparently
shared several of the properties of the aspirin-like drugs which
were thought to be due to inhibition of prostaglandin biosynthesis;
thus there was a lingering impression that the steroidal anti-
inflammatory agents could in some way interfere with the prostaglandin
biosynthetic pathway. Table 1 (based on data published in 1972)
compares the anti-cyclo-oxygenase activity of four aspirin-like
drugs with four anti-inflammatory steroids. Both types of drug
are effective in the anti-inflammatory (rat paw edema) test, but
only the aspirin-like drugs block the cyclo-oxygenase. These
findings posed a problem because the steroids are very powerful
anti-inflammatory agents, and yet apparently had no effect on PG

TABLE 1

Differences in antienzyme activity between
steroid and nonsteroid anti-inflammatory drugs*

Drug	Cyclo-Oxygenase		Rat Paw Edema ED_{50} (mg/kg)
	I_{50} (µg/ml)	% Inhibition at 100 µg/ml	
Meclofenamic acid	0.03	100	15
Niflumic acid	0.03	100	47
Indomethacin	0.06	100	6
Mefenamic acid	0.17	100	68
Dexamethasone	–	10	< 0.001
Triamcinolone acetonide	–	0	0.08
Fludrocortisone	–	5	≃ 0.15
Hydrocortisone	–	3	13

*Data from Flower , et al. 1972

biosynthesis: did this mean they had a completely separate mode
of action or that PGs were not important in inflammation after all?
Several papers were soon to be published which strongly suggested
that steroids could block PG formation, althought their mechanism
of action was completely different from the aspirin-like drugs.

    The first reports came from Herbaczynska-Cedro and Staszewska-
Barczak (14) who demonstrated a reduction by hydrocortisone of
PG-like substances, released into the venous effluent of the
dog hind limb during muscular exercise. The mechanism of action
of the drug was not elucidated although other workers had been
unable to inhibit PG production in tissue homogenates or other
cell-free cyclo-oxygenase preparations, suggesting some mechanism
of action other than a direct effect on the enzyme itself. Lewis
and Piper (18) studied ACTH-induced lipolysis in the fat pad of
rabbits. In this system, lipolysis was accompanied by vasodilatation and the formation of PGs. An infusion of hydrocortisone,
prior to ACTH, reduced the vasodilatation and PG release. Since

the hydrocortisone neither prevented the formation of PGs in fat
tissue homogenates, nor antagonised the vasodilatation induced
by exogenous PGE_2, it was proposed that corticosteroids
inhibited the release of PGs preventing their transport from
inside the fat cell to the extracellular space. However,
experiments by other workers suggested a different interpretation:
Gryglewski and his colleagues (11) found that two corticosteroids,
hydrocortisone and dexamethasone, prevented the noradrenaline-
induced release of PGs from the rabbit perfused mesenteric
vascular bed, as well as the release of PGs from guinea-pig
perfused lungs induced by antigen. However, the direct conversion
of arachidonic acid in these preparations was not affected by
the steroids indicating that the site of inhibition was not the
cyclo-oxygenase or a "release mechanism". Indeed, these workers
concluded that the corticosteroids acted by limiting substrate
availability. This view was soon to receive confirmation from
the work of Levine's group (16,24). Some elegant experiments
published later by Levine's group (15,23) using cell cultures
labelled with tritiated arachidonic acid added considerable
experimental support to this idea as did the work of other groups
(7,20).

What follows is an account of the pharmacological activity
of anti-inflammatory steroids in one model system - the guinea-
pig perfused lung. The work reviewed here is based on experimental
results recently published by my coworkers and myself (19,3,
9).

The Guinea Pig Lung as a Model System for Examining the Effects of Steroids

Since the experiments of Vane and Piper (26), the guinea pig
perfused lung used in conjunction with a bioassay cascade has
been a favourite preparation in our laboratory for studying the
generation and release of prostaglandins. The idea of the
preparation is simple: oxygenated Krebs' solution at 37°C is
perfused at 5 to 10 ml/min through the pulmonary artery of a
guinea pig isolated lung. The pulmonary venous effluent is
diverted over a selection of bioassay tissues in cascade. For
the detection of prostaglandin endoperoxides and thromboxanes,
a typical choice of tissues would be a rabbit aortic strip plus
a rat stomach strip, a rat colon, guinea pig trachea, or a
chick rectum. The specificity of the tissues for prostaglandin
products is further increased by the infusion into the pulmonary
venous effluent of antagonists to other smooth muscle contractile
substances.

In 1976, this preparation was used by us to determine the
activity of rabbit aorta contracting substance-releasing factor
(RCS-RF), a low molecular weight principle extracted from shocked

lung effluent. As Fig. 1 shows, injection into the pulmonary artery of purified RCS-RF results in the liberation from the lungs of smooth muscle contractile substances (which may be identified by differential bioassay and other techniques as a mixture of prostaglandin endoperoxides and thromboxane A_2). Indomethacin (and other aspirin-like drugs) inhibit this generation as expected; but, while looking at the inhibitory activity of some other types of drugs, we noticed that the anti-inflammatory steroid dexamethasone prevented the effect of RCS-RF but did not inhibit the conversion of arachidonic acid to prostaglandin products by the lung (see Fig. 1).

The lack of effect of dexamethasone on the conversion of arachidonic acid by the lung clearly showed that there was no inhibitory action by the drug on the cyclo-oxygenase. Other steroids were tried and it was soon discovered that almost all the anti-inflammatory agents were effective against RCS-RF-induced release, and that furthermore, their rank order and ratio of potency against RCS-RF was very similar to their anti-inflammatory activity (see Table 2). Another interesting point emerged: the I_{50} concentration for each steroid depended on the duration of the infusion. This meant, for example, that an infusion of 1 µg/ml dexamethasone for long periods of time produced the same or greater inhibition than 20 µg/ml infused for much shorter periods. In any case there was a time delay of 15-30 min before the onset of the effect. Further experiments quickly established that steroids also inhibited the releasing activity of histamine and serotonin; curiously, however, bradykinin-induced release was unaffected by the steroid blockade.

Mode and Site of Action of Steroid Blockade

How and where were the steroids acting? When arachidonic acid was injected or infused into the pulmonary artery of the guinea pig lung preparation, it was immediately converted into hydroxy-acids and prostaglandin endoperoxide transformation products (that this was a conversion and not a release was easily demonstrated by using labelled arachidonate). We therefore inferred that the availability of the substrate was an important rate-limiting step in prostaglandin generation by this preparation. Thus it could be that releasing agents, such as RCS-RF, act by releasing substrate from some intracellular store. We decided to test this hypothesis by measuring the release of arachidonate from lungs during challenge by these agents. Unfortunately, the lungs avidly metabolize arachidonate and it was necessary to prevent this by infusing into the lungs, 5,8,8,11,14-eicosatetraynoic acid (TYA), an acetylenic arachidonic acid analogue that inhibits both the lipoxygenase and cyclo-oxygenase pathways (12). Control experiments using labelled arachidonate demonstrated that TYA at 20 µg/min completely

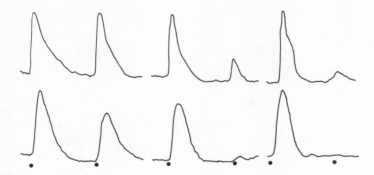

Fig. 1. Bioassay of guinea pig perfused lung effluent by rabbit
         aortic strip (RA) and rat stomach strip (RSS) showing
         the conversion of arachidonic acid (AA) to prostaglandin
         products with smooth muscle contractile activity and
         generation of these products by injection of RCS-RF (RF).
         The action of RF is blocked in a dose-dependent fashion by
         dexamethasone (DEX) infused into the pulomonary artery.

inhibited the metabolism of arachidonate by the lungs. During
the infusion of TYA, an injection of RCS-RF was made and the
perfusate collected. This was extracted, methylated, the methyl
arachidonate isolated by TLC, and the amount estimatee by
GLC. Table 3 shows the results of some experiments. In each
case, injections of RCS-RF caused (variable) releases of arachidonic
acid from the lungs. When steroids were infused, however, this
action was blocked, although it was quickly restored when the
steroid infusion was stopped.

    It seemed that the anti-inflammatory steroids somehow
prevented the release of substrate from an intracellular lipid
store - but which one? Free arachidonic acid is present in
rather low amounts in cells (13,17,21) but is present in very
large amounts in phospholipids, mono-, di-, or triglycerides, or
cholesterol esters. Most attention has been focused on the
first of these possibilities. We have demonstrated in spleen and
platelets that the majority of the arachidonic acid substrate
utilized for prostaglandin biosynthesis is derived from the
phosphatide fraction (8,2). A conceptual advantage of the
phosphatide fraction as a source of the arachidonate is that it
provides a ready explanation for the ability of so many membrane-
linked events to trigger the generation of prostaglandins.   If
the cellular source of arachidonate is the phosphatide pool, then
it follows that a phospholipase plays an important role. In the
particular case of arachidonic acid (which is generally esterified
in the 2' position), phospholipase A_2 is presumably the hydrolytic
enzyme.

TABLE 2

Effect of some anti-inflammatory steroids on the release of PG
endoperoxides and TXA$_2$ from perfused guinea pig lungs in response
to RCS-RF injections.

Steroid	I$_{50}$*(µg/ml)	Relative† potency	Relative anti-inflammatory potency†
Dexamethasone	1.4	31.2	25
Betamethasone	1.4	31.2	25
Triamcinolone	4.2	10.4	5
Fludrocortisone	5.1	8.5	10
Prednisolone	6.4	6.8	4
Corticosterone	33.6	1.3	0.4
Cortisone	43.5	1	0.8
Hydrocortisone	43.8	1	1

*Expressed as base

†Hydrocortisone = 1

    Do prostaglandin-releasing agents, such as RCS-RF, stimulate
phospholipase, and if so, is this the enzymatic step which is
steroid sensitive? To try and answer these questions, we devised
a method for assaying phospholipase activity in perfused lungs.
This depends on the metabolism by lungs of a specifically labelled
phosphatide. An aliquot of a mixture 2'(^{3}H-oleoyl) phosphatidylcholine and ^{14}C-oleic acid was injected as a bolus through the
lungs and the effluent was collected and extracted with hexane.
The ^{14}C/^{3}H ratio was determined and the hydrolysis of the
phosphatide was calculated. We found that the timing of these
experiments was critical; when the lung preparation was first
perfused, the basal (i.e. unstimulated) hydrolysis was very high;
but this soon declined (within about 30 min) reaching a
relatively stable level (which was maintained for approximately
2 hr), after which the basal hydrolysis rapidly began to rise. In
our experience, this second phase (which occurs after about 3 hr)

TABLE 3

Release of arachidonic acid from lungs
by RCS-RF and inhibition by steroids

Steroid	nmoles/min Dose	RCS-RF injected (units)	Arachidonic efflux from lung (μg)				
			Basal	RCS-RF alone	RCS-RF +steroid	RCS-RF alone	Net release by RCS-RF
None	–	5	0.15	0.22	–	–	0.07
None	–	5	0.18	0.24	–	–	0.06
None	–	5	0.26	0.31	–	–	0.05
Betamethasone	14	8	1.13	5.99	0.78	–	4.86
Dexamethasone	14	8	0.38	1.63	0.43	1.24	1.35
Fludrocortisone	57	4.5	0.78	1.16	0.65	0.78	0.38
Hydrocortisone	438	4.5	–	1.56	0.52	1.92	≈ 1.04

was irreversible, and may be connected with cytolysis and cell death. All the experiments described hereafter were performed on the relatively stable "plateau" phase.

The background hydrolytic activity of the lung was blocked by several agents, such as mepacrine (I_{50} 20 µg/ml perfusing fluid), chlorpromazine (I_{50} 33.5 µg/ml), and procaine (I_{50} 73.4 µg/ml). Aspirin and indomethacin had I_{50} values of 400 µg/ml or even greater, demonstrating that these drugs are virtually inactive against this enzyme. The steroids, betamethasone, dexamethasone and hydrocortisone were very active (I_{50}s 1.4, 1.5 and 48 µg/ml, respectively). Alderstone was inactive at concentrations of up to 80 µg/ml.

Unlike mepacrine, chlorpromazine, and procaine, the steroids did not act against phospholipase A_2 activity in cell-free lung homogenates, and their mode of inhibition is different from the nonsteroids in a temporal sense too. Figure 2 shows an experiment in which the phosphatide hydrolysis was measured every 10 min before, during, and after an infusion of dexamethasone (2 µg/ml). Before the steroid infusion began, the basal hydrolysis was rising (rather atypically). Soon after the infusion commenced, the rate of hydrolysis began to fall and had almost reached nil 50 min later. As soon as the infusion was terminated, the hydrolysis began to increase again and had returned to control values 40 to 50 min later.

The basal hydrolysis could be stimulated as well as inhibited. A variety of agents "activated" phospholipase A_2 activity, the most potent being mechanical trauma (in this case equivalent to 15 sec gentle mechanical vibration of the lung parenchyma with an electrical vibrator). This observation corresponds well with biological data previously obtained showing that a massive release of prostaglandin endoperoxide occurs after mechanical vibtation of the lung. The phospholipase-stimulating activity of histamine, RCS-RF, and antigen was blocked in a dose-dependent fashion by both mepacrine and dexamethasone.

We had shown that the anti-inflammatory steroids prevented the release of thromboxanes by preventing arachidonic acid mobilisation secondary to phospholipase stimulation. How exactly did they accomplish this, and why did they only work in intact cells?

In many types of target cells, the steroid must first combine with a cytosolic receptor protein. This drug-receptor complex is then translocated to the nucleus where it initiates protein biosynthesis ultimately resulting in a biological effect (4,5,1). In the lung a similar situation seems to obtain: we have demonstrated that guinea pig lung contains proteinaceious glucocorticoid receptors capable of binding ^{3}H-dexamethasone.

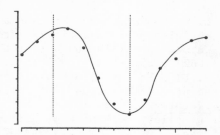

Fig. 2.   Time course of the inhibition of lung phospholipase
          A_2 activity by dexamethasone (DEX).

Interestingly, cortexolone, a glucocorticoid analogue which
prevents the combination of dexamethasone with the receptor in
these binding assays,also inhibits the action of dexamethasone
in the perfused lung. Our experiments do not enable us to say
definitely that the steroid-receptor complex migrates to the
nucleous, but presumably it does because we have also found that
an inhibition of RNA synthesis (actinomycin D), protein synthesis
(puromycin)or inhibition of both (cycloheximide) reduce or
abolish the anti-phospholipase activity of dexamethasone in the
perfused lungs.

     These findings strongly suggest that, despite the short
latency of action, the steroids produce their anti-phospholipase
effect by initiating transcriptional and translational activity
within the target cells of the lung. Presumably a new enxyme
or polypeptide was being produced in response to the steroid.

     Our most recent experiments appear to bear this out: we
have observed that the effluent of lung's which are stimulated
with steroids contains a factor which has steroid-like effects
on phospholipase activity in the perfused lung. This factor
is distinct from the steroid itself and is apparently polypeptide
in nature. Obviously, if it is true that this factor is a
"second messenger" of steroid hormone action then this finding is
extremely valuable, for it opens up a path towards the
development of a drug which has steroid-like activity, but none
of the side effects which often curtail the clinical use of
such drugs.

REFERENCES

1.   J. D. Baxter and G. M. Tomkins, Specific cytoplasmic
     glucocorticoid hormone receptors in hepatoma tissue culture
     cells. Proc. Nat. Acad. Sci., USA, 68:932-937 (1971).
2.   G. J. Blackwell, W. G. Duncombe, R. J. Flower, M. F. Parsons
     and J. R. Vane, The distribution and metabolism of arachidonic
     acid in rabbit platelets during aggregation and its
     modification by drugs. Br. J. Pharmac., 59:353-366 (1977).

3. G. J. Blackwell, R. J. Flower, F. P. Nijkamp and J. R. Vane, Phospholipase A_2 activity of guinea pig isolated perfused lungs: stimulation and inhibition by anti-inflammatory steroids. Br. J. Pharmacol., 62:79-89 (1978).

4. R. E. Butler and B. W. O'Malley, he biology and mechanism of steroid hormone receptor interaction with the eukaryotic nucleus. Biochem. Pharmac., 25:1-12 (1976).

5. L. Chan and B. W. O'Malley, Mechanism of action of the sex steroid hormones. New. Engl. J. Med., 294:1372-1379 (1976).

6. S. H. Ferreira, S. Moncada and J. R. Vane, Indomethacin and aspirin abolish prostaglandin release from the spleen. Nature New Biol., 231:237-239 (1971).

7. N. Floman and U. Zor, Mechanism of steroid action in ocular inflammation: Inhibition of prostaglandin production. Invest. Ophthalmol. Visual Sci., 16:69-73 (1977).

8. R. J. Flower and G. J. Blackwell, The importance of phospholipase A_2 in prostaglandin biosynthesis. Biochem. Pharmac., 25:285-291 (1976).

9. R. J. Flower and G. J. Blackwell, Anti-inflammatory steroids induce biosynthesis of a phospholipase A_2 inhibitor which prevents prostaglandin generation. Nature, 278:456-459 (1979).

10. R. J. Flower, R. Gryglewski, K. Herbaczynska-Cedro and J. R. Vane, The effects of anti-inflammatory drugs on prostaglandin biosynthesis. Nature New Biol., 238:104-106 (1972).

11. R. J. Gryglewski, B. Panczenko, R. Korbut, L. Grodzinska and A. Ocetkiewicz, Corticosteroids inhibit prostaglandin release from perfused mesenteric blood vessels of rabbit and from perfused lungs of sensitized guinea-pigs. Prostaglandins, 10:343-355 (1975).

12. M. Hamberg and B. Samuelsson, Prostaglandin endoperoxides VII. Novel transformations of arachidonic acid in guinea-pig lung. Biochem. biophys. Res. Commun., 16:942-949 (1974).

13. B. Haye, S. Champion and C. Jacquemin, Control by TSH of a phospholipase A_2 activity, a limiting factor in the biosynthesis of prostaglandins in the thyroid. FEBS Letters, 30:253-260 (1973).

14. K. Herbaczynska-Cedro and J. Staszewska-Barczak, Adrenocortical hormones and the release of prostaglandin-like substances (PLS). Abstract of II Congress of Hungarian Pharmacological Society, p.19, Budapest (1974).

15. S-C.L. Hong and L. Levine, Inhibition of arachidonic acid release from cells as the biochemical action of anti-inflammatory steroids. Proc. Natn. Acad. Sci., USA., 73:1730-1734 (1976).

16. F. Kantrowitz, D. C. Robinson, M. B. McGuire and L. Levine, Corticosteroids inhibit prostaglandin production by rheumatoid synovia. Nature, Lond., 258:737-739 (1975).

17. H. Kunze and W. Vogt., Significance of phospholipase A for prostaglandins formation. Ann. N.Y. Acad. Sci., 180:123-125 (1971).

18. G. P. Lewis and P. J. Piper, Inhibition of release of prostaglandins as an explanation of some of the actions of anti-inflammatory steroids. Nature, Lond., 254:308-311 (1975).

19. F. P. Nijkamp, R. J. Flower, S. Moncada and J. R. Vane, Partial purification of rabbit aorta contracting substance - releasing factor and inhibition of its activity by anti-inflammatory steroids. Nature, Lond., 263:479-482 (1976).

20. L. Parente, G. Ammendola, P. Persico and M. Di Rosa, Glucocorticosteroids, prostaglandins and the inflammatory process. Pol. J. Pharmacol. Pharm., 30:141-155 (1978).

21. B. Samuelsson, Biosynthesis of prostaglandins Fed. Proc., 31:1442-1450 (1972).

22. J. B. Smith and A. L. Willis, Aspirin selectively inhibits prostaglandin production in human platelets. Nature, New Biol., 231:235-237 (1971).

23. S. Tam, S-C. L. Hong and L. Levine, Relationships among the steroids of anti-inflammatory properties and inhibition of prostaglandin production and arachidonic acid release by transformed mouse fibroblasts. J. Pharmacol. Exp. Therap., 203:162-168 (1977).

24. A. H. Tashjian, E. F. Voelkel, J. McDonough and L. Levine, Hydrocortisone inhibits prostaglandin production by mouse fibrosarcoma cells. Nature, Lond., 258:739-741 (1975).

25. J. R. Vane, Inhibition of prostaglandin synthesis as mechanism of action for aspirin-like drugs. Nature, New Biol., 231:232-235 (1971).

26. J. R. Vane and P. J. Piper, Release of additional factors in anaphylaxis and its antagonism by anti-inflammatory drugs. Nature (London), 233: 29-35 (1969).

INHIBITION OF PROSTAGLANDIN BIOSYNTHESIS BY ANTI-INFLAMMATORY STEROIDS

Massimo Di Rosa

Institute of Experimental Pharmacology
Faculty of Pharmacy, University of Naples
via L. Rodinò 22, 80138, Italy

Few years ago it was reported that in vitro prostaglandin (PG) release from rabbit mesenteric artery stimulated by norepinephrin, as well as from sensitized guinea pig lungs challenged with antigen, was inhibited by anti-inflammatory steroids (11).

Since then the inhibition of PG biosynthesis or release by anti-inflammatory steroids has been demonstrated in a variety of tissues and cultured cells such as rabbit adipose tissue (15), human and rat inflamed synovia (14,5), mouse fibrosarcoma cells (19), guinea pig and mouse macrophages (1,9), human fibroblasts (21), rat leucocytes (16).

In these experiments arachidonic acid was able to revert the inhibition of PG release induced by steroids, which resulted ineffective when the inhibition was induced by indomethacin.

Since anti-inflammatory steroids do not inhibit the conversion of arachidonic acid to PGs,it has been suggested that cortico-steroids may prevent the activation of phospholipase A_2, possibly by a direct interaction with biomembranes (10), thus limited the availability of arachidonic acid, i.e. the substrate for microsomal cyclo-oxygenase (6).

Recent findings have shown that corticosteroids inhibit PG output from rat renal papillae by a mechanism involving RNA and proteins synthesis (2).

Furthermore the existence of specific steroid binding sites as well as a close correlation between receptor affinity and ability

to inhibit PG generation by various steroids have been demonstrated
(7,18).

These findings support the hypothesis that the mechanism of
inhibiton of PG biosynthesis by anti-inflammatory steroids is in
good agreement with the classical mode of action of steroid
hormones which act primarily by stimulating transcription, thus
controlling the rate of synthesis of certain key proteins (20).

A steroid-induced factor which mimics the anti-phospholipase
effect of anti-inflammatory steroids has been discovered in the
effluent of guinea pig lungs perfused with dexamethasone (7).

In this paper we present evidence that (i) the mechanism of
inhibition of PG biosynthesis by hydrocortisone in rat leucocytes
depends on transcription and protein synthesis; (ii) hydrocortisone induces in leucocytes the release of a factor which
inhibits PG generation.

METHODS

General Procedure

Male Wistar rats (weighing 150-200 g) were killed by
exposure to ether and bleeded. The peritoneal cavity was washed
with 20 ml of heparinized Krebs solution. The cell rich fluid
was removed and centrifuged (50xg). The cells pooled from 8-10
animals were washed twice by resuspending in Krebs solution
enriched with bovine serum albumin (100 μg/ml). The final
suspension contained 5-10 million of cells per ml(80% mononuclears
and 20% polymorphonuclears).

Samples of the cell suspension were incubated for various
times (30-60-90-120 min) in a metabolic shaker at 37°C with
killed bacteria (Bordetella Pertussis) in a ratio of 1,000
bacteria per cell (13).

Various drugs were added, separately or in various combinations,
to the medium when incubation was started (see Results). After
the incubation the cells were removed by centrifugation. The
supernatant was acidified to pH 3.0 with 0.1 N HCl, extracted
twice with equal volume of ethyl acetate and evaporated. The
residue was dissolved in 1 ml of Krebs solution and PG bioassayed
using rat stomach strips suspended in Krebs solution containing
a mixture of antagonists to prevent the action of other mediators
(8). The recovery of this procedure, evaluated with synthetic
PGE_2 (Upjohn), was about 80%.

Generator and Test Leucocytes

Rat peritoneal cells (generator leucocytes) were collected, pooled and suspended as above. The final suspension was divided in two samples. Hydrocortisone sodium phosphate (10 µg/ml) was added to one sample. No drug was present in the other sample. Incubation was carried out for 90 min at 37°C in a metabolic shaker.

After the incubation cells were removed by centrifugation and the supernatants were separately dialyzed overnight at 4°C against a large volume of Krebs solution   replaced three times (supernatant/Krebs final ratio 1:300).

PG in the supernatants were occasionally determined before and after the dialysis. In some experiments a small amount of labelled hydrocortisone ({1,2,6,7 (n) ^{3}H}-hydrocortisone, 90 mCi/nmol, C.E.A., France) was added to supernatants and the radioactivity measured before and after the dialysis.

A second pool of freshly collected peritoneal cells (test leucocytes) was suspended in Krebs-albumine. A series of 3 ml samples was prepared by mixing 1 ml of cell suspension with 2 ml of dialyzed supernatant from control or steroid-treated leucocytes and incubated for 120 min as described in the general procedure. After incubation,PGs were extracted and assayed as above.

In some experiments cycloheximide (1 µg/ml) or arachidonic acid (1 µg/ml) were also added to the incubation medium of either generator or test leucocytes (see Results).

RESULTS

1.   Inhibition of Prostaglandin Production

Rat peritoneal leucocytes release small quantities of PGs(about 3 ng per 1.10^6 cells in 2 hrs.). When the cells phagocytose killed bacteria the PG release rises to about 10 ng (Table 1).

Hydrocortisone when added to the medium in concentration ranging from 1.25 to 10 µg/ml is able to reduce the PG release. The inhibitory effect of hydrocortisone is dose dependent.

Hydrocortisone, prednisolone and dexamethasone inhibit the PG release from phagocytosing leucocytes according to their anti-inflammatory potency in vivo (1:4:25). In fact an inhibition of about 70% is induced by equiactive steroid concentrations (µg/ml):hydrocortisone 10, prednisolone 2.5, dexamethasone 0.4.

TABLE 1

Effect of corticosteroids on PG release by
rat peritoneal leucocytes phagocytosing killed bacteria

Drugs	μg/ml	PG release (ng) (o)	% inhibition
None (controls)	-	10.9±1.1 (20)	-
Hydrocortisone	1.25	8.9±0.2 (3)	18
"	2.5	7.4±0.7 (5)	32
"	5.0	5.2±0.9 (6)	52
"	10.0	3.4±0.5 (10)	68
Prednisolone	2.5	3.6±0.2 (4)	67
Dexamethazone	0.4	2.8±0.1 (4)	74
Desoxycorticosterone	100	8.4±0.8 (3)	23
Aldosterone	100	9.0±0.2 (3)	17

(o) Results are expressed in terms of PGE_2 equivalents per
1×10^6 cells (mean ± s.e. of (n) values).

Desoxycorticosterone and aldosterone, agents devoid of
anti-inflammatory properties, are ineffective on PG release
when added in a concentration of 100 μg/ml.

The time course shows that prostaglandins are produced
at rather constant rate during incubation (Fig. 1).

Hydrocortisone (10 μg/ml) fails to inhibit the
prostaglandin production occurring at 30 min, while it
virtually abolishes the prostaglandin generation at
subsequent times.

Indomethacin (1 μg/ml) greatly suppresses prostaglandin
formation throught the time course considered.

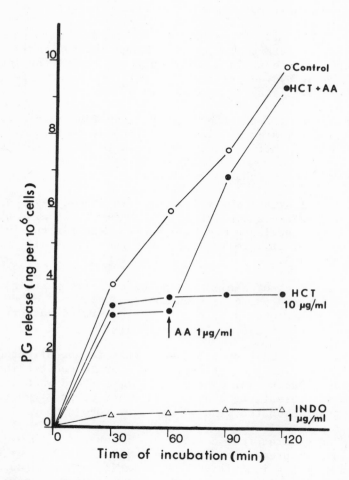

Fig. 1. The inhibitory effect of hydrocortisone (HCT) on the PG
         release from rat peritoneal leucocytes phagocytosing
         killed bacteria. HCT was added to the cell medium when
         incubation was started; arachidonic acid (AA) was added
         60 min later. Indomethacin (INDO) has been used as
         reference inhibitor. Results are expressed in terms of
         PGE_2 equivalents. Each point represents the mean value
         of 4-6 experiments.

2.   Reversion of Hydrocortisone Inhibition

        Arachidonic acid (1 µg/ml) is able to rapidly revert
established hydrocortisone inhibition (Fig. 1).

        Cycloheximide (1 µg/ml), added to the medium when
incubation is started, does not change prostaglandin
production while it is able to entirely revert the inhibition
exhibited by hydrocortisone (Fig. 2). The same effect is
exhibited by 0.5 µg/ml actinomycin D.

        However either actinomycin D or cycloheximide, when
added to the medium 15 min after hydrocortisone, fail to
revert the inhibition occurring at 2h (data not shown).

3.   Hydrocortisone - Induced Inhibitor

        After dialysis supernatants of incubated cells do not
contain detectable amounts of PGs. Dailysis is also able to
remove hydrocortisone from the supernatant for the initial
radioactivity of labelled hydrocortisone after dialysis is
reduced by 99%.

        The effect of dialyzed supernatants from either control
or steroid-treated cells (generator leucocytes) on PG
production by leucocytes phagocytosing killed bacteria
(test leucocytes) is summarized in Fig. 3.

        The PG release by test leucocytes is not affected by
the dialyzed supernatant from generator leucocytes incubated
in Krebs-albumine while it is greatly reduced when in the
medium is present the dialyzed supernatant from generator
leucocytes incubated with 10 µg/ml hydrocortisone.

        When generator leucocytes are incubated with hydro-
cortisone in presence of cycloheximide (1 µg/ml) the supernatant does not inhibit the PG formation by test leucocytes.
In contrast cycloheximide added to the medium of test
leucocytes fails to modify the inhibition of PG formation
exhibited by the supernatant from generator leucocytes
incubated with hydrocortisone. On the other hand the
inhibition exhibited by this supernatant does not occur
when arachidonic acid (1 µg/ml) is present into the medium
of test leucocytes.

DISCUSSION

        The above results show that PG biosynthesis by rat peritoneal
leucocytes phagocitosing killed bacteria is inhibited by anti-
inflammatory steroids. In contrast, mineralcorticoid agents are
ineffective.

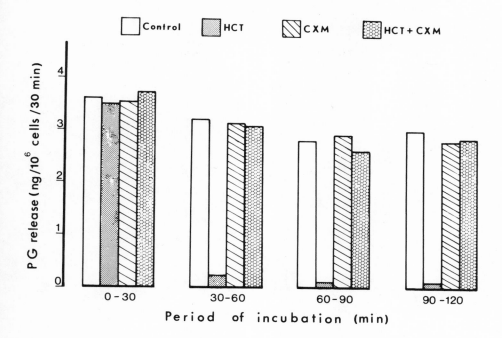

Fig. 2.   Time course of PG release from rat peritoneal
          leucoytes phagocytosing killed bacteria. The effect of
          hydrocortisone (HCT, 10 μg/ml) was tested in the presence
          of cycloheximide (CXM, 1 μg/ml). Results are expressed
          in terms of PGE_2 equivalents. Bars represent the
          mean value of 4-6 experiments.

     The inhibition of PG biosynthesis exhibited in vitro by
hydrocortisone, prednisolone and dexamethasone is closely
related to their anti-inflammatory potency in vivo (12).

     In our experiments effective concentrations of hydrocortisone
are in the same range as human blood levels observed following
oral administration of 200 mg of the drug (17).

     The time course of hydrocortisone inhibition shows that PG
formation is suppressed after an initial latency of 30 min. A
latency was also reported to occur in the inhibition of PG production
exhibited by corticosterone in rat inflamed synovia (5) and by
hydrocortisone in rat renal papillae (2).

     The lag period, according to recent hypothesis and views on
the mode of action of corticosteroids (10,20), could depend on
the availability of preformed substrates for cyclo-oxygenase and/or
the time required for protein synthesis.

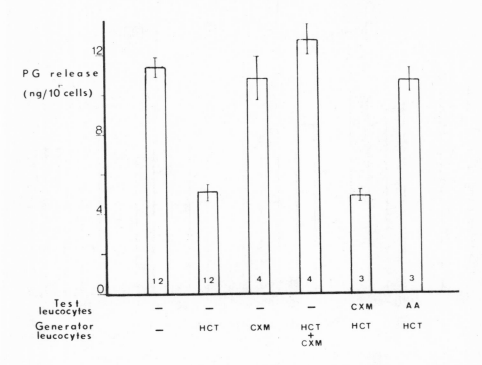

Fig. 3.   Effect of the dialyzed supernatant from rat leucocytes
          incubated with hydrocortisone (generator leucocytes) on
          the prostaglandin (PG) release by rat leucocytes
          phagocytosing killed bacteria (test leucocytes).
          Generator leucocytes ($5-10 \times 10^6$ per ml) were incubated
          for 90 min at 37°C. At the end of the incubation cells
          were removed by centrifugation and supernatants dialyzed
          overnight at 4°C against Krebs solution. Test leucocytes
          suspension (1 ml) and dialyzed supernatant from
          corresponding generator leucocytes (2 ml) were incubated
          for 120 min at 37°C with killed bacteria.

          Results are expressed in terms of PGE_2 equivalents. Bars
          represent the mean value ±s.e. Numbers inside the bars
          refer to number of experiments.

          HCT: hydrocortisone 10 µg/ml; CXM: cycloheximide 1µg/ml;
          AA: arachidonic acid 1 µg/ml.

The ability of arachidonic acid to promptly revert
hydrocortisone inhibition supports the concept that anti-
inflammatory steroids induce a shortage of PG percursors.

On the other hand the complete reversion of hydrocortisone
inhibition exhibited by either actinomycin D or cycloheximide
demonstrates for the first time that RNA synthesis and protein
synthesis are involved in the hydrocortisone inhibition of PG
biosynthesis by leucocytes. These two antibiotics are in fact
well known inhibitors of RNA synthesis and protein synthesis,
respectively.

The reversion of hydrocortisone inhibition occurs only
when actinomycin D is added to the incubation medium simultaneously
with hydrocortisone, while the antibiotic fails in its effect
when added 15 min after the steroid. A similar lack of the
reversion is observed when cycloheximide is added after hydrocortisone.

These data indicate that in rat leucocytes hydrocortisone
stimulation of RNA synthesis occurs within few minutes as well
as that the synthesis of protein/s,which might be responsible
for the inhibition of PG biosynthesis, is quite rapid.

In this light the latency in hydrocortisone inhibition, may
not be entirely explained on the basis of the time required for
RNA and protein synthesis. Possibly cell stores of preformed
arachidonic acid may contribute to delay the onset of hydrocortisone
inhibition (3).

Anti-inflammatory steroids inhibit PG biosynthesis by
preventing the release and/or the activation of phospholipase
A_2, the enzyme which releases fatty acids from phospholipids and
therefore supplies the substrates for cyclo-oxigenase (6).

Recent findings have shown that the inhibition of phospholipase
A_2 by anti-inflammatory steroids works through the same mechanism
exhibited by steroid hormones on their target cells, i.e.
stimulation of transcription and consequent induction of specific
proteins (2,7,4,18).

Rat peritoneal leucocytes incubated with hydrocortisone
release a not dialyzable inhibitor which mediates the anti-
phospholipase effect of anti-inflammatory steroids. Arachidonic
acid is in fact able to revert the inhibition of PG biosynthesis
exhibited by the hydrocortisone-induced inhibitor in rat leucocytes.

The steroid-induced inhibitor of phospholipase A_2 may be
a protein or a polypeptide since its formation is prevented by
cycloheximide.

The discovery of a steroid-induced inhibitor of PG biosynthesis in leucocytes, because of the key role played in inflammation by both PG
mechanisms of inflammatory response.

A steroid-induced phospholipase A_2 inhibitor has been recently reported to occur in guinea pig lungs (7). It will be of great interest to further explore and compare the properties of these steroid-induced inhibitors, generated respectively by guinea pig lungs and rat leucocytes.

REFERENCES

1. M. A. Bray and D. Gordon, Effects of anti-inflammatory drugs on macrophage prostaglandin biosynthesis. Br. J. Pharmacol., 57:466P-467P (1976).
2. A. Danon and G. Assouline, Inhibition of prostaglandin bio-synthesis by corticosteroids requires RNA and protein synthesis. Nature, 273:552-554 (1978).
3. M. Di Rosa and P. Persico, Latency and reversion of hydro-cortisone inhibition of prostaglandin biosynthesis in rat leucocytes. Agents and Actions Suppl.4,pp63-68 (1979a).
4. M. Di Rosa and P. Persico,Mechanism of inhibition of prostaglandin biosynthesis by hydrocortisone in rat leucocytes. Br. J. Pharmacol., 66:161-163 (1979b).
5. Y. Floman and U. Zor, Mechanism of steroid action in inflammation: inhibition of prostaglandin synthesis and release. Prostaglandins, 12:403-413 (1976).
6. R. J. Flower and G. J. Blackwell, The importance of phospholipase A_2 in prostaglandin biosynthesis. Biochem. Pharmacol., 25:285-291 (1976).
7. R. J. Flower and G. J. Blackwell, Anti-inflammatory steroids induce biosynthesis of a phospholipase A_2 inhibitor which prevents prostaglandin generation. Nature, 278:456-459 (1979).
8. N. Gilmore, J. R. Vane and J. H. Wyllie, Prostaglandin release by the spleen. Nature, 218:1135-1140 (1968).
9. M. Glatt, H. Kälin, K. Wagner and K. Brune, Prostaglandin release from macrophage: an assay system for anti-inflammatory drugs in vitro. Agents and Actions, 7:321-326 (1977).
10. R. J. Gryglewski, Steroid hormones, anti-inflammatory steroids and prostaglandin. Pharm. Res. Commun., 8:337-348 (1976).
11. R. J. Gryglewski, B. Panczenko, R. Korbut, L. Grodzinska and A. Ocetkiewicz, Corticosteroids inhibit prostaglandin release from mesenteric blood vessels of rabbit and from perfused lungs of sensitized guinea pig. Prostaglandins, 10:343-355 (1975).
12. R. C. Haynes and J. Larner, Adrenocorticotropic hormone; adrenocortical steroids and their synthetic anal inhibitors of adrenocortical steroid biosynthesis. In "The Pharmacological Basis of Therapeutics", pp. 1472-1506,

L. S. Goodman and A. Gilman, eds., 5th edition, New York
MacMillan (1975).

13. G. S. Higgs, E. McCall and L. J. F. Youlten, A chemotactic role
for prostaglandins released from polymorphonuclear leucocytes
during phagocytosis. Br. J. Pharmacol., 53:539-546 (1975).

14. F. Kantrowitz, D. R. Robinson, M. B. McGuire and L. Levine,
Corticosteroids inhibit prostaglandin by rheumatoid synovia.
Nature, 258:737-739 (1975).

15. G. P. Lewis and P. J. Piper, Inhibition of release of
prostaglandins as an explanation of some of the action of
anti-inflammatory corticosteroids. Nature, 254:308-311
(1975).

16. L. Parente, G. Ammendola, P. Persico and M. Di Rosa,
Glucocortico steroids, prostaglandins and the inflammatory
process. Pol. J. Pharmacol. Pharm., 30:141-155 (1978).

17. R. E. Peterson, J. B. Wyngaarden, S. L. Guerra, B. B. Brodie,
and J. J. Bunim, The physiological disposition and metabolic
fate of hydrocortisone in man. J. Clin. Invest., 34:1779-
1795 (1955).

18. F. Russo-Marie, Involvement of glucocorticoid receptors in
steroid-induced inhibition of prostaglandin secretion.
J. Biol. Chem., in press (1979).

19. A. H. Rashjian, E. F. Voelkel, J. McDonough and L. Levine,
Hydrocortisone inhibits prostaglandin production by mouse
fibrosarcoma cells. Nature, 258:739-741 (1975).

20. B. E. Thompson and M. E. Lippman, Mechanism of action of
glucocorticoids. Metabolism, 23:159-202 (1974).

21. M. Yaron, I. Yaron, D. Gurari-Rotman, M. Revel, H. R. Lindner
and U. Zor, Stimulation of prostaglandin E production in
cultured human fibroblasts by poly (I), poly (C) and human
interferon. Nature, 267:457-459 (1977).

PROSTAGLANDINS AND IMMUNITY

M. A. Bray* and J. Morley

Clinical Pharmacology, Cardio-throacic Institute
Fulham Road
London, SW3 6PH, U.K.

INTRODUCTION

Immune mechanisms fall into two major classes: firstly, reactions of humoral immunity involving the generation of anti-bodies by bone marrow derived thymus independent lymphocytes (B-lymphocytes); secondly, reactions of cellular immunity involving the generation of lymphokines, by thymus dependent lymphocytes (T-lymphocytes). Lymphokines are macromolecular agents, probably glycoprotein, which affect a range of cell types, including macro-phages, neutrophils, lymphocytes, osteoclasts and vascular endothelium. Within this general framework there exists a range of cell/cell interactions to both specific antigens and non-specific stimuli of lymphocyte function leading to the generation of antibodies or lymphokines. As well as mediator release in response to antigen stimulus T-lymphocytes are involved in the control of antibody secretion. Macrophages also play a role in the allergic response serving to regulate the secretion of lymphokines or antibodies. Neutrophils, eosinophils and basophils are more usually considered to be involved in immediate hypersensitivity anaphylactic type reactions though involvement in other responses may be more than incidental (e.g. basophils in Jones-Mote responses).

*Present address: Biochemical Pharmacology Research Unit, Department of Chemical Pathology, King's College Hospital Medical School, Denmark Hill, London, SE5 8RX.

Prostaglandins and Lymphocyte Interactions

Interest in the possible role of prostaglandins in immunological
processes was initially stimulated by observations that E-type
PGs were potent activators of intracellular adenyl cyclase so
modifying intracellular cAMP levels. During the early 1970s several
groups showed that PGs (particularly PGE_1) elevated cAMP and in
so doing inhibited the ability of human T-lymphocytes to respond
to a mitogenic stimulant such as the plant mitogen phyto-
haemagglutinin (PHA) (40,25). It may be inferred that this
inhibition of lymphocyte mitogenesis is a T-lymphocyte response
since the B-lymphocyte stimulant (pokeweek mitogen) was unaffected
by PGE_2 (41). Other products of arachidonic acid metabolism
might be anticipated to affect lymphocyte activation, since a
variety of fatty acids will inhibit human lymphocyte responses
to PHA or tuberculin PPD in vitro, with arachidonic acid being
the most active (26). The role of both cyclo-oxygenase and
lipoxygenase products in lymphocyte activation has recently been
explored by Parker and his colleagues who showed that within 10
minutes to 1 hour following stimulation of human T-cells by PHA
there is considerable release of arachidonic acid and generation
of thromboxanes, PGE_2, PGI_2, 5HETE and 12 HETE (31-32). On the
basis of experiments using selective inhibitors of AA
metabolism these workers concluded that inhibition of thromboxane
or lipoxygenase synthesis inhibited mitogenesis (16). It appears,
therefore, that in addition to the generally inhibitory effect of
the classic prostaglandins, other AA metabolites such as
thromboxane or lipoxygenase products may also contribute to
modulation of lymphocyte activation. The phenomenon is of some
interest as inhibition of cyclo-oxygenase is a feature of a
number of drugs used in clinical medicine (particularly NSAIDs)
and since there is extensive interest in defining the various pathways
of arachidonic acid metabolism and in so doing identifying selective
inhibitors of various components of this metabolic cascade.

Prostaglandins and Lymphokines

Lymphokine activity may be measured both in vitro and in vivo,
reflecting the activity of these mediators on different target
tissues (4,28). For instance LKs will inhibit the emigration of
guinea-pig peritoneal exudate macrophages in tissue culture and
will cause differentiation of lymphocytes measured by uptake of
radio-labelled thymidine. In vivo injection of LKs causes increased
vascular permeability in guinea-pig skin as measured by leakage of
iodine labelled serum albumin into the injection site and is
associated with increased capillary permeability. These three
techniques have been used to test the effect of E-type PGs on
lymphokine generation in response to antigen stimulation (2-3).
The presence of concentration of PGE_1 or PGE_2 as low as 10ng/ml

was shown to inhibit the ability of tuberculin PPD antigen to
cause macrophage migration inhibition of mixed peritoneal
exudate cell population   containing T-lymphocytes sensitised to
tuberculin. Similarly both PGE_1 and PGE_2 caused dose-related
reduction in the incorporation of tritiated thymidine by sensitised
lymphocytes responding to tuberculin. The vascular permeability
response, however, may be enhanced by the presence of E-type PGs
reflecting either a non-specific consequence of increased blood
flow or a modification of the action of lymphokines on vascular
endothelium. These results show E-type PGs to be capable of
modifying responses to antigen both in vitro and in vivo, however
they do not establish the site of action of these compounds.
Because of the considerable potency of E-type PGs as stimulants
of adenyl cyclase, in a variety of cells, it became necessary to
consider whether they were affecting the production or action of
lymphokines. In the guinea-pig PGE_2 was not observed to modify
the response of migrating macrophages to preformed lymphokines,
although the response of the same cell population to antigen was
inhibited (Figure 1). As a corollary when sensitised lymphocytes
were cultured in the presence of tuberculin and increasing doses
of E-type PGs with harvesting of the lymphokine enriched
supernatants, a dose-related reduction in the generation of LKs
causing macrophage migration inhibition and hymphocyte thymidine
incorporation was observed though not for LK active in the guinea
pig skin. These results imply that PGs may act as homeostatic
regulators of generation f LKs by T-lymphocytes. For such a
proposition to have physiological and pathological significance
levels of PGs capable of affecting LK secretion would need to be
generated in vivo. We have been able to demonstrate: firstly,
that peritoneal inflammatory macrophages were capable of generating
substantial amounts of PGE_2 in culture (see below) and, secondly,
that preformed LK or antigen reacting with T-lymphocytes present
in PEC cultures from sensitised guinea-pigs enhanced the generation
of PGE_2 to levels approaching those shown in bulk solution to be
capable of modifying LK secretion. The presence of endogenous PGE
generation by PEC populations responding to specific antigen has
been further examined by the addition of indomethacin, a relatively
specific cyclo-oxygenase inhibitor. Indomethacin caused enhanced
generation of LKs implying that there was sufficient endogenous
PG production by these macrophage rich PEC populations to inhibit
the production of LKs by responding T-cells. Such results
are consistent with the hypothesis that LK generation is regulated
by PGE_2 production from macrophages, a feedback inhibition system
that may bear considerable potential importance in both physiology,
and more especially, pathology of diseases with a cellular immune
component (Figure 2). Generation of the lymphokine osteoclast-
activating factor (OAF) which mediates bone resorption may be
enhanced by macrophage derived PGs (47) and thus whilst our
results indicate that PGs generally suppress LK generation it
appears that in some circumstances (e.g. OAF generation and

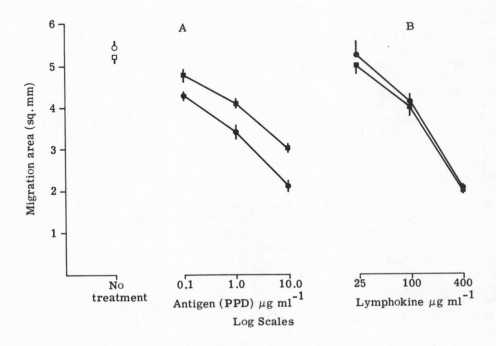

Fig. 1.   Action of prostaglandin E_1 (100 ng/ml) on (A) antigen
          (PPD) and (B) lymphokine induced cell migration
          inhibition. Mean ± SEM (n=5). By analysis of variance:
          slopes are not significantly different. P values
          compare the dose response data ±PGE_1. Antigen: P<0.001.
          Lymphokine: not significant (P>0.05). (0) Response in the
          absence of treatment. (⊡) Response in the presence of
          PGE_1 (100 ng/ml). (●) Response in the presence of
          increasing doses of antigen or lymphokine. (■) Response
          in the presence of increasing doses of antigen or
          lymphokine plus PGE_1 (100 ng/ml).

          Taken from: M. A. Bray, D. Gordon and J. Morley.
          Prostaglandins and Medicine, 1978).

possibly inflammatory LK generation) PGs enhance the production
of LK. Such results could reflect the presence of different
lymphocyte subpopulations responding to PGs either by enhanced or
reduced secretion of particular LK activities.

The ability of PGs to modulate LK generation raises the
possibility that a defect in PG regulation could lead to an
uncontrolled immulogical response and may readily encompass a
number of features of chronic inflammation where there exists a
predominantly lymphocyte/macrophage granulomatous lesion with high
levels of both LK and E-type PGs (27). Recent studies have
demonstrated that a breakdown in T-lymphocyte responsiveness to
PGE_2 may contribute to the pathology of multiple sclerosis (MS)
for peripheral blood cells from MS patients fail to respond to PGs
in the cell migration inhibition test to a comparable degree to
those of normal individuals (17). In another situation Goodwin and
his colleagues have been able to show that patients with Hodgkin's
disease have an adherent monocyte capable of producing relatively
high levels of PGE during culture leading these workers to propose
over-production of PGs by these cells as an explanation of the
lack of cellular immune responsiveness in such patients (12). As
an extension of this concept Goodwin has been able to partially
reverse the anergic response to delayed skin tests in immunodepressed
patients by administration of moderate doses of indomethacin (11).
Whilst there appears to be mounting evidence for a PG modulated
cellular immune system of importance in some disease processes
there is as yet little information on the possible role of such a
system in the physiological regulation of cellular immunity.

Prostaglandins and Other T-Lymphocyte Functions

Apart from the secretion of LKs T-lymphocytes perform several
other functions and now evidence exists that PGs may modify these
activities. Thus there is a subpopulation of T-cells known as
killer cells, which are able to directly lyse target cells in
response to antigen. Such killing is reduced in the presence of
E-type PGs (22). T-cells are thought to play a role in graft
rejection and graft versus host (GVH) reactions and there is
some evidence that high PG levels will enhance both rejection and
GVH (24). Similarly there appears to be some in vivo evidence
of PG involvement as there are changes is serum PGE levels with
the severity of graft rejection processes (1). In an experimental
mouse model PGE_1 has been found to be synergistic with the
immunosuppressive drug procarbazine in enhancing the survival of
heterologous murine skin grafts (37).

T-cells are known to be capable of modifying the response of
B-cells to antigen, the suppressor T-cell causing a reduction of
antibody secretion and the helper T-cell augmenting antibody production Webb and his colleagues have recently demonstrated that T-cell

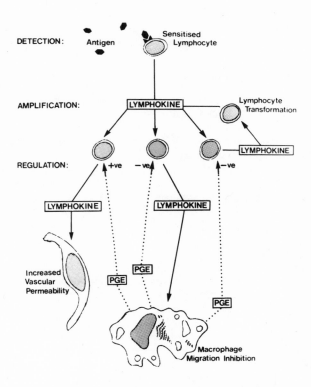

Fig. 2.   Modulation of lymphokine secretion by E-type prostaglandins.

dependent antigens will cause an increase in splenic PG levels
and that PG inhibitors such as indomethacin will increase 19S
antibody secretion and enhance mixed lymphocyte responses
implying an effect on both T and B cell responses to antigen
(44,48).   Such data point to an involvement of E-type PGs in the
regulation of T-suppressor cell modulation of antibody secretion.

Prostaglandins and Antibody Secretion

        There has been little work on the action of PGs on antibody
secretion or responses and most of the reports of PG effects have
been related to changes in cyclic nucleotide levels.   Thus PGEs
will enhance lymphocyte cAMP levels and so inhibit antibody-
dependent cell-mediated cell lysis (42).   Similarly, PGE_1 will
inhibit the generation of IgC and IgM antibodies in response to
DNP-hapten conjugated antigen (18). PGE_1 has been found to
suppress the haemagglutinin response to sheep red blood cells,
suggesting an inhibition of the appearance of antibody forming
cells (49).   Finally, as mentioned above, PGs may modify antibody
secretion via an action on T-helper or T-suppressor cell function.

Prostaglandins and Other Cells Involved in Immune Responses

(a) Macrophages: The macrophage has several roles in immunological
     process as well as that of scavenger of invading organisms
     or materials. Since the demonstration in 1974 that guinea-pig
     macrophages were capable of generating E-type PGs several
     other groups have made similar observations, some having
     reported the generation of other AA metabolites including
     $PGF_{2\alpha}$ by human uterine macrophages (30)and murine peritoneal
     macrophages (9); $PGF_{1\alpha}$ by murine macrophages (14);
     thromboxane B_2 by human and guinea-pig macrophages (29) and
     mouse peritoneal cells (5) with finally 5 HETE and 11 HETE
     from rabbit alveolar macrophages (43).

     Such generation of PGs could explain the reports of low
     molecular weight materials derived from macrophages which
     modify the processing of antigen prior to recognition by
     specifically sensitised lymphocytes (6). The non-specific
     generation of lysosomal enzymes by macrophages provides a
     mechanism of some pathological importance and reports that
     elevation of cAMP results in an inhibition of lysosomal
     hydrolase secretion by mouse macrophages (45),provides the
     basis for proposing that macrophage PG generation may act as
     an autoregulator of enzyme secretion. Indeed suppression of
     PG generation by indomethacin enhanced collagenase secretion
     from synovial cell explants (7) although, in contrast, 5μM
     PGE_2 suppressed the generation of collagen by lung fibroblasts
     in tissue culture (8). Finally the clonal proliferation of
     committed granulocyte-macrophage stem cells due to the
     presence of colony stimulating factor (CSF) can be inhibited
     by PGE which is itself generated following CSF stimulation of
     monocyte-macrophage populations, providing evidence for PG
     modulation of macrophage maturation and limiting myelopoesis
     (21,33).

     The ability of macrophages to generate PGs and lipoxygenase
     products may be of importance in the regulation of cell
     movement, as E-type PGs inhibit neutrophil chemotaxis toward
     bacterial products (38) whilst HETE and thromboxane are known
     to be chemotactic for human neutrophils (10,19).

(b) Neutrophils: These cells have been reported to generate
     E-type PGs and $PGF_{2\alpha}$ during phagocytosis so that the possibility
     exists that such PG generation may have a regulatory function
     on the accumulation of neutrophils at sites of immune-
     inflammatory reactions and on lysosomal enzyme secretion by
     these cells. The inhibitory actions of PGs on neutrophil
     function are thought to be mediated via intracellular cAMP as
     raising cAMP levels inhibit neutrophil movement (39) and
     enzyme release (46).

(c) Other cells: There is considerable evidence for the involve-
     ment of AA metabolites in mast cell and basophil function.
     For instance PGE_1 will inhibit IgE mediated histamine
     secretion from basophils (23) whilst Hubscher has proposed that
     eosinophil generation of PGE may act as a feedback inhibitor
     of basophil histamine secretion (13). The ability of TYA
     to fully suppress histamine release from basophils suggests
     a central role for the involvement of the arachidonic acid
     cascade in this process.

Prostaglandins and Cancer

     High levels of E-type PGs have been found in a variety of
tumours of different organs in both animals and man as well as a
variety of cultured tumour cell lines (34,20). The involvement
of such PGs in tumour survival perhaps by depressing immune
surveillance is suggested by experiments showing that treatment
with indomethacin suppressed the growth of tumours in anti-lymphocyte
serum treated mice (15) and that indomethacin could also enhance
the mitogenic responses of splenic lymphocytes from tumour bearing
mice (35). Similar experiments have demonstrated that tumour
derived PGs will suppress the immunological responses of mice to
sheep red blood cells, a suppression reversible by treatment
with indomethacin.

CONCLUSIONS

     Experimental data from a number of groups suggest the
proposition that classical prostaglandins act as intercellular
messengers in a variety of immunological responses a process
possibly depending upon changes in intracellular cyclic nucleotide
levels. In general the PGs can be regarded as assuming an
immunomodulatory role.

REFERENCES

1. C. B. Anderson, W. T. Newton and B. M. Jaffe. Transplantation,
    19:527 (1975).
2. M. A. Bray, D. Gordon and J. Morley. Agents and Actions,
    6:171 (1976).
3. M. A. Bray, D. Gordon and J. Morley. Prostaglandins and Med.,
    1:183 (1978).
4. M. A. Bray and J. Morley. In: "Immunology in Medicine"
    E. Holborow and W. G. Reeves, eds., Academic Press, London,
    265 (1977).
5. K. Brune, M. Glatt, H. Kalin and B. A. Peskar. Nature, 274:261
    (1978).
6. J. Calderon and E. R. Unanue. Nature, 253:359 (1975).

7. J. F. Dayer, S. R. Goldring and S. M. Krane. In: "Proc. Mech.
    Localised Bone Loss", J. E. Horton, T. M. Tarpley and W. F.
    Davis, eds., Inf. Res. Inc. U.S.A., 181 (1978).
8. M. DuComb, P. Polgar and C. Franzblau. Prostaglandins,
    15:708 (1978).
9. A. Farzad, A. S. Penneys, A. Ghaffar, V. A. Ziboh and J.
    Schlossberg. Prostaglandins, 14:829 (1979).
10. E. J. Goetzl, J. A. Wood and R. R. Gorman. J. Clin.Invest.,
    59:179 (1977).
11. J. S. Goodwin, A. D. Bankhurst, S. A. Murphy, D. S. Selinger,
    R. P. Messner and R. C. Williams. J. Clin. Lab. Immunol.,
    1:197 (1978).
12. J. S. Goodwin, R. P. Messner, A. D. Bankhurst, G. T. Peake,
    J. H. Saiki and R. C. Williams. New Eng. J. Med., 297:963
    (1977).
13. T. J. Hubscher. J. Immunol., 114:1389 (1975).
14. J. L. Humes, R. J. Bonney, L. Pelus, M. E. Dahlgren,S.J. Vsadowski,
    F. A. Keuhl and P. Davies. Nature, 269:149 (1977).
15. J. L. Humes and H. R. Strausser. Prostaglandins, 5:183 (1974).
16. J. P. Kelly, M. C. Johnson and C. W. Parker. J. Immunol.,
    122:1563 (1979).
17. P. J. Kirby, J. Morley, J. R. Ponsford and W. I. McDonald.
    Prostaglandins, 11:621 (1976).
18. T. Kishimoto and K. Ishizaka. J. Immunol., 116:534 (1976).
19. E. A. Kitchen, J. R. Boot and W. Dawson. Prostaglandins, 16:
    239 (1978).
20. F. A. Kuehl. Comprehensive Immunology, 3:145 (1977).
21. J. I. Kurland, R. S. Bockman, H. E. Broxmeyer and M. A. Moore.
    Science, 199:552 (1978).
22. L. M. Lichtenstein, E. Gillespie, H. R. Bourne and C. S.
    Henney. Prostaglandins, 2:519 (1972).
23. L. M. Lichtenstein and S.Margolis. Science, 161:902 (1968).
24. L. D. Loose and N. R. Di Luzio. J. Retic. Soc., 13:70 (1973).
25. J. Mendelsohn, M. M. Multer and R. F. Boone. J. Clin. Invest.,
    52:2129 (1973).
26. J. Mertin and D. Hughes. Int. Arch. Allergy Appl. Immunol.,
    48:203 (1975).
27. J. Morley. Prostaglandins, 8:315 (1974).
28. J. Morley. In: "Inflammation" (eds. J. R. Vane and S. H.
    Ferreira, Handbook of Exp. Pharm., 50/1. 314 (1¼78).
29. J. Morley, M. A. Bray, R. W. Jones, D. H. Nugteren and D. A.
    Van Dorp. Prostaglandins, 17:730 (1979).
30. L. Myatt, M. A. Bray, D. Gordon and J. Morley. Nature,
    257:227 (1975).
31. C. W. Parker, J. P. Kelly, S. F. Falkenheim and M. G. Huber.
    J. Exp. Med., 149:1487 (1979).
32. C. W. Parker, W. F. Stenson, M. G. Huber and J. P. Kelly.
    J. Immunol., 122:1572 (1979).
33. L. M. Pelus, H. E. Broxmeyer, J. I. Kurland and M. A. Moore.
    J. Exp. Med., 150:277 (1979).

34. L. M. Pelus and H. R. Strausser. <u>Life Sciences</u>, 20:903
     (1977).
35. L. M. Pelus and H. R. Strausser. <u>Int. J. Cancer</u>, 18: in
     press.
36. O. J. Plescia, A. Smith and K. Grinwich. <u>Proc. Nat. Acad. Sci.</u>
     U.S.A., 72:1848 (1975).
37. F. Quagliata, V. S. W. Lawrence and J. M. Philips-
     Quagliata. <u>Cell. Immunol.</u>, 6:457 (1973).
38. I. Rivkin and E. L. Becker. <u>Fed. Proc.</u>, 31:657 (1972).
39. I. Rivkin, J. Rosenblatt and E. L. Becker. <u>J. Immunol.</u>,
     115:1126 (1975).
40. J. W. Smith, A. L. Steiner and C. W. Parker. <u>J. Clin. Invest.</u>,
     50:442 (1971).
41. G. D. Stockman and D. M. Mumford. <u>Exp. Haematol.</u>, 2:65
     (1974).
42. K. F. Trofatter and C. A. Daniels. <u>J. Immunol.</u>, 122:1363
     (1979).
43. F. H. Valone, M. Franklin and E. J. Goetzl. <u>Clin. Res.</u>, 27:
     476A (1979).
44. D. R. Webb and P. L. Osheroff. <u>Proc. Nat. Acad. Sci. U.S.A.</u>,
     73:1300 (1976).
45. G. Weissmann, P. Dukor and R. B. Zurier. <u>Nature</u> (New Biol.),
     231:131 (1971).
46. G. Weissmann, R. B. Zurier and S. Hoffstein. <u>Am. J. Pathol.</u>,
     68:539 (1972).
47. T. Yoneda and G. R. Mundy. <u>J. Exp. Med.</u>, 150:338 (1979).
48. M. Zimecki and D. R. Webb. <u>J. Immunol.</u>, 117:2158 (1976).
49. R. B. Zurier and F. Quagliata. <u>Nature</u>, 234:304 (1971).

PROSTACYCLIN

S. Moncada and J. R. Vane

Wellcome Research Laboratories
Langley Court, Beckenham
Kent, U.K.

In 1976, the Wellcome group discovered that prostaglandin endoperoxides were transformed by a microsomal enzyme from blood vessels into an unstable substance which is a potent vasodilator and an inhibitor of platelet aggregation (13,14, 75,76, 42). This compound originally called PGX was later chemically identified as an intermediate in the formation of 6-oxo-$PGF_{1\alpha}$, a compound described earlier (95). PGX was then renamed prostacyclin and given the abbreviation of PGI_2 (61).

Prostacyclin is formed by vascular tissues from all species so far studied including rabbit, ox and human (13,27,78). and is the main metabolic product of arachidonic acid in vascular tissue (61,102). Clearly, the postulated participation of PGEs or PGFs (or their unstable intermediates) in the regulation of vascular tone has to be reinterpreted. Moreover, since PGI_2 is a potent inhibitor of platelet aggregation and its generation is reduced or abolished by cyclo-oxygenase inhibitors such as aspirin (112) the use of aspirin as an anti-thrombotic agent needs to be reexamined.

Prostacyclin is the most potent endogenous inhibitor of platelet aggregation yet discovered, being 30-40 times more potent than PGE_1 (81). Prostacyclin applied locally in low concentrations inhibits thrombus formation due to ADP in the microcirculation of the hamster cheek pouch (52) and given systemically to the rabbit it prevents electrically-induced thrombus formation in the carotid artery and increases bleeding time(111). These effects in vivo disappear within 30 min of dosing. A property of prostacyclin which has potential therapeutic importance is that it disaggregates platelets in vitro (76), in vivo (111) in

203

extracorporeal circulations where platelet clumps have been formed
on collagen strips (43,45) or in the circulation of man (47).

Prostacyclin protects the vessel wall against deposition of
platelet aggregates and its discovery provides a comprehensive
explanation of the long recognised fact that contact with healthy
vascular endothelium is not a stimulus for platelet clumping.

Prostacyclin is unstable and its activity disappears within
15 s on boiling or within 10 min at 22°C at neutral pH. In blood
at 37°C prostacyclin has a half life of 2-3 min (28). Alkaline pH
increases the stability of PGI_2 (61).

Prostacyclin inhibits platelet aggregation by stimulating
adenylate cyclase, leading to an increase in cAMP levels in the
platelets (38,110). In this respect prostacyclin is much more
potent than either PGE_1 or PGD_2(110). 6-oxo-$PGF_{1\alpha}$ has very weak
anti-aggregating activity and is almost devoid of activity on
platelet cAMP (110).

In contrast to prostacyclin, prostaglandin endoperoxides
and thromboxane A_2 reduce cAMP activity in platelets (39). Because
of these opposing effects we and others have suggested that a
balance between TXA_2 and prostacyclin formation regulates platelet
cAMP in vivo and therefore platelet aggregability (38,110,82).
This proposition has been reinforced by the recent finding that
prostacyclin is a circulating hormone. Unlike other prostaglandins
such as PGE_2 and $PGF_{2\alpha}$, prostacyclin is not inactivated on passage
through the pulmonary circulation. Indeed, the lungs constantly
release small amounts of prostacyclin into the passing blood
(44,80) perhaps because of the huge mass of endothelial cells
present. The concentration of prostacyclin is higher in arterial
than in venous blood for there is about 50% overall inactivation
in one circulation through peripheral tissues (28,30).

Platelets, therefore, may be constantly influenced by
circulating prostacyclin and consequently they can have higher
cAMP levels and be less aggregable than has ever been detected by
in vitro measurements which are only made after a 10-30 min
delay during which the blood is processed. In this period,
prostacyclin and its effects will decay. This concept explains
the differences in reactivity between platelets in vitro and in vivo
reported by many authors and might throw light on recent controversies
about control of cAMP levels in platelets.

Vasodilatation

In the anaesthetized dog, prostacyclin is hypotensive in
doses ranging from 50-1000 ng/kg/min (4). Intravenously in
anaesthetized rabbit or rat, prostacyclin causes a fall in blood

pressure and is 4-8 times more potent than PGE_2. Prostacyclin is at least 100 times more active than its degradation product, $6\text{-}oxo\text{-}PGF_{1\alpha}$ (4). Since it is not inactivated by the pulmonary circulation, prostacyclin is equipotent as a vasodilator when given either intra-arterially or intravenously in the rat, rabbit or dog (5,28,30). This is an important difference from PGE_1 or PGE_2 which, because of strong pulmonary metabolism, are much less active when given intravenously (34). Many authors have suggested a vasolilator role for locally generated PGE_2 in the vascular wall and others have suggested that PGE_1 is released. There is little evidence that PGE_1 is a naturally occurring prostaglandin in the cardiovascular system of mammals.

In the heart, local injections of arachidonic acid into the coronary circulation of the dog cause vasodilatation, and because this effect was abolished by indomethacin (50) it was assumed that PGE_2 was the likely mediator. However, there were some major difficulties with this proposal. In isolated Langendorff-perfused hearts of the rabbit, arachidonic acid dilated the coronary vasculature, but PGE_2 was inactive (9,87). Isolated strips of bovine, canine and human coronary artery were relaxed by arachidonic acid but PGE_2 contracted them (67). Arachidonate-induced relaxation of these strips was abolished by indomethacin and it was suggested, therefore, that the metabolite responsible must be the endoperoxide intermediate PGH_2 (67).

Later, Dusting et al. (27) showed that bovine coronary arteries were relaxed by prostacyclin and PGH_2 (which sometimes induced an initial transient contraction), and after treatment with 15-HPAA (an inhibitor or prostacyclin synthetase) the relaxation induced by arachidonic acid was abolished, whilst that induced by PGH_2 was reversed to a contraction. Thus, relaxation of coronary arteries induced by arachidonic acid as PGH_2 is due to intramural metabolism to prostacyclin. This study further confirmed that the intrinsic activity of PGH_2 on isolated blood vessels is contractile (27). Similar results have been published by Needleman and associated (88,98).

In isolated Langendorff-perfused hearts of the guinea pig and rabbit, not only is prostacyclin a potent vasodilator but it is also the predominant metabolite of arachidonic acid (103). Similarly, using chromatographic procedures, others have identified $6\text{-}oxo\text{-}PGF_{1\alpha}$, the degradation product of prostacyclin, as the major product from rat and rabbit hearts perfused with arachidonic acid (24). We and others have investigated the coronary actions of prostacyclin in the intact heart of open chest dogs (4,26,60). Local injection of prostacyclin (50-500 ng) into the coronary circulation increased coronary blood flow without systemic effects and it was a more potent coronary dilator than PGE_2. Furthermore, profound and prolonged coronary vasodilatation was rapidly elicited

by prostacyclin (20-100 µg) absorbed through the myocardium after
dripping a solution on to the surface of the left ventricle (26).
Interestingly, the coronary circulation is sensitised to the
vasodilator effects of exogenous prostacyclin, but not to those of
PGE_2, when endogenous synthesis is inhibited by indomethacin or
meclofenamate (56,26). These inhibitors of cyclo-oxygenase
decrease resting coronary blood flow in anaesthetised, open chest
dogs. Although this is not seen in conscious dogs without acute
surgery (94), it does indicate that the generation of a vasodilator
metabolite of arachidonic acid increases or maintains coronary
blood flow during mildly traumatic conditions. It is clear that
this metabolite is prostacyclin.

Bradycardia accompanying the hypotension induced by prostacyclin
has been observed in anaesthetised dogs (4,26,57) and only transient
weak tachycardia accompanied prostacyclin infusion in anaesthetised
cats (69). In contrast, the hypotension induced by PGE_2 always
causes tachycardia, which presumably, is mediated by baroreceptors
(73). Although there is no clear difference in the overall systemic
vasodilator effects of these two prostaglandins as assessed by
total peripheral resistance, PGE_2 has a more pronounced effect on
cardiac output and myocardial contractility (as indicated by maximum
acceleration of aortic blood flow). These observations indicate
that in equi-hypotensive doses, prostacyclin reduces cardiac work
more than PGE_2.

Recent experiments (16,17) suggest that bradycardia induced
by prostacyclin is a reflex response mediated at least partially
by vagal pathways since atropine reduces or abolishes the bradycardia. However, the afferent arc is also subserved by vagal
fibres, for vagotomy (but not atropine treatment) reduces the hypotensive effects of prostacyclin. Therefore, the hypotension induced
by prostacyclin has at least two components: direct arteriolar
vasodilatation and reflex, non-cholinergic vasodilatation.
Similar resutls have been obtained by Hintze et al. (57).

In the renal circulation of the dog, prostacyclin infused
intravenously reduces renal vascular resistance and increases
blood flow and urinary excretion of sodium, potassium and chloride
ions at doses below those needed for a systemic effect (10,55).
There is increasing evidence that prostacyclin mediates the
release of renin from the renal cortex. Arachidonic acid,
prostaglandin endoperoxides or prostacyclin all stimulate renin
release from slices of rabbit renal cortex, but PGE_2 has no such
effect (113,116). Furthermore, indomethacin reduces renin release
in animals and man (68,23,35). Prostacyclin-like activity and
$6-oxo-PGF_{1\alpha}$ have been identified in incubates of PGG_2 or PGH_2 with
renal cortical microsomes (117,119,100).. Thus, prostacyclin may
be the obligatory endogenous mediator of renin secretion by the kidney
Indeed,Gerber et al(36) have demonstrated that prostacyclin induces rer

release when infused intrarenally into dogs, and Hill, Moncada and Vane (54) have demonstrated increased concentrations of angiotension II in arterial blood during intrarenal infusions of prostacyclin. 6-oxo-PGF$_{1\alpha}$ is also formed by collecting tubule cells isolated from rabbit papillae (40). Interestingly, angiotension II releases prostacyclin from the rat kidney in vitro (104) and the dog kidney in vivo (86).

Prostacyclin is also a strong vasodilator in the mesenteric and hind limb circulations of the dog (where TXA$_2$ is a vasoconstrictor) (31) and on the precapillary side of the microcirculation of the hamster cheek pouch (53), where it also reverses catecholamine-induced vasoconstriction. In this preparation 6-oxo-PGF$_{1\alpha}$ had 1/20th the vasodilator activity of prostacyclin and was more potent than PGE$_2$. In the pulmonary circulation of the dog, prostacyclin is the only product of arachidonic acid which produces strong vasocilatation (63,85). It also dilates the pulmonary vascular bed of the foetal lamb where its potency is greater than PGE$_1$ but less than PGE$_2$ (70). Prostacyclin also induces vasocilatation and hypotension in man when given either intravenously or by inhalation (47, 108,93). This is accompanied by tachycardia.

Prostacyclin relaxes in vitro most vascular strips including rabbit coeliac and mesenteric arteries (13), bovine coro arteries (27,88), human and baboon cerebral arteries(11)and lamb ductus arteriosus (19). Exceptions to this include the porcine coronary arteries (29) and some strips of rat venous tissue and isolated human saphenous vein (71) which are weakly contracted by prostacyclin. Whether these same effects are induced in the corresponding circulations in the intact animal or man has not been studied. In the human umbilical arterial strip, prostacyclin induces a dose-dependent relaxation at low concentrations ($< 10^{-6}$M) and a dose-dependent contraction at higher concentrations ($> 10^{-5}$M) (96). As mentioned earlier, prostacyclin and not PGE$_2$ is the main metabolite of arachidonic acid in isolated vascular tissue, and this has led to an intense study to reassess the effects and role of arachidonic acid and its metabolites on vascular tissue and the cardiovascular system.

Prostacyclin in Vascular Homeostasis

Vessel microsomes in the absence of cofactors can utilise prostaglandin endoperoxides but not arachidonic acid to synthesise prostacyclin (75). Fresh vascular tissue can utilise both precursors although it is far more effective in utilising prosta-glandin endoperoxides (13). Moreover, vessel microsomes, fresh vascular rings or endothelial cells treated with indomethacin can, when incubated with platelets, generate a prostacyclin-like anti-aggregating activity (13,14,42). The release of this substance is inhibited by 15-hydroperoxy arachidonic acid (15-HPAA) a selective inhibitor of prostacyclin formation (42,76). From all

these results it was concluded that the vessel wall can synthesise
prostacyclin from its own endogenous procursors, but that it can
also utilise prostaglandin endoperoxides released by the platelets,
thus suggesting a biochemical cooperation between platelets and
vessel wall (82,83).

This latter hypothesis has proved to be controversial.
Needleman and associates (88) demonstrated that while arachidonic
acid was rapidly converted to prostacyclin by perfused rabbit
hearts and kidneys, PGH_2 was not readily used. The authors concluded
that some degree of vascular damage is necessary for the
endoperoxide to be utilised by prostacyclin synthetase. On the
other hand, incubation of PRP with fresh indomethacin-treated
arterial tissue leads to an increase in platelet cAMP which
parallels the inhibition of the aggregation (7) and which can be
abolished by previous treatment of the vascular tissue with
tranylcypromine,a less active inhibitor of prostacyclin
formation (42). Additionally, Tansik, Namm and White (109) showed
that lysed aortic smooth muscle cells could be fed prostaglandin
endoperoxides by lysed human platelets, and Nordoy, Svensson and
Hoak (90) have demonstrated that endothelial cells can be fed
with endoperoxides released from platelets during collagen-induced
aggregation. Further, undisturbed endothelial cell monolayers
readily utilise PGH_2 to transform it into prostacyclin (74).

In contrast, recent work by Needleman, Wyche and Raz (89) and
Hornstra, Haddeman and Don (59) using vessel microsomes and fresh
vascular tissue, suggests that the feeding of endoperoxides from
platelets does not take place under their experimental circumstances.
However, Needleman et al. (89) made the observation that when
platelets were treated with a TXA_2 synthetase inhibitor then
endoperoxides were available for utilisation by the vessel wall.
Interestingly in the presence of a thromboxane synthetase inhibitor,
arachidonic acid or collagen added to blood in vitro lead to the
formation of 6-oxo-$PGF_{1\alpha}$ rather than TXB_2, showing that some cell
other than platelets has synthesised prostacyclin (8). These
results support our suggestion that thromboxane synthetase
inhibitors might have a superior antithrombotic effect to simple
cyclo-oxygenase inhibitors (81). It is important to realize at
this stage however, that all these observations have been made in in
vitro systems and that in vivo experiments are necessary in order
to clarify further the nature of the interaction between platelets
and normal or damaged vessel wall.

In arteries the enzyme which metabolises prostaglandin endoperoxides to prostacyclin (prostacyclin synthetase) is most highly
concentrated in the intimal surface and progressively decreases in
activity towards the adventitial surface (77). Production of
prostacyclin by cultured cells from vessel walls also shows that
endothelial cells are the most active producers of prostacyclin

(48,72,115); moreover, this production persists after numerous sub-cultures in vitro (18).

Clearly, generation of prostacyclin is an active mechanism by which the vessel wall could be protected from deposition of platelet aggregates. Thus, prostacyclin formation provides a comprehensive explanation of the long recognised fact that contact with healthy vascular endothelium is not a stimulus for platelet clumping. An imbalance between formation of prostacyclin and TXA_2 could be of dramatic consequence.

Vascular damage leads to platelet adhesion but not necessarily to thrombus formation. When the injury is minor, platelet thrombi are formed which break away from the vessel wall and are washed away by the circulation. The degree of injury is an important determinant, and there is general agreement that for the development of thrombosis, severe damage or physical detachment of the endothelium must occur. All these observations are in accord with the distribution of prostacyclin synthetase, for it is abundant in the intima and progressively decreases in concentration from the intima to the adventitia. Moreover, the proaggregating elements increase from the sub-endothelium to the adventitia. These two opposing tendencies render the endothelial lining anti-aggregatory and the outer layers of the vessel wall thrombogenic (77).

It is not yet clear whether or not prostacyclin is responsible for all the thromboresistant properties of the vascular endothelium. However, recent work by Czervionke, et al (21) with endothelial cell cultures has demonstrated that platelet adherence in the presence of thombin increases from 4% to 44% after treatment with 1 mM aspirin. This increase was parallelled by a decrease in 6-oxo-$PGF_{1\alpha}$ formation from 107 nM to < 3 nM and could be reversed by addition of 25 nM of exogenous PGI_2. This work suggests that prostacyclin, although probably not responsible for all the thromboresistant properties of vascular endothelium, plays a very important role in the control of platelet aggregability.

The fact that prostacyclin inhibits platelet aggregation (platelet-platelet interaction) at much lower concentrations than those needed to inhibit adhesion (platelet-collagen interaction) (51), suggests that, indeed, prostacyclin allows platelets to stick to vascular tissue and to interact with it, while at the same time preventing or limiting thrombus formation. Certainly, platelets adhering to a site where prostacyclin synthetase is present could well feed the enzyme with endoperoxide, thereby producing prostacyclin and preventing other platelets from clumping onto the adhering platelets, limiting the cells to a monolayer. Recently, Weiss and Turitto (114) have observed some

degree of inhibition of platelet-subendothelium interactions with
low concentrations of prostacyclin at high shear rates, but at none
of the concentrations used could they observe total inhibition of
platelet adhesion.

Prostacyclin, Thromboxane A_2, Thrombosis and Haemostasis

Prostacyclin and thromboxane A_2 represent in biological terms,
the opposite poles of the same general homeostatic mechanism for
regulation of platelet aggregability in vivo. Manipulation of this
control mechanism will, therefore, affect thrombus and haemostatic
plug formation. Selective inhibition of the formation of TXA_2
should lead to an increased bleeding time and inhibition of thrombus
formation, whereas inhibition of or loss or prostacyclin formation
should be propitious for a "pro-thrombotic state". The amount of
control exerted by this system can be tested, for selective
inhibitors of each pathway have been described (81,82).

There is ample evidence showing that aspirin is very active
against platelet cyclo-oxygenase in vivo and in vitro. Moreover,
this effect is irreversible. Platelets are unable to synthesise
new protein and do not replace the cyclo-oxygenase; therefore the
inhibition is long-lasting and will only be overcome by new
platelets coming into the circulation after the blockade of
synthesis in megakaryocytes has worn off (15).

Vessel wall cyclo-oxygenase at least in vitro, is much less
sensitive to aspirin than that of platelets (6) and there is also
the suggestion that the endothelial cells recover from aspirin
inhibition by regeneration of their cyclo-oxygenase (20,64).

Recent studies in rabbits (79) suggest that low doses of
aspirin reduce TXA_2 formation to a greater extent than prostacyclin
formation. These experiments also showed that inhibition of
thromboxane A_2 formation is longer lasting than that of prostacyclin.
Indeed, infusions of arachidonic acid into rabbits and cats lead
to an anti-thrombotic effect and to an increase in bleeding time
which can be potentiated by low doses of aspirin and blocked by
large doses which inhibit prostacyclin and TXA_2 formation (2,66).

The anti-thrombotic activity of dipyridamole depends mainly
on its inhibition of phosphodiesterase, so amplifying the increase
in cAMP induced by circulating prostacyclin (79). It is most
effective when there is a favourable PGI_2/TXA_2 ratio, after a
small dose of aspirin or more than 24 h after a high dose. These
experiments have provided the explanation for the well
recognised synergism of small doses of aspirin and dipyridamole
in experimental models or clinical experience (49,58). A
selective inhibitor of thromboxane formation and a phosphodiesterase
inhibitor should now be tested for anti-thrombotic efficacy, since

theoretically this provides an advantage over aspirin in leaving
endoperoxides from platelets available for the vessel walls or
other cells to synthesise prostacyclin.

These results also suggest that, as an anti-thrombotic agent,
aspirin should be given in a small daily dose or large doses
at weekly intervals alone or in combination with a phosphodiesterase
inhibitor such as dipyridamole. Clearly, it is important
not to use too high a dose of aspirin, for that will neutralise
the whole system, including prostacyclin formation and might
lead to the opposite effect.

Until the discovery of prostacyclin the use of aspirin as
an anti-thrombotic agent was based on its effect on thromboxane
formation. Now, however, the situation needs further clarification,
especially with respect to the optimal dose of aspirin. Aspirin
in high doses (200 mg/kg) increases thrombus formation in a
model of venous thrombosis in the rabbit (64) and in vitro
treatment of endothelial cells with aspirin enhances thrombin-
induced platelet adherence to them (20). Interestingly, recent
studies in humans have demonstrated that small doses of aspirin
(0.3 g) increase cutaneous bleeding time while large doses are
devoid of such an effect (92). Some authors have supported these
observations (97) but others have been unable to confirm them (37).
The possible explanation for this discrepancy lies in the different
response to aspirin with age (62). Moncada and colleagues (3) have
also shown that after a single large oral dose of aspirin the
cutaneous bleeding time increases only after 24 h and recovers after
several days in a way reminiscent of the renewal of the platelet
population in the circulation.

Therapeutic Potential of Prostacyclin

We have suggested that chemical analogues of prostacyclin
could be used as a "hormone replacement" therapy in conditions in
which platelet aggregation is involved, such as acute myocardial
infarction or crescendo angina and other conditions in which
excessive platelet aggregation takes place in the arterial as well
as in the venous side of the circulation (84). Moreover, we
have suggested the use of prostacyclin in extracorporeal circulation
systems such as cardio-pulmonary bypass and renal dialysis (84).
In these systems there is a substantial fall in platelet count,
accompanied by the formation of micro-aggregates which, when
returning to the patient, are responsible for the cerebral and renal
impairment observed after bypass (1,12). Side effects are also
produced by the chronic use of heparin, especially the development
of osteoporosis (41,101).

Several anti-platelet drugs have been tried to deal with these
two problems and some have been used with moderate success. We have

recently used prostacyclin in both systems in experimental animals
and demonstrated that it can replace heparin altogether; moreover,
there is no formation of microaggregates or platelet loss.
Although the long-term effects of this substance are still to be
studied and its evaluation in humans has not been completed, its
clinical possibilities are at the moment bright.

Fatty Acids and Thrombosis

Before the discovery of prostacyclin, it was suggested that
the use of dietary dihomo-γ-linolenic acid, the precursor of
the E_1 series of prostaglandins could be an approach to the prevention
of thrombosis, for PGG_1 and TXA_1 are not pro-aggregating and PGE_1
is anti-aggregating (118). Other reports tend to agree with this
proposal (105) but there is some controversy, for feeding rabbits
with dihomo-γ-linolenic acid leads to increase in the tissue content
of this acid without change in platelet responsiveness, at least
to ADP (91). The main criticism of all this work, including that
on human platelets (65), is that the conclusions are based on studies
performed in vitro in which platelets are studied as isolated
cells without contact with vessel walls.

It is now evident that the use of dihomo-γ-linolenic acid
in an attempt to direct the synthetic machinery of the platelets
is not the most rational approach for prevention of thrombosis.
This is because the endoperoxides PGG_1 and PGH_1 are not substrates
for prostacyclin synthetase; indeed they or their precursor
might adversely affect the prostacyclin protective mechanism.
Eicosapentaenoic acid (C20:5ω3), the precursor of the trienoic
prostaglandins, can, however, act as a precursor for an anti-
aggregating agent, Δ^{17} prostacyclin (PGI_3), and it is known that
C20:5ω3 is a weak anti-aggregating agent. TXA_3 if found, is a
weak pro-aggregating agent (99,46). Thus, the use of this fatty
acid could afford a dietary protection against thrombosis.
Indeed, it has been suggested that the low incidence of myocardial
infarction in Eskimos and their increased tendency to bleed could
be due to the high eicosapentaenoic acid and low arachidonate
content of their diet and consequently of their tissue lipid (32).
In Greenland Eskimos, there is an elevated content of C20:5ω3
(as compared to Danes) in the platelet lipids and a prolonged
bleeding time. Furthermore, their platelets are resistant to
aggregation (33).

Lipid peroxides, and their methyl esters, are strong and
selective inhibitors of the formation of PGI_2 (102). Lipid
peroxidation induced by free radical formation is known to occur
in several pathological conditions (107). Indeed, lipid peroxidation takes place in plasma as a non-enzymic reaction in the presence
of a high partial pressure of oxygen and metal ions as catalysts
(50). Hence, lipid peroxides present in these conditions could

inhibit PGI_2 formation by the vascular wall without impairing TXA_2 generation by platelets, thus predisposing to thrombus formation.

Gryglewski and collaborators have found that there is a substantial reduction of PGI_2 formation in the vascular tissue of rabbits made atherosclerotic (25) and more recently, there is a report that human tissue obtained from an atherosclerotic plaque does not produce prostacyclin whereas tissue obtained from a normal vessel does (22). Sinzinger, Feigl and Silberbauer (106) have also shown that different types of atherosclerotic lesions ranging from fatty streaks to complicated lesions all produced much less prostacyclin than normal arteries.

The understanding of the role of fatty acids and their oxidised products in thrombosis and/or atherosclerosis is however at an early stage and much experimental and clinical work is needed before a full picture is completed.

REFERENCES

1. R. M. Abel, M. J. Buckley, W. G. Austen, G. O. Barrett, C. H. Beck and J. E. Fischer, Etiology, incidence and prognosis of renal failure following cardiac operations. J. Thorac. Cardiovasc. Surg., 71:323-333 (1976).
2. J. L. Amezcua, M. Parsons and S. Moncada, Unstable metabolites of arachidonic acid, aspirin and the formation of the haemostatic plug. Thromb. Res., 13:477-488 (1978).
3. J. L. Amezcua, J. O'Grady, J. A. Salmon and S. Moncada, Prolonged paradoxical effect of aspirin on platelet behavious and bleeding time in man. Thromb. Res., 16:69-79 (1979).
4. J. M. Armstrong, D. J. Chapple, G. J. Dusting, R. Hughes, S. Moncada and J. R. Vane, Cardiovascular actions of prostacyclin (PGI2) in chloralose anaesthetized dogs. Br. J. Pharmac., 61: 136P (1977).
5. J. M. Armstrong, N. Lattimer, S. Moncada and J. R. Vane, Comparison of the vasodepressor effects of prostacyclin and 6-oxo-prostaglandin $F_{1\alpha}$ with those of prostaglandin E_2 in rats and rabbits. Br. J. Pharmac., 62:125-130 (1978).
6. N. L. Baenziger, M. J. Dillender and P. W. Majerus, Cultured human skin fibroblasts and arterial cells produce a labile platelet-inhibitory prostaglandin. Biochem. Biophys. Res. Commun., 78:294-301 (1977).
7. L. C. Best, T. J. Martin, R. G. G. Russell and F. E. Preston, Prostacyclin increases cyclic AMP levels and adenylate cyclase activity in platelets. Nature (Lond.), 267:850-851 (1977).
8. G. J. Blackwell, R. J. Flower, N. Russell-Smith, J. A. Salmon, P. B. Thorogood and J. R. Vane, 1-n-Butylimidazole: a potent and selective inhibitor of "Thromboxane Synthetase". Br. J. Pharmac., 64:436P (1978).

9. A. J. Block, H. Feinberg, K. Herbaczynska-Cedro and J. R. Vane,
    Anoxia induced release of prostaglandins in rabbit isolated
    heart. Circ. Res., 36:34-42 (1975).

10. P. M. Bolger, G. M. Eisner, P. W. Ramwell and L. M. Slotkoff,
    Renal actions of prostacyclin. Nature (Lond.), 271:457-469
    (1978).

11. D. J. Boullin, S. Bunting, W. P. Blaso, T. M. Hunt and S.
    Moncada, Responses of human and baboon arteries to prostaglandin
    endoperoxides and biologically generated and synthetic
    prostacyclin: their relevance to cerebral arterial spasm in
    man. Br. J. Clin. Pharmac., 7:139-147 (1979).

12. M. A. Branthwaite, Neurological damage related to open heart
    surgery. Thorax, 27:748-753 (1972).

13. S. Bunting, R. Gryglewski, S. Moncada and J. R. Vane, Arterial
    walls generate from prostaglandin endoperoxides a substance
    (prostaglandin X) which relaxes strips of mesenteric and
    coeliac arteries and inhibits platelet aggregation.
    Prostaglandins, 12:897-913 (1976).

14. S. Bunting, S. Moncada and J. R. Vane, Antithrombotic properties
    of vascular endothelium. Lancet, ii:1075-1076 (1977).

15. J. W. Burch, N. Stanford and P. W. Majerus, Inhibition of
    platelet prostaglandin synthetase by oral aspirin. J. Clin.
    Invest., 61:314-319 (1978).

16. D. J. Chapple, G. J. Dusting, R. Hughes and J. R. Vane, A vagal
    reflex contributes to the hypotensive effect of prostacyclin
    in anaesthetized dogs. J. Physiol., 281:43-44P (1978).

17. D. J. Chapple, G. J. Dusting, R. Hughes and J. R. Vane, Some
    direct and reflex cardiovascular actions of prostacyclin
    (PGI$_2$) and PGE$_2$ in anaesthetized dogs. Br. J. Pharmac., in
    press (1979).

18. G. J. Christofinis, S. Moncada, C. MacCormick, S. Bunting and
    J. R. Vane, Prostacyclin (PGI$_2$) release by rabbit aorta and
    human umbilical vein endothelial cells after prolonged sub-
    culture. Weibel-Palade bodies were observed in low and high
    passages of these cells. In: Prostacyclin, J. R. Vane and S.
    Bergstrom, eds., Raven Press, New York, in press (1979).

19. F. Coceani, I. Bishai, E. White, E. Bodack and P. M. Olley,
    Action of prostaglandins, endoperoxides and thromboxanes on
    the lamb ductus arteriosus. Am. J. Physiol., 234:H117-H112
    (1978).

20. R. L. Czervionke, J. C. Hoak, and G. Fry, Effect of aspirin on
    thrombin-induced adherence of platelets to cultured cells
    from the blood vessel wall. J. Clin. Invest., 62:847-856
    (1978).

21. R. L. Czervionke, J. B. Smith, G. L. Fry and J. C. Hoak,
    Inhibition of prostacyclin by treatment of endothelium with
    aspirin. J. Clin. Invest., 63:1089-1092 (1979).

22. V. D'Angelo, S. Villa, M. Mysliwiec, M. B. Donati and G. De
    Gaetano, Defective fibrinolytic and prostacyclin-like activity
    in human atheromatous plaques. Thromb. Haem., 39:535-536
    (1978).

23. J. L. Data, W. J. Crump, J. W. Hollifield, J. C. Frolich and
     A. S. Nies, Prostaglandins: a role in baroreceptor control of
     renin release. Clin. Res., 24:397A (1976).
24. E. A. M. De Dekere, D. H. Nugteren and F. Ten Hoor, Prosta-
     cyclin is the major prostaglandin released from the isolated
     perfused rabbit and rat heart. Nature (Lond.), 268:160-163
     (1977).
25. A. Dembinska-Kiec, T. Gryglewska, A. Zmuda and R. J.
     Gryglewski, The generation of prostacyclin by arteries and
     by the coronary vascular bed is reduced in experimental
     atherosclerosis in rabbits. Prostaglandins, 14:1025-1054
     (1977).
26. G. J. Dusting,D. J. Chapple, R. Hughes, S. Moncada and
     J. R. Vane, Prostacyclin induces coronary vasodilatation in
     anaesthetized dogs. Cardiovasc. Res., 12:720-730 (1978c).
27. G. J. Dusting, S. Moncada and J. R. Vane, Prostacyclin (PGX)
     is the endogenous metabolite responsible for relaxation of
     coronary arteries induced by arachidonic acid. Prostaglandins,
     13:3-15 (1977a).
28. G. J. Dusting, S. Moncada and J. R. Vane, Disappearance of
     prostacyclin in the circulation of the dog. Br. J. Pharmac.,
     62:414-415P (1977b).
29. G. J. Dusting, S. Moncada and J. R. Vane, Prostacyclin is a
     weak contractor of coronary arteries in the pig. Eur. J.
     Pharmac., 45:301-304 (1977c).
30. G. J. Dusting, S. Moncada and J. R. Vane, Recirculation of
     prostacyclin (PGI$_2$) in the dog. Br. J. Pharmacol., 64:315-
     320 (1978a).
31. G. J. Dusting, S. Moncada and J. R. Vane, Vascular actions of
     arachidonic acid and its metabolites in perfused mesenteric
     and femoral beds of the dog. Eur. J. Pharmac., 49:65-72
     (1978b).
32. J. Dyerberg, H. O. Bang, E. Stoffersen, S. Moncada and J. R.
     Vane, Polyunsaturated fatty acids, atherosclerosis and
     thrombosis. Lancet, ii:117-119 (1978).
33. J. Dyerberg and H. O. Bang, Haemostatic function and platelet
     polyunsaturated fatty acids in Eskimos. Lancet, ii:433-435
     (1979).
34. S. H. Ferreira and J. R. Vane, Prostaglandins: their
     disappearance from and release into the circulation. Nature
     (Lond.), 216:868-873 (1967).
35. J. C. Frolich, J. W. Hollifield, J. C. Dormois, B. L. Frolich,
     H. Seyberth, A. M. Michelakis and J. A. Oates, Suppression
     of plasma renin activity by indomethacin in man. Circ. Res.,
     39:447-452 (1976).
36. J. G. Gerber, R. A. Branch, A. S. Nies, J. F. Gerkens, D. G.
     Shand, J. Hollifield and J. A. Oates, Prostaglandins and renin
     release: II.assessment of renin secretion following
     infusion of PGI$_2$, E$_2$ and D$_2$ into the renal artery of
     anaesthetized dogs. Prostaglandins, 15:81-88 (1978).

37. H. C. Godal, C. Eika, J. H. Dybdahl. L. Daae and S. Larsen,
     Aspirin and bleeding time. Lancet, i:1236 (1979).
38. R. R. Gorman, S. Bunting and O. V. Miller, Modulation of
     human platelet adenylate cyclase by prostacyclin (PGX).
     Prostaglandins, 13:377-388 (1977).
39. R. R. Gorman, F. A. Fitzpatrick and O. V. Miller, A selective
     thromboxane synthetase inhibitor blocks the cAMP lowering
     activity of PGH$_2$. Biophys. Biochem. Res. Commun., 79:305-313
     (1977).
40. F. C. Grenier and W. L. Smith, Formation of 6-keto-PGF$_1$ by
     collecting tubule cells isolated from rabbit renal papillae.
     Prostaglandins, 16:759-772 (1978).
41. G. C. Griffith, C. Nichols, J. D. Asher and B. Flanagan,
     Heparin osteoporosis. J. Am. Med. Ass., 193:91-94 (1965).
42. R. Gryglewski, S. Bunting, S. Moncada, R. J. Flower and J.
     R. Vane, Arterial walls are protected against deposition of
     platelet thrombi by a substance (prostaglandin X) which
     they make from prostaglandin endoperoxides. Prostaglandins
     12:685-714 (1976).
43. R. J. Gryglewski, R. Korbut and A. C. Ocetkiewicz, De-
     aggregatory action of prostacyclin in vivo
     and its enhancement by theophylline. Prostaglandins, 15:
     637-644 (1978a).
44. R. J. Gryglewski, R. Korbut and A. Ocetkiewicz, Generation of
     prostacyclin by lungs in vivo and its release into the arterial
     circulation. Nature (Lond.), 273:637-644 (1978b).
45. R. J. Gryglewski, R. Korbut, A. Ocetkiewicz and T. Stachwa,
     In vivo method for quantitation of anti-platelet potency of
     drugs. Naunyn-Schmiedeberg's Arch. Pharmac., 302:25 (1978).
46. R. J. Gryglewski, J. A. Salmon, F. B. Ubatuba, B. C.
     Weatherly, S. Moncada and J. R. Vane, Effects of all cis-5,8,
     11,14,17 eicosapentaenoic acid and PGH$_3$ on platelet aggrega-
     tion. Prostaglandins, in press (1979).
47. R. J. Gryglewski, A. Szczeklik and R. Nizankowski, Anti-
     platelet action of intravenous infusion of prostacyclin in
     man. Thromb. Res., 13:153-163 (1978).
48. L. A. Harker, N. Joy, R. T. Wall, L. Quadracci and G. Striker,
     Inhibition of platelet reactivity by endothelial cells.
     Thromb. Haem. (Abstract), 38:137 (1977).
49. L. A. Harker and S. J. Slichter, Platelet and fibrinogen
     consumption in man. New Eng. J. Med., 287:999-1005 (1972).
50. D. Harman and L. H. Piette, Free radical theory of ageing:
     Free radical reaction in serum. J. Gerontol., 21:560 (1966).
51. E. A. Higgs, S. Moncada, J. R. Vane, J. P. Caen, H. Michel and
     G. Tobelem, Effect of prostacyclin (PGI$_2$) on platelet
     adhesion to rabbit arterial subendothelium. Prostaglandins,
     16:17-22 (1978).

52. G. A. Higgs, S. Moncada and J. R. Vane, Prostacyclin (PGI_2) inhibits the formation of platelet thrombi induced by adenosine diphosphate (ADP) in vivo. Br. J. Pharmacol., 61:137P (1977).

53. G. A. Higgs, S. Moncada and J. R. Vane, Microcirculatory effects of prostacyclin (PGI_2) in the hamster cheek pouch. Microvasc. Res., in press (1979).

54. T. W. K. Hill, S. Moncada and J. R. Vane, Stimulation of renin release of protacyclin (PGI_2) in anaesthetized dogs. Abstract for 7th International Congress of Pharmacology, Paris, July, 1978.

55. T. W. K. Hill and S. Moncada, The renal haemodynamic and excretory actions of prostacyclin and 6-oxo-$PGF_{1\alpha}$ in anaesthetized dogs. Prostaglandins, 17:87-98 (1979).

56. T. H. Hintze and G. Kaley, Prostaglandins and the control of blood flow in the canine myocardium. Circ. Res., 40:313-320 (1977).

57. T. H. Hintze, G. Kaley, E. G. Martin and E. J. Messina, PGI_2 induces bradycardia in the dog. Prostaglandins, 15:p712 (1978).

58. A. J. Honour, T. D. R. Hockaday and J. I. Mann, The synergistic effect of aspirin and dipyridamole upon platelet thrombi in living blood vessels. Br. J. Exp. Path., 58:268-272 (1977).

59. G. Hornstra, E. Haddeman and J. A. Don, Blood platelets do not provide endoperoxides for vascular prostacyclin production. Nature, 279:66-68 (1979).

60. A. L. Hyman, P. J. Kadowitz, W. E. M. Lands, C. G. Crawford, J. Fried and J. Barton, Coronary vasodilator activity of 13,14-dehydro prostacyclin methyl ester: comparison with prostacyclin and other prostanoids. Proc. Natl. Acad. Sci., USA, 75:3522-3526 (1978).

61. R. A. Johnson, D. R. Morton, J. H. Kinner, R. R. Gorman, J. C. McGuire, F. F. Sun, N. Whittaker, S. Bunting, J. A. Salmon, S. Moncada and J. R. Vane, The chemical structure of prostaglandin X (prostacyclin), Prostaglandins, 12:915-928 (1976).

62. K. A. Jorgensen, A. S. Olesen, J. Dyerberg and E. Stoffersen, Aspirin and bleeding time: Dependency of Age. Lancet, ii: 302 (1979).

63. P. J. Kadowitz, B. M. Chapnick, L. P. Feigen, A. L. Hyman, P. K. Nelson and E. W. Spannhake, Pulmonary and systemic vasodilator effects of the newly discovered prostaglandin, PGI_2. J. Appl. Physiol., 45:408-413 (1978).

64. J. G. Kelton, J. Hirsh, C. J. Carter and M. R. Buchanan, Relationship to inhibition of vessel wall synthesis of prostaglandin I_2-like activity. J. Clin. Invest., 62:892-895 (1978).

65. P. B. A. Kernoff, A. L. Willis, K. J. Stone, J. A. Davies and G. P. McNicol, Antithrombotic potential of dihomo-gamma-linolenic acid in man. Br. Med. J., 2:1441-1444 (1977).

66. R. Korbut and S. Moncada, Prostacyclin (PGI$_2$) and thromboxane A$_2$ interaction in vivo. Regulation by aspirin and relationship with anti-thrombotic therapy. Thromb. Res., 13:489-500 (1978).

67. P. S. Kulkarni, R. Roberts and P. Needleman, Paradoxical endogenous synthesis of a coronary dilating substance from arachidonate. Prostaglandins, 123:337-353 (1976).

68. C. Larsson, P. Weber and E. Anggard, Arachidonic acid increases and indomethacin decreases plasma renin activity in the rabbit. Eur. J. Pharmac., 28:391-394 (1974).

69. A. M. Lefer, M. L. Ogletree, J. B. Smith, M. J. Silver, K. C. Nicolaou, W. E. Barnette and G. P. Gasic, Prostacyclin: A potentially valuable agent for preserving myocardial tissues in acute myocardial ischaemia. Science, 200:52-54 (1978).

70. C. W. Leffler and J. R. Hessler, Pulmonary and systemic vascular effects of exogenous prostaglandin I$_2$ in fetal lambs. Eur. J. Pharmac., 54:37-42 (1979).

71. S. V. Levy, Contractile responses to prostacyclin (PGI$_2$) of isolated human saphenous and rat venous tissue. Prostaglandins, 16:93-97 (1978).

72. D. E. MacIntyre, J. D. Pearson and J. L. Gordon, Localisation and stimulation of prostacyclin production in vascular cells. Nature, 271:549-551 (1978).

73. K. U. Malik and J. C. McGiff, Cardiovascular actions of prostaglandins. Prostaglandins: Physiological, Pharmacological and Pathological Aspects, S.M.Karim,ed., pp.103-200,MTP, Lancaster.

74. A. J. Marcus, B. B. Weksler and E. A. Jaffe, Enzymatic conversion of prostaglandin endoperoxide H$_2$ and arachidonic acid to prostacyclin by cultured human endothelial cells. J. Biol. Chem., 253:7138-7141 (1978).

75. S. Moncada, R. Gryglewski, S. Bunting and J. R. Vane, An enzyme isolated from arteries transforms prostaglandin endoperoxides to an unstable substance that inhibits platelet aggregation. Nature (Lond.), 263:663-665 (1976a).

76. S. Moncada, R. J. Gryglewski, S. Bunting and J. R. Vane, A lipid peroxide inhibits the enzyme in blood vessel microsomes that generates from prostaglandin endoperoxides the substance (prostaglandin X) which prevents platelet aggregation. Prostaglandins,12:715-733 (1976b).

77. S. Moncada, A. G. Herman, E. A. Higgs and J. R. Vane, Differential formation of prostacyclin (PGX or PGI$_2$) by layers of the arterial wall. An explanation for the anti-thrombotic properties of vascular endothelium. Thromb. Res., 11:323-344 (1977).

78. S. Moncada, E. A. Higgs and J. R. Vane, Human arterial and venous tissues generate prostacyclin (prostaglandin X), a potent inhibitor of platelet aggregation. Lancet, i:18-20 (1977).

79. S. Moncada and R. Korbut, Dipyridamole and other phospho-
    diesterase inhibitors act as anti-thrombotic agents through
    potentiating endogenous prostacyclin. Lancet, i:1286-1289
    (1978).
80. S. Moncada, R. Korbut, S. Bunting and J. R. Vane, Prostacyclin
    is a circulating hormone. Nature (Lond.), 273:767-768 (1978).
81. S. Moncada and J. R. Vane, The discovery of prostacyclin
    (PGX); a fresh insight into arachidonic acid metabolism.
    In: Biochemical Aspects of Prostaglandins and Thromboxanes,
    N. Kharasch and J. Fried, eds., pp.155-177, Academic Press,
    New York, San Francisco, London (1977).
82. S. Moncada and J. R. Vane, Unstable metabolites of
    arachidonic acid and their role in haemostasis and thrombosis.
    Br. Med. Bulletin, 34:129-135 (1978).
83. S. Moncada and J. R. Vane, Arachidonic acid metabolites and
    the interactions between platelets and blood vessel walls.
    New Eng. J. Med., 300:1142-1147 (1979a).
84. S. Moncada and J. R. Vane, The role of prostacyclin in
    vascular tissue. Fed. Proc., 38:62-66 (1979b).
85. K. M. Mullane, G. J. Dusting, J. A. Salmon, S. Moncada and
    J. R. Vane, Biotransformation and cardiovascular effects
    of arachidonic acid in the dog. Eur. J. Pharmac., 54:217-
    228 (1979).
86. K. M. Mullane, S. Moncada and J. R. Vane, Prostacyclin
    release induced by bradykinin may contribute to the anti-
    hypertensive action of angiotensin converting enzyme
    inhibitors. 4th Int. Prostaglandin Congress, Washington,
    27-31st May, 1979, p.84.
87. P. Needleman, The synthesis and function of prostaglandins
    in the heart. Fed. Proc., 35:2376-2381 (1976).
88. P. Needleman, S. D. Bronson, A. Wyche, M. Sivakoff and
    K. C. Nicolaou, Cardiac and renal prostaglandin I_2. J. Clin.
    Invest., 61:839-849 (1978).
89. P. Needleman, A. Wyche and A. Raz, Platelet and blood vessel
    arachidonate metabolism and interactions. J. Clin. Invest.,
    63:345-349 (1979).
90. A. Nordoy, B. Svensson and J. C. Hoak, The inhibitory effect
    of human endothelial cell monolayers on platelet reactions
    and its inhibition by aspirin. Thromb. Res., 12:597-608
    (1978).
91. O. Oelz, H. W. Seyberth, H. R. Knapp, B. J. Sweetman and
    U. A. Oates, Effects of feeding ethyl-dihomo-γ-linolenate on
    prostaglandin biosynthesis and platelet aggregation in the
    rabbit. Biochim. Biophys. Acta., 431:268-277 (1976).
92. J. O'Grady and S. Moncada, Aspirin: A paradoxical effect
    on bleeding time. Lancet, ii:780P (1978).

93. J. O'Grady, S. Warrington, M. J. Moti, S. Bunting, R. J.
     Flower, A. S. E. Fowle, E. A. Higgs and S. Moncada, Effects
     of intravenous prostacyclin infusions in healthy volunteers -
     some preliminary observations. In: Prostacyclin, J. R.
     Vane and S. Bergstrom, eds., Raven Press, New York, in
     press (1979).

94. T. L. Owen, I. C. Ehrhart, W. J. Weidner, J. B. Scott and F. J.
     Haddy, Effects of indomethacin on local blood flow regulation
     in canine heart and kidney. Proc. Soc. Exp. Biol. Med.,
     149:871-876 (1975).

95. C. Pace-Asciak, Isolation, structure and biosynthesis of
     6-keto-prostaglandin $F_{1\alpha}$ in the rat stomach. J. Am. Chem.
     Soc., 98:2348-2349 (1976).

96. K. Pomerantz, A. Sintetos and P. Ramwell, The effect of
     prostacyclin on the human umbilical artery. Prostaglandins,
     15:1035-1044 (1978).

97. S. M. Rajah, S. Penny and R. Kester, Aspirin and bleeding
     time. Lancet, ii:1104 (1978).

98. A. Raz, P. C. Isakson, M. S. Minkes and P. Needleman,
     Characterisation of a novel metabolic pathway of arachidonate
     in coronary arteries which generates a potent endogenous
     coronary vasodilator. J. Biol. Chem., 252:1123-1126 (1977).

99. A. Raz, M. S. Minkes and P. Needleman, Endoperoxides and
     thromboxanes. Structural determinants for platelet
     aggregation and vasoconstriction. Biochim. Biophys. Acta.,
     488:305-311 (1977).

100. G. Remuzzi, A. E. Cavenaghi, G. Mecca, M. B. Donati and G.
     De Gaetano, Human renal cortex generates prostacyclin-like
     activity. Thromb. Res., 12:363-366 (1978).

101. J. P. Sackler and J. Liu, Heparin induced osteoporosis.
     Br. J. Radiol., 46:548-550 (1973).

102. J. A. Salmon, D. R. Smith, R. J. Flower, S. Moncada and
     J. R. Vane, Some characteristics of the prostacyclin
     synthesizing enzyme in porcine aorta, Biochim. Biophys. Acta.,
     523:250-262 (1978).

103. K. Schror, S. Moncada, F. B. Ubatuba, and J. R. Vane, Trans-
     formation of arachidonic acid and prostaglandin endoperoxides
     by the guinea-pig heart. Formation of RCS and prostacyclin.
     Eur. J. Pharmac., 47:103-114 (1978).

104. K. Silberbauer, H. Sinzinger and M. Winter, Prostacyclin
     activity in rat kidney stimulated by angiotensin II. Br. J.
     Exp. Path., 60:38-44 (1979).

105. A. K. Sim and A. P. McCraw, The activity of γ-linolenate and
     dihomo-γ-linolenate methyl esters in vitro and in vivo on
     blood platelet function in non-human primates and in man.
     Thromb. Res., 10:385-397 (1977).

106. H. Sinzinger, W. Feigl and K. Silberbauer, Prostacyclin
     generation in atherosclerotic arteries, Lancet, ii:469 (1979).

107. T. J. Slater, Free Radical Mechanisms in Tissue Injury,
      Pion Ltd., London (1972).
108. A. Szczeklik, R. J. Gryglewski, E. Nizankowska, R.
      Nizankowski and J. Musial, Pulmonary and antiplatelet effects
      of intravenous and inhaled prostacyclin in man. Prostaglandins,
      16:654-660 (1978).
109. R. L. Tansik, D. H. Namm and H. L. White, Synthesis of
      prostaglandin 6-keto-$F_{1\alpha}$ by cultured aortic mooth muscle
      cells an d stimulation of its formation in a coupled system
      with platelet lysates. Prostaglandins, 15:399-408 (1978).
110. J. E. Tateson, S. Moncada and J. R. Vane, Effects of
      prostacyclin (PGX) on cyclic AMP concentrations in human
      platelets. Prostaglandins, 13:389-399 (1977).
111. F. B. Ubatuba, S. Moncada and J. R. Vane, The effect of
      prostacyclin (PGI$_2$) on platelet behaviour, thrombus formation
      in vivo and bleeding time. Thromb. Haem., 41:425-434 (1979).
112. J. R. Vane, Inhibition of prostaglandin synthesis as a
      mechanism of action for aspirin-like drugs. Nature New Biol.,
      231:232-235 (1971).
113. P. C. Weber, C. Larsson, E. Anggard, M. Hamberg, E. J. Corey,
      K. C. Nicolaou and B. Samuelsson, Stimulation of renin
      release from rabbit renal cortex by arachidonic acid and
      prostaglandin endoperoxides. Circ. Res., 39:868-874 (1976).
114. H. J. Weiss and V. T. Turitto, Prostacyclin (prostaglandin
      I$_2$, PGI$_2$) inhibits platelet adhesion and thrombus formation
      on subendothelium. Blood, 53:244-250 (1979).
115. B. B. Weksler, A. J. Marcus and E. A. Jaffe, Synthesis of
      prostaglandin I$_2$ (prostacyclin) by cultured human and bovine
      endothelial cells. Proc. Natl. Acad. Sci. USA, 74:3922-
      3926 (1977).
116. A. R. Wharton, K. Misono, J. Hollifield, J. C. Frolich,
      T. Inagami and J. A. Oates, Prostaglandins and renin release:
      I Stimulation of renin release from rabbit renal cortical
      slices by PGI$_2$. Prostaglandins, 14:1095-1104 (1977).
117. A. R. Wharton, M. Smigel, J. A. Oates and J. C. Frolich,
      Evidence for prostacyclin production in renal cortex.
      Prostaglandins, 13:1021 (1977)
118. A. L. Willis, K. Comai, D. C. Kuhn and J. Paulsrud,
      Dihomo-γ-linolenate suppresses platelet aggregation when
      administered in vitro or in vivo. Prostaglandins, 8:509-
      519 (1974).
119. T. V. Zenser, C. A. Herman, R. R. Gorman and B. B. Davis,
      Metabolism and action of the prostaglandin endoperoxide
      PGH$_2$ in rat kidney. Biochem. Biophys. Res. Commun.,
      79:357-363 (1977).

PROSTACYCLIN AS AN ANTI-ATHEROSCLEROTIC HORMONE - A HYPOTHESIS

Ryszard J. Gryglewski

Department of Pharmacology
Copernicus Academy of Medicine, 31-531 Cracow
16 Grzegórzecka, Poland

INTRODUCTION

Although many factors in pathogenesis of atherosclerosis still remain unknown, intravascular activation of blood platelets seems to play an important role in the development of this disease. The thrombogenic hypothesis of atherosclerosis (the so called "incrustation theory") was proposed as early as in 1842 by Carl von Rokitansky (1), but Virchow's "infiltration theory" prevailed and dominated the academic community for many years, owing greatly to Anichkov's experimental demonstration (2) that atherosclerosis in rabbits could be induced by a diet high in lipids and cholesterol content. The yellow streaks of lipids which "infiltrated" the rabbit aorta could be seen with the naked eye.

More than a century after von Rokitansky put forward his hypothesis, pathologists could see that myointimal cells of arteries were growing over mural thrombi and thus forming an atherosclerotic plaque (3,4). Indeed, platelets and fibrin seemed to "incrustate" the arterial wall. Intra-arterial platelet adhesion and aggregation is the key event in the initiation of arterial thrombosis (5,6). Platelets react avidly with polymerizing fibrin (7). Activated platelets release a factor that stimulates proliferation of arterial myocytes and promotes their migration to an arising atheromatic plaque (8,9). The experimental intimal thickening due to myocyte hyperplasia following injury to the arterial endothelium is mediated most probably by a platelet-derived growth factor which is released from beneath a carpet of platelets which cover the site of the injury (10). Homocysteine-induced atherosclerosis in baboons starts from focal vascular lesions of endothelium and an immense

223

increase in platelet consumption. This is followed by arterial
myocyte proliferation (11). These and other facts allowed to
develop the most attractive concept of pathogenesis of
atherosclerosis by Ross and Glomset (12,13), according to which the
platelet-induced proliferation of arterial myocytes is a crucial
event. However, the basic question was - why in atherosclerotic
subjects platelets start to release their growth factor inside
arteries? This question can be reversed - why platelets do not
release their growth factor (as well as other factors) inside
arteries of healthy subjects? We postulate that in healthy
humans and animals platelets are prevented from activation by
prostacyclin (PGI$_2$) which is generated by vascular endothelium
(14,15), lungs (16,17) and kidneys (18,19,20). By rising cAMP
levels in platelets (21) prostacyclin keeps them in "non-
aggressive" state. We also suggest that atherosclerosis develops
when the secretory function of endothelial cells is impaired.
It is proposed that atherosclerosis is a disease from deficiency
of prostacyclin (22).

PLATELET - ENDOTHELIUM INTERACTION

Ten years ago it was recognized that endothelial cell
function appears to be dependent on the presence of blood platelets
in the fluid that perfuses arteries (23,24). Endothelial "supporting"
function of the platelets has been confirmed by ultrastructural
studies (25).

Little is known about the biochemical character of this
platelet-endothelium interaction. Certainly, it is a complex
phenomenon. We have proposed that platelets can "feed"
endothelium with their prostaglandin endoperoxides and thus
promote the generation of prostacyclin (26,27). This mode of
biochemical interaction between platelets and vascular walls was
confirmed in one laboratory (28) and disproved in another (29).

There is no doubt that arterial walls generate prostacyclin
without any help of platelets (14,15,26,27), however, our concept
of the biochemical interaction between platelets and vascular walls
offers a reasonable explanation for the following phenomena.
Arterial microsomes reverse ADP-induced platelet aggregation
in vitro (30) and in certain circumstances ADP shows a slight
thrombolytic effect in vivo (31). ADP-induced platelet
aggregation is associated with the release of minute amounts of
TXA$_2$ and prostaglandin endoperoxides (32,33). This activation of
arachidonic metabolism is not sufficient to contribute to the
aggregatory response to ADP, but it may be sufficient to feed
arterial prostacyclin synthetase with endoperoxides. Arterial
prostacyclin synthetase avidly converts 80 - 100% of available
endoperoxides to PGI$_2$ (14,34), whereas the arterial cyclo-
oxygenase converts not more that 1% of available arachidonic acid

to endoperoxides. Therefore, the external supply with endoperoxides to endothelium may be of a significance, irrespectively how modest it is.

Endothelium may increase its synthetic capability of prostacyclin during a mild injury. In vitro platelets do no adhere to endothelium scraped from rabbit aorta (35) and in vivo there is little platelet adhesion to patches of remaining endothelium in mechanically injured aorta (6). Spirally cut strips of rabbit aorta are not covered with platelet clumps when superfused with heparinized blood, unless the aortic strips are prepared from atherosclerotic animals (36,37). All these phenomena may be ascribed to the accelerated rate of prostacyclin generation by endothelium as the consequence of cutting, squeezing, scraping, etc. In vivo the release of prostacyclin into circulation is stimulated by angiotensin II (18,19), bradykinin (20), hyperventilation (16) and pulmonary embolism (38).

There are, however, certain limits beyond which physical or chemical trauma no longer stimulates endothelium but rather destroys its prostacyclin synthetizing apparatus. This effect is probably reached after an injury from a laser beam directed into the arterial wall (39). We believe that a chemical stimulus that leads to a similar damage to endothelial prostacyclin synthetase is the chronic intoxication with lipid peroxides. This intoxication results in a deficiency in prostacyclin, followed by an increased platelet aggressiveness, their pathological interaction with endothelium and finally the formation of an atheromatic plaque.

LIPID PEROXIDES AND ATHEROSCLEROSIS

In one of the pioneering papers on the discovery of prostacyclin (14) we have described that 15-hydroperoxyarachidonic acid is a potent inhibitor (IC_{50} = 1.5 µM) of prostacyclin synthetase in porcine aortic microsomes. Otherwise, the enzyme is resistant to intoxication by many other chemicals. 15-hydroperoxyarachidonic acid inhibits also the generation of prostacyclin by arterials strips (27), and by cultured endothelial cells (40). A powerful inhibition of prostacyclin synthetase by a number of other linear peroxides of poly-unsaturated fatty acids has been also reported (34). An atherogenic diet consisting of oleic acid and cholesterol causes an early and dramatic suppression of prostacyclin generation by arteries in rabbits (22,41,42) as well as a diversion of endoperoxide metabolism to PGE_2 in arteries (43) and to TXA_2 in platelets (44). These findings promted us to put forward a hypothesis on the pathogenesis of atherosclerosis. We believe that hyperlipidemia induces an increased lipid peroxidation. Lipid peroxides or corresponding free radicals inactivate prostacyclin synthetase in arteries. A deficiency in prostacyclin is responsible for development of atherosclerosis.

There is no direct evidence that in experimental or human atherosclerosis lipid peroxidation is the earliest sign of development of the disease. Methodological difficulties in evaluation of intensity of lipid peroxidation in vivo (45) do not help in solving this important problem. Nonetheless, lipid peroxides have been found in human atheromatic arteries (46,47), in retina during ocular siderosis (48), and in ceroid atheromateous plaques of human arteries (49). At the same time in human atheromatic plaques prostacyclin is hardly generated (50), although experimental venous thrombosis is not associated with a decrease in prostacyclin production by the damaged rat veins (51). Interestingly, feeding rabbits a diet enriched with safflower oil causes a marked suppression of prostacyclin generation by their vascular endothelium (52). Safflower oil is the richest plant source of polyunsaturated fatty acids (53), which can be the substrates for the formation of lipid peroxides. A potential hazard of overfeeding with unsaturated lipids has been also demonstrated in another experiment. Swines kept on a corn soybean diet free of cholesterol and saturated fatty acids develop atherosclerosis identical to that seen in humans (54). On the other hand antioxidants protect rats against the vascular damage of acute choline deficiency - a damage which is resulted in by an increased lipid peroxidation in the body (55).

In summary, there exists a number of circumstantial evidence that atherosclerosis may be initiated by an increased lipid peroxidation, however, a direct evidence has not been produced.

EXPERIMENTAL ATHEROSCLEROSIS AND PROSTACYCLIN

At the early stage of experimental atherosclerosis in rabbit (one week (42) or one month (22) of an atherogenic diet) there occurs a severe depression (by 70 - 90%) in generation of prosta- cyclin by heart, aorta, mesenteric arteries (41), lungs and kidney (56). The suppression of prostacyclin generation is detected before any anatomical changes in arteries are visible (22) and before the metabolism of arachidonic acid in platelets is activated (22,44). In parallel to the development of atherosclerosis a tendency to recovery of prostacyclin synthetizing capacity by arteries appears (22) and platelets are activated (44). This generalized suppression of the prostacyclin synthetizing system in athero- sclerosis is associated with an increased susceptibility of platelet adenylate cyclase and endothelial adenylate cyclase to the stimulatory action of exogenous prostacyclin (57,58). This atherosclerosis-induced hypersensitivity of the "second messenger system" towards the primary mediator may be a consequence of prostacyclin deficency, similarly as it has been observed in other biological systems deprived of a primary physiological mediator. The fact that functioning of prostacyclin-stimulated adenylate cyclase not impaired in atherosclerosis - on contrary,

it is activated – creates a sound basis for administration of
prostacyclin in the treatment of the disease. Animal models of
atherosclerosis are subdued to a rightful criticism. Their
relevance for human atherosclerosis is questioned. It should be
added that in another model of experimental atherosclerosis – in
minipigs – the generation of prostacyclin by vascular tissue is
increased (59). However, the coronary arteries of pigs, unlike
those of other species, are contracted by prostacyclin. Our
hypothesis on pathogenesis of atherosclerosis is based on the rabbit
model of atherosclerosis. In aim to check its validity for humans
we decided to administer prostacyclin into atherosclerotic human
subjects.

CLINICAL EVIDENCE

When we established the effective and safe doses of prostacyclin in healthy volunteers (60,61), the synthetic hormone
(Wellcome Research and Upjohn Co product) was administered into
five patients with advanced arteriosclerosis obliterans of
lower extremities. Prostacyclin was infused upstream into femoral
artery at a dose of 5–10 ng/kg/min during 72 hours (62). All
patients had chronic ischemic ulcers, in three focal necrosis was
present. The lesions were painful and had resisted healing from
3 months to 3 years. In past various types of conservative
treatment were tried. No further treatment could be offered except
for amputation. In all patients two days after prostacyclin therapy
pain extinguished, and 4 – 8 weeks later in three patients the
regression of necrosis and healing of ischemic ulcers occurred. In
two others a remarkable improvement was observed. The striking
clinical improvement after prostacyclin therapy was accompanied
by a persistant increase in capillary blood flow through the calf
muscle, as measured by the clearance of ^{133}Xe. The anatomical
obstruction to major arteries remained unchanged as evidenced by
angiograms. Until now, fourteen patients with advanced
arteriosclerosis obliterans were treated with intra–arterial or
intravenous infusions of prostacyclin. The reported results of
prostacyclin therapy (62) were confirmed (Dr. A. Szczeklik,
personal communication). Since the pharmacological treatment of
advanced obstructive vascular disease with various vasodilators
was totally unsuccessful (63), we believe that the prostacyclin
therapy was indeed the hormonal substitution therapy. The only
other effective drug in the treatment of advanced arteriosclerosis
obliterans is PGE_1 (64). The therapeutical efficacy of PGE_1 can
be explained by its biological similarity to the natural hormone
– PGI_2. It may well be that owing to the powerful anti-
aggregating and dis-aggregating properties of prostacyclin the non-
obstructed small arteries and capillaries were cleared from platelet
microaggregates. Thus atherogenesis was arrested, peripheral
blood flow increased, and possibly the vascular endothelium which
had been deprived of prostacyclin synthetase had a chance to re-
build the lacking enzyme. A transient vasodilatation produced by

prostacyclin during the infusion period seems an unlikely cause of clinical improvement, since increased capillary blood flow was observed 6 weeks after termination of prostacyclin infusion and the curative effects of prostacyclin persisted for at least 3 months of the observation period. Prostacyclin might, however, act directly on blood vessels by stimulation proliferation of new capillaries into the ischemic area. The successful therapy of advanced arteriosclerosis obliterans with prostacyclin supports ex iuvantibus our concept that atherosclerosis is a disease from deficiency of prostacyclin.

HYPOTHESIS

We postulate that atherosclerosis is a disease from deficiency of prostacyclin. This hormonal defect is resulted in by intoxication of prostacyclin synthetase with lipid peroxides or with corresponding free radicals which are likely to be generated during hyperlipidemia (Fig. 1). Deficiency of prostacyclin leads to a decrease in cAMP levels both in platelets and in arterial walls, thus increasing platelet aggregability and endothelial permeability (65). Arterial endothelium when deprived of its capacity to synthetize prostacyclin (22,50) becomes a surface prone to platelet adhesion and aggregation. Aggregating platelets are activated not only by lack of "prostacyclin resistance" at the endothelial surface, but also by low concentrations of circulating prostacyclin and by diversion of arachidonic acid metabolism from prostacyclin to pro-aggregatory metabolites. Activated platelets adhere and aggregate on the endothelial cells and release harmful substances that cause endothelial damage, mural inflammatory response, migration of myocytes and formation of atheromatic plaque (13,66). The aggressive behaviour of platelets in atherosclerosis is facilitated by low levels of cAMP in arterial walls (67). Both phenomena are growing from the same stem, i.e. a damage to an enzymatic system which synthetizes prostacyclin (Fig. 1).

CONCLUSIONS

The above laboratory and clinical data encourage the following lines of research. Protection against atherosclerosis by anti-oxidants, substitution therapy with prostacyclin or its stable analogs and stimulation of endogenous generation of prostacyclin by various releasers.

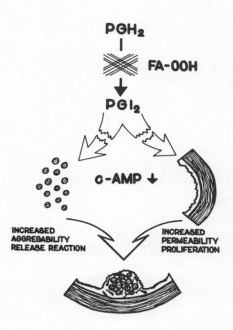

Fig. 1.   Schematic representation of a hypothesis on the role of
          prostacyclin in development of atherosclerosis. Athero-
          sclerosis is initiated by intoxication of prostacyclin
          synthetase ($PGH_2 \rightarrow PGI_2$) with lipid peroxides (FA-OOH) or
          with corresponding free radicals. A reduction in
          amount of PGI_2 which is synthetized by vascular endothelium,
          lungs and kidneys leads to lowering of cAMP in platelets,
          in arterial walls, and consequently to an increased
          aggregability and stimulation of the release reaction in
          platelets. The above activation of platelets in
          conjunction with an increased permeability of endothelium
          and a susceptibility of myocytes to proliferation
          promotes a pathological interaction between platelets and
          endothelium. Platelets invade arterial wall, destroy
          endothelium, induce proliferation of myocytes and an
          atheromatic plaque is formed.

REFERENCES

1. C. Von Rokitansky, Handbuch der Patologischen Anatomie, Bd.
   4 1842, English translation by G. E. Day, Sydenham
   Society, London, 1852:261.
2. N. Anitschkow, Über Veranderungen der Kaninchen-Aorta bei
   experimenteller Cholesterinsteatose, Beitr. Anat. Allg.
   Path., 56:379 (1913).
3. W. C. Roberts and V. J. Ferrans, The role of thrombosis in
   the etiology of atherosclerosis (a positive one) and in
   precipitating fatal ischemic heart disease (a negative one).
   In: "Current Cardiovascular Topics",Vol.2., "Thrombosis,
   Platelets, Anticoagulation and Acetylsalicylic Acid", E. Donoso
   and J. I. Haft, eds., Georg Thieme Pub., Stuttgart, (1976).
4. J. I. Haft, Platelets, coronary artery disease and stress,
   In: "Current Cardiovascular Topics, Vol. II, Thrombosis,
   Platelets, Anti-Coagulation and Acetylsalicylic Acid", E. Donoso
   and J. I. Haft, eds., Georg Thieme, Stuttgart 97 (1976).
5. J. F. Mustard and M. A. Packham, Platelet thrombosis and
   drugs, Drugs, 9:19 (1975).
6. H. R. Baumgartner, Platelet interaction with vascular
   structures. Thromb. Diath. Haemorrh. Suppl., 43:161 (1971).
7. S. Niewiarowski, F. Regoeczi, G. J. Stewart, A. Senyi and
   J. F. Mustard, Platelet interaction with polymerizing fibrin.
   J. Clin. Invest., 51:685 (1972).
8. R. Ross, J. Glomset, R. Kariya and L. Harker, A platelet-
   dependent serum factor that stimulates the proliferation of
   arterial smooth muscle sells in vitro. Proc. Natl. Acad.
   Sci. USA, 71:1207 (1974).
9. H. N. Antoniades, C. D. Scher and C. D. Stiles, Purification
   of human platelet-derived growth factor, Proc. Natl. Acad. Sci.
   USA, 76:1809 (1979).
10. A. W. Clowes and M. J. Karnowsky, Failure of certain anti-
    platelet drugs to affect myointimal thickening following
    arterial endothelial injury in the rat. Lab. Invest., 36:452
    (1977).
11. L. A. Harker, S. J. Slichter, R. Scott and R. Ross, Homo-
    cystinemia - vascular injury and arterial thrombosis.
    N. Engl. J. Med., 291:537 (1974).
12. R. Ross and J. A. Flomset, Atherosclerosis and the arterial
    smooth muscle cell. Science, 180:1332 (1973).
13. R. Ross and J. A. Glomset, The pathogenesis of atherosclerosis
    (two parts). New Engl. J. Med., 295:369 and 420 (1976).
14. R. J. Gryglewski, S. Bunting, S. Moncada, R. J. Flower and
    J. R. Vane, Arterial walls are protected against deposition of
    platelet thrombi by a substance (Prostaglandin X) which they
    make from prostaglandin endoperoxide. Prostaglandins, 12:685
    (1976).
15. S. Moncada, R. J. Gryglewski, S. Bunting and J. R. Vane, An
    enzyme isolated from arteries transforms prostaglandin

endoperoxides to an unstable substance that inhibits platelet
aggregation. Nature, 263:663 (1976).

16. R. J. Gryglewski, R. Korbut and A. Ocetkiewicz; Generation of
    prostacyclin by lungs in vivo and its release into the
    arterial circulation. Nature, 273:765 (1978).
17. S. Moncada, R. Korbut, S. Bunting and J. R. Vane, Prostacyclin
    is a circulating hormone. Nature, 273:767 (1978).
18. R. J. Gryglewski, R. Korbut and J. Splawinski, Endogenous
    mechanisms which regulate prostacyclin release. Haemostasis
    in press.
19. R. J. Shebuski and J. W. Aiken, Angiotensin II induced renal
    prostacyclin release suppresses platelet aggregation in the
    anaesthetized dog. Abstracts of IVth International
    Prostaglandin Conference, Washingotn, D.C. May 27-31, 1979.
20. K. M. Mullane, S. Moncada and J. R. Vane, Prostacyclin
    release induced by bradykinin may contribute to the anti-
    hypertensive action of angiotensin converting enzyme inhibitors.
    Abstracts of IVth International Prostaglandin Conference,
    Washington, D.C. 27-31 May, 1979.
21. R. R. Gorman, S. Bunting and O. V. Miller, Modulation of human
    platelet adenylate cyclase by prostacyclin (PGX), Prostaglandins,
    13:377 (1977).
22. R. J. Gryglewski, A. Dembinska-Kiec, A Chytkowski and T.
    Gryglewska, Prostacyclin and thromboxane A_2 biosynthesis
    capacities of heart, arteries and platelets at various stages
    of experimental atherosclerosis in rabbits. Atherosclerosis,
    31:385 (1978).
23. J. D. Wojcik, D. L. Vanhorn and A. J. Weber, Mechanism whereby
    platelets support endothelium. Transfusion, 9:324 (1969).
24. M. A. Gimbrone, R. H. Aster and R. S. Cotran, Preservation of
    vascular integrity in organs perfused in vitro with platelet-
    rich medium. Nature (London), 222:33 (1969).
25. S. A. Johnson, Endothelial supporting function of platelets,
    In: "The Circulating Platelets", S. A. Johnson, ed.,
    Academic Press, New York (1971).
26. S. Moncada, R. J. Gryglewski, S. Bunting and J. R. Vane, A
    lipid peroxide inhibits the enzyme in blood vessel microsomes
    that generates from prostaglandin endoperoxides the substance
    (prostaglandin X) which prevents platelet aggregation.
    Prostaglandins, 12:715 (1976).
27. S. Bunting, R. J. Gryglewski, S. Moncada and J. R. Vane,
    Arterial walls generate from prostaglandin endoperoxides
    a substance (Prostaglandin X) which relaxes strips of
    mesenteric and coeliac arteries and inhibits platelet
    aggregation. Prostaglandins, 12:897 (1976).
28. R. L. Tansik, D. H. Namm and H. L. White, Synthesis of
    prostaglandin 6-keto PGF_1 by cultured aortic smooth muscle
    cells and stimulation of its formation in a coupled system
    which platelet lysates. Prostaglandins, 15:399 (1978).

29. G. Hornstra, E. Haddeman and J. A. Don, Some investigations
     into the role of prostacyclin in thromboregulation. Thromb.
     Res., 12:367 (1978).

30. P. P. K. Ho, R. G. Herrmann, R. D. Towner and C. P. Walters,
     Reversal of platelet aggregation by aortic microsomes.
     Biochem. Biophys. Res. Commun., 74:514 (1977).

31. N. Begent and G. V. R. Born, Growth rate in vivo of platelet
     thrombi, produced by ionophoresis of ADP as a function of mean
     blood flow velocity, Nature (London) 227:926 (1970).

32. E. Marcinkiewicz, L. Grodzinska and R. J. Gryglewski, Platelet
     aggregation and thromboxane A_2 formation in cat platelet rich
     plasma. Pharmacol. Res. Commun., 10:1 (1978).

33. L. Grodzinska and E. Marcinkiewicz, The generation of TXA_2
     in human platelets rich plasma and its inhibition by
     nictindole and prostacyclin. Pharmacol. Res. Commun., 11:133
     (1979).

34. J. A. Salmon, D. R. Smith, R. J. Flower, S. Moncada and
     J. R. Vane, Further studies on the enzymatic conversion of
     prostaglandin endoperoxide into prostacyclin in porcine
     aorta microsomes. Biochim. Biophys. Acta., 523:250 (1978).

35. T. H. Spaet and R. B. Erichson, The vascular wall in the
     pathogenesis of thrombosis. Thromb. Diath. Haemorrh. Suppl.
     21:67 (1966).

36. R. J. Gryglewski, R. Korbut and A. Ocetkiewicz, De-
     aggregatory action of prostacyclin in vivo and its enhancement
     by theophylline. Prostaglandins, 15:637 (1978).

37. R. J. Gryglewski, R. Korbut and A. Ocetkiewicz, Reversal of
     platelet aggregation by prostacyclin. Pharmacol. Res. Commun.
     10:185 (1978).

38. R. J. Gryglewski, Prostacyclin as a circulatory hormone.
     Biochem. Pharmacol. in press (1979).

39. K. E. Arfors, H. C. Hint, D. P. Dhall and N. A. Matheson,
     Counteraction of platelet activity at sites of laser-induced
     endothelial thrauma. Br. Med. J., 4:430 (1968).

40. A. J. Marcus, B. B. Weksler and E. A. Jaffe, Enzymatic
     conversion of prostaglandin endoperoxide H_2 and arachidonic
     acid to prostacyclin by cultured human endothelial cells.
     J. Biol. Chem., 253:7138 (1978).

41. A. Dembinska-Kieć, T. Gryglewska, A. Zmuda and R. J. Gryglewski,
     The generation of prostacyclin by arteries and by the
     coronary vascular bed is reduced in experimental athero-
     sclerosis in rabbits. Prostaglandins, 14:1025 (1977).

42. G. Masotti, G. Galanti, L. Poggesi, A. Curcio and G. G.
     Neri Serneri, Early changes of the endothelial antithrombotic
     properties in cholesterol fed rabbits. III-decreased PGI_2
     production by aortic wall. Thrombos. Haemostas., 42:423
     (1979).

43. P. A. Berberian, V. A. Ziboh, S. L. Hsia, Prostaglandin E_2
     biosynthesis: changes in rabbit aorta and skin during
     experimental atherosclerosis. J. Lipid Res., 17:46 (1976).

44. A. Zmuda, A. Dembinska-Kieć, A. Chytkowski and R. J. Gryglewski, Experimental atherosclerosis in rabbits: Platelet aggregability, thromboxane A_2 generation and anti-aggregatory potency of prostacyclin. Prostaglandins, 14:1035 (1977).

45. G. Cohen, Lipid peroxidation: detection in vivo and in vitro through the formation of saturated hydrocarbon gases. In: Ciba Foundation Symposium 65 "Oxygen Free Radicals and Tissue Damage", Excerpta Medica, Amsterdam, Oxford, New York (1979).

46. J. Glavind, S. Hartman, J. Clemensen, K. E. Jessen and H. Dam, Studies on the rôle of lipid peroxides in human pathology. II. The presence of peroxidized lipids in the atherosclerotic aortas. Acta.Pathm.Microbiol. Scand., 30:1 (1952).

47. K. Fukuzumi, Lipids of atherosclerotic artery. The cause of atherosclerosis from the view point of fat chemistry. Fette. Seifen, Anstrichmittel, 11:953 (1969).

48. T. Hiramitsu, Y. Majima, Y. Hasegava, K. Hirata and K. Yaki, Lipidperoxide formation in the retina in ocular siderosis. Experientia, 32:1324 (1976).

49. W. S. Hartroft and E. A. Prta, Ceroid. Amer. J. Med. Sci., 250:324 (1965).

50. V. Angelo, M. Mysliwiec, M. B. Donati and G. Gaetano, Defective fibrinolytic and prostacyclin-like activity in human atheromateus plaques. Thrombos. Haemostas., 39:535 (1978).

51. M. Mysliwiec, S. Villa, G. de Gaetano and M. B. Donati, Decreased plasminogen activator (PA) but normal prostacyclin (PGI_2) activity in veins with experimental thrombosis. Thrombos. Haemostas., 42:7 (1979).

52. P. D. Vinocour, H. M. Groves, E. Dejana, R. L. Kinlough-Rathbone and F. J. Mustard, The effects of dietary fats in rabbits on platelet survival, platelet turnover, platelet density, PGI_2 production and thrombus formation in response to an aortic indwelling cannula. Thrombos. Haemostas., 42: 423 (1979).

53. J. L. Weihrauch, C. A. Brignoli, J. N. Reeves and L. Iverson, Fatty acid composition of margarines, processed fats and oils. Food Technol., 1:80 (1977).

54. S. Taura, M. Taura and F. A. Kummerow, Human arterio- and atherosclerosis; identical to that in 6 and 36 month old swine fed a corn soy diet free of cholesterol and saturated fat. Artery, 4:100 (1978).

55. R. B. Wilson, N. S. Kula, P. M. Newberne and M. W. Conner, Vascular damage and lipid peroxidation in choline-deficient rats. Exper. Molecul. Path., 18:357 (1973).

56. A. Dembinska-Kieć, W. Rücker, P. S. Schönhöfer, Atherosclerosis decreases prostacyclin synthesis in rabbit lungs and kidneys. Prostaglandins in press (1979).

57. A. Dembinska-Kieć, W. Rücker, P. S. Schönhöfer, Effects of dipyridamole in vivo on ATP and cAMP content in platelets and arterial walls and on atherosclerotic plaque formation. Naunyn-Schmiedeberg's Arch. Pharmacol., in press (1979).

58. A. Dembinska-Kieć, W. Rücker, P. S. Schönhöfer, Effects of dipyridamole in experimental atherosclerosis: Action of PGI_2, platelet aggregation and atherosclerotic plaque formation. Atherosclerosis, in press (1979).

59. H. Sinzinger, P. Clopath and K. Silberbauer, Increased prostacyclin generation in minipig vascular tissue after atherogenic diet. Thrombos. Haemostas., 42:424 (1979).

60. A. Szczeklik, R. J. Gryglewski, R. Nizankowski, J. Musial, R. Pieton and J. Mruk, Circulatory and anti-platelet effects of intravenous prostacyclin in healthy men. Pharmacol. Res. Commun., 10:545 (1978).

61. R. J. Gryglewski, A. Szczeklik and R. Nizankowski, Anti-platelet action of intravenous infusion of prostacyclin in man. Thrombos. Res., 13:153 (1978).

62. A. Szczeklik, R. Nizankowski, S. Skawinski, J. Szczeklik, P. Gluszko and R. J. Gryglewski, Successful therapy of advanced arteriosclerosis obliterans with prostacyclin. Lancet, 1:1111 (1979).

63. J. D. Coffman, Drug therapy; vasodilator drugs in peripheral vascular disease. New Engl. J. Med., 300:713 (1979).

64. A. G. Olsson and T. Jogestrand, Effects of prostaglandin E_1 in peripheral vascular disease. In: International Conference on Atherosclerosis, Milan 1977, L. A. Carlson, R. Paoletti, Siroti and G. Weber, eds., Raven Press, New York (1978).

65. F. Numano, Progression and regression of atherosclerosis. Asian Med. J., 20:625 (1977).

66. R. Ross, L. Harker, Hyperlipidemia and atherosclerosis. Science, 193:1094 (1976).

67. F. Numano, H. Maezawa, T. Shimamoto, K. Adachi, Changes of cyclic AMP and cyclic AMP phosphodiesterase in the progression and regression of experimental atherosclerosis. Ann. NY Acad. Sci., 275:311 (1976).

PROSTAGLANDIN MECHANISMS IN BLOOD PRESSURE

REGULATION AND HYPERTENSION

John C. McGiff, Eric G. Spokas and Patrick Y-K Wong

Departments of Pharmacology and Medicine
New York Medical College
Valhalla, New York 10595, U.S.A.

In 1970, three studies were published which provided the basis
for the proposal that prostaglandins are modulators of pressor
hormones and adrenergic nervous activity (1,2,3). In the first
two studies, infusion of either angiotensin II or norepinephrine
was shown to cause release of PGE-like material into renal venous
blood; the latter was associated with attenuation of the
vasoconstrictor and anti-diuretic actions of these pressor
hormones (1,2). In the third study, it was demonstrated that
within minutes after induction of unilateral renal ischemia,
prostaglandins were released into the venous blood of both kidneys.
Release from the contralateral kidney was mediated by angiotensin
II, which, presumably, also contributed to the release from the
ischemic kidney (3). This study offered an explanation for the antihypertensive function of the contralateral kidney in terms of a
possible prostaglandin mechanism. Thus, activation of the renin-
angiotensin system by renal ischemia can effect enhanced
prostaglandin production in the ischemic and contralateral kidneys.
A related study on the effects of norepinephrine infusion and
renal nerve stimulation on renal function (4) strongly supported
the proposal that renal prostaglandins act as a component of an intrarenal negative feedback control system which moderates anti-diuretic
and vasoconstrictor systems. Thus, norepinephrine, in contrast to
moderate intensity renal nerve stimulation, released prostaglandins
into the venous effluent of the kidney; restoration of renal blood
flow occurred only with norepinephrine and was associated with
release of prostaglandin-like material, identified tentatively
on the basis of its chromatographic properties as primarily PGE_2.
As this study was completed before the discovery of prostacyclin,
it is important to recognize that 6-keto-$PGF_{1\alpha}$, the hydrolysis
product of prostacyclin (PGI_2), would have been measured as PGE-like

235

material as it co-migrates with PGE_2 in the solvent system used
for separation of prostaglandins on thin-layer plates prior to
their assay. Further, this study should not be interpreted to
mean that renal nerve stimulation cannot release prostaglandins
from the kidney as such release has been demonstrated in response
to more intense nerve stimulation, particularly when renal
perfusion pressure is greatly increased (5).

Prostacyclin, discovered recently by Moncada, Gryglewski,
Bunting and Vane (6), is the most potent known inhibitor of
platelet aggregation; it also relaxes vascular smooth muscle.
PGI_2 is the principal arachidonic acid metabolite of blood vessels
and, unlike PGE_2, may act as a circulating hormone because it is
not removed from the blood on passage through the pumonary
circulation (7). The first study which suggested that a prostaglandin could function as a circulating hormone was published
more than 10 years ago; we demonstrated that PGA_2 was not
removed from the venous blood on passage across the lung (8).
However, PGA_2 has since been shown to be an artifact, arising from
PGE_2 during extraction and purification of blood (9). PGE_2 is
also an important product of arachidonic acid metabolism in blood
vessels in some blood vessels PGE_2 is produced in greater amounts
than prostacyclin (10). Further, PGE_2 appears to possess properties
required of a modulator of pressor hormones not possessed by
prostacyclin (11).

In all these studies, release of prostaglandins during
application of a pressor stimulus is associated with attenuation
of the vasoconstrictor action of the stimulus. These observations
suggest possibly links to the development of hypertenstion. A
generalized increase in vascular reactivity often precedes the
onset of hypertension in man; moreover, as the disease evolves,
there tends to be increased reactivity to pressor stimuli (12).
If one or more prostaglandins determine vascular reactivity,
limitation of their production or activity could contribute to
the evolution of hypertension. The participation of prostaglandins
in the regulation of vascular responsiveness relates to the
consideration of a prostaglandin mechanism which protects organ
function against excessive activity of pressor hormones and
contributes to the control of regional blood flows and, thereby,
the allocation of cardiac output. Presumably, in most organs the
prostaglandin system remains relatively dormant until challenged
(13).

ASPIRIN-LIKE DRUGS MAY CAUSE HYPERTENSION

Since increased vascular reactivity precedes the onset of
hypertension (12), the contribution of prostaglandins to changes
in vascular reactivity should be of importance to the pathogenesis
of hypertension. Specifically, if a deficiency in prostaglandin

production initiates or exaggerates hypertension, chronic administration of cyclo-oxygenase inhibitors should result in hypertension. An elevated blood pressure has not been reported in heavy users of non-steroidal anti-inflammatory agents. However, acute administration of indomethacin can produce hypertension in the anesthetized dog (14). The immediate hemodynamic effects of indomethacin in the anesthetized dog resemble those of uncomplicated essential hypertension: elevated blood pressure, unchanged cardiac output, marked increase in the vascular resistance of the kidneys and a smaller increase in the vascular resistance of the limbs (14). Nonetheless, most attempts to reproduce chronic hypertension with aspirin-like drugs have failed, probably because the dose was too small or they were not given for a long enough period.

In a recent study, administration of a non-steroidal anti-inflammatory drug to the conscious rabbit resulted in sustained elevation in blood pressure; it was several days before the full effect was evident (15). Thus, indomethacin, 15 mg/kg administered sub-cutaneously each day, caused elevation of the average mean arterial pressure in seven rabbits from 88 ± 3 mm Hg on the last day of the control period to 105 ± 3 mm Hg and 107 ± 2 mm Hg on the 6th and 14th day of indomethacin treatment, respectivley. Urinary excretion of a PGE-like substance was reduced when measured on days zero and twelve, respectively, from 1.06 ± 0.26 to 0.17 ± 0.05 nmol of PGE_2/day. The dose of indomethacin is critical as prostaglandin synthesis must be suppressed by more than 80% as evidenced by reduced urinary excretion of prostaglandins and decreased conversion of arachidonic acid to prostaglandins by renomedullary slices. This dose of indomethacin is lethal to the rat and produces severe toxicity in the dog. Indomethacin did not affect the intake of water, the 24 hour urine volume, the cumulative difference between sodium intake and urinary sodium excretion, or the plasma volume. The results of the study support the hypothesis that one or more prostaglandins act to maintain normotension by an effect(s) independent of changes in extracellular fluid volume.

ARACHIDONIC ACID METABOLISM IN VASCULAR TISSUES

The proposed role of prostaglandins as antihypertensive agents received important support with the demonstration of prostaglandin synthesis by blood vessels. The first study, based on biochemical evidence, to demonstrate synthesis of prostaglandins by blood vessels was reported in 1975 (16). In this study, radio-labelled arachidonic acid was shown to be transformed to prosta-glandins by these blood vessels. The principal product in blood vessels of enzymic transformation of the prostaglandin endoperoxides was later shown to be prostacyclin (17). Terragno et al. (18) have shown that all renal arteries, irrespective of size, are capable of transforming arachidonic acid to prostacyclin, primarily;

lesser amounts of PGE_2 and $PGF_{2\alpha}$ were generated by these arteries. Further, there is a naturally occurring inhibitor which modulates the rate of prostacyclin formation in the renal cortex. The role of this inhibitor in the regulation of renal vascular resistance and in the control of renin release by affecting prostaglandin formation within renal blood vessels is potentially important.

METABOLISM OF PROSTACYCLIN

Blood Vessels

The vascular wall is also an important source of the major prostaglandin catabolizing enzyme, 15-hydroxyprostaglandin dehydrogenase (19), which is a possible point of hormonal control. Wong et al. (20) were the first to show that prostacyclin metabolism can proceed via the 15-hydroxy dehydrogenase. Several important metabolites of prostacyclin have been identified in other tissues such as the liver and kidney. These metabolites must be considered in future studies directed towards measuring changes in prostacyclin release into the circulation.

As the activity of 15-hydroxyprostaglandin dehydrogenase has been shown to be high in both mesenteric arteries and veins, these vascular tissues were used to study metabolism of prostacyclin (20). The cytoplasmic fractions of bovine mesenteric arteries and veins were incubated with radiolabelled PGI_2 in the presence of cofactor, either NAD^+ or $NADP^+$. Prostacyclin was rapidly converted to a product identified as 6, 15-diketo $PGF_{1\alpha}$, by thin-layer chromatography and gas chromatography-mass spectrometry. The initial reaction rate began to level off after less than 1 minute of incubation at 37°C. When radiolabelled 6-keto-$PGF_{1\alpha}$ a stable hydrolysis product of PGI_2, was used as substrate under the same condition, 97% was recovered unmetabolized after 2 minutes of incubation. Catabolism of PGI_2 may be a major determinant of the levels in blood vessels and, therefore, may be important to regulating its vascular actions. Whether prostacyclin is released intact or metabolized may be determined by the ratio of reduced to oxidized pyridine nucleotides in the tissue. This study suggests that estimation of PGI_2 generation by a tissue may be misleading if only 6-keto-$PGF_{1\alpha}$ is measured.

Liver

We have recently obtained evidence that a potent metabolite of either prostacyclin or 6-keto-$PGF_{1\alpha}$ is generated in the rabbit isolated liver (21). A highly active and stable material, 6-keto-PGE_1, may be derived from the biologically inactive hydrolysis product of prostacyclin, 6-keto-PG $_{1\alpha}$. As prostacyclin is unstable, its conversion to a stable product, having similar biological potency, is of considerable importance. Thus, 6-keto-PGE$_1$ was found to be equally potent to PGI$_2$ as an inhibitor of platelet aggregation (22). PGI$_2$ may be transformed in the liver to 6-keto-PGE$_1$ via the 9-hydroxyprostaglandin dehydrogenase pathway (Fig. 1). Whether 6-keto-PGF$_{1\alpha}$ is an obligatory intermediate is unknown. The generation of 6-keto-PGE$_1$ from PGI$_2$ may explain the unexpectedly long duration of biological activity of PGI$_2$ observed in some studies.

We have also found that the cardiovascular properties of authentic 6-keto-PGE$_1$ are similar to those of PGI$_2$ (23). The hypotensive effect of 6-keto-PGE$_1$ is equipotent by either intra-aortic or intravenous administration suggesting that it, like PGI$_2$, escapes pulmonary metabolism. Another important similarity to PGI$_2$, which also distinguishes 6-keto-PGE$_1$ from other prostaglandins, is the capacity to lower vascular resistance in the rat kidney. These studies suggest that 6-keto-PGE$_1$ could be a circulating vasodilator hormone and may account for some of the in vivo effects of prostacyclin; 6-keto-PGE$_1$ could be more important than PGI$_2$ because of its greater stability at physiological pH.

PROSTAGLANDINS: PROHYPERTENSIVE IN THE RAT?

We have questioned the suitability of the rat as a model for investigating the role of vasodepressor systems in regulating blood pressure, as a principal renal prostaglandin,PGE$_2$, has been shown in the rat to augment the renal vasoconstrictor responses of the isolated perfused kidney to nerve stimulation and to constrict the renal vasculature (24). Under identical conditions in the isolated perfused kidney of the rabbit, PGE$_2$ inhibited adrenergic vasoconstriction and dilated blood vessels. The anomalous response of the isolated kidney of the rat to PGE$_2$ takes on greater significance in view of the more recent demonstration in studies conducted in vivo that PGE$_2$ constricts the renal vasculature of the rat, whereas prostacyclin (PGI$_2$) has a weak dilator effect in this vascular bed (25). Renal blood flow and systemic blood pressure were measured before and during infusion of PGE$_2$ (2-20 ug/min) or PGI$_2$ (1-5 ug/min) into the aorta just proximal to the renal arteries. Both prostaglandins significantly decreased blood pressure and renal blood flow, but had dissimilar effects on renal vascular resistance. At low doses, PGI$_2$ usually reduced renal vascular resistance, whereas PGE$_2$ increased it. PGI$_2$ was thought to be the only vasodilator prostaglandin in the rat kidney until the finding that 6-keto-PGE$_1$, the putative stable metabolite of PGI$_2$, could also lower vascular resistance in the rat kidney (23). In this species, infusion of PGI$_2$ did not alter GFR, urine composition or renal function (26). It should be emphasized that the renal vascular bed of the rat is relatively resistant to prostaglandins when compared to other species as dog and rabbit.

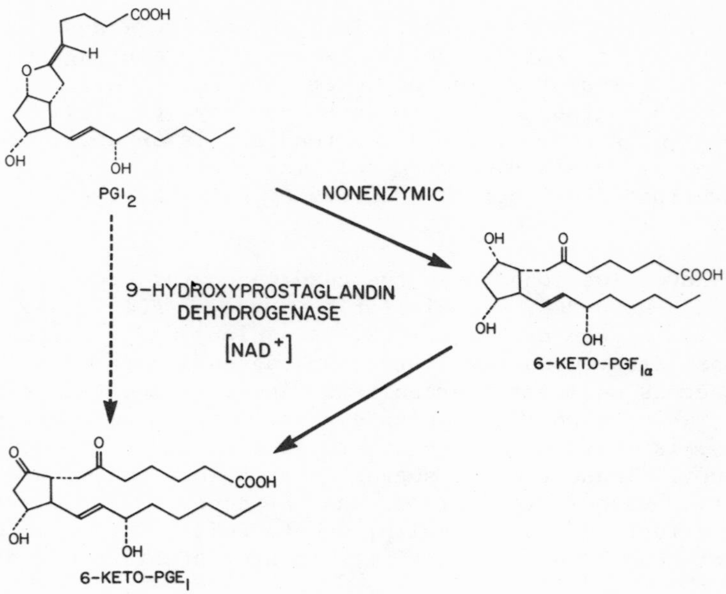

Fig. 1. Chemical structures of PGI$_2$, 6-keto PGF$_{1\alpha}$ and 6-keto
         PGE$_1$. Spontaneous hydrolysis of PGI$_2$ forms 6-keto PGF$_{1\alpha}$
         which differs from 6-keto PGE$_1$ in the substituent at
         C-9. The enzyme 9-hydroxyprostaglandin dehydrogenase
         is probably responsible for transforming the hydroxyl
         group to a ketone. Alternatively, 6-keto PGE$_1$ may be
         formed from PGI$_2$ through an unknown intermediary pathway.

     Renal prostaglandins could contribute to the development of
hypertension in the rat, as an increase in renal vascular resistance
produced by PGE$_2$ might be an initiating factor in the pathogenesis
of the disease. This hypothesis has received support from a study
in the New Zealand genetic hypertensive rat (27); a deficiency in
the principal prostaglandin catabolizing enzyme, 15-hydroxy-
dehydrogenase, has been shown. The latter, has been suggested
to result in elevated renal vascular resistance due to increased
levels of PGE$_2$ intrarenally. This was the first demonstration of
an abnormality in a prostaglandin catabolizing enzyme; it was
suggested to be the inherited abnormality primarily responsible
for the development of hypertension in this strain of genetically
hypertensive rat. An endogenous inhibitor of 15-hydroxyprosta-
glandin dehydrogenase has been recovered from the kidneys of the
New Zealand hypertensive rat (28), a finding which may account for
decreased activity of the enzyme. It should be noted that the
original conclusion resulting from the initial study (24), that
the rat may not be a suitable model for human hypertensive disease,
remains unchallenged.

A VASODEPRESSOR SYSTEM: KALLIKREIN-KININ-PROSTAGLANDIN

We first demonstrated that bradykinin evokes release of prostaglandins (29). This study is the basis for all subsequent studies linking some actions of kinins to prostaglandin mechanisms and provides the conceptual framework for a vasodepressor network present in the kidneys, vasculature and, very likely, in the central nervous system: the kallikrein-kinin-prostaglandin system. This major vasodepressor system can antagonize the effects of the blood pressure-elevating system, the adrenergic nervous-renin-angiotensin-aldosterone (30).

Excretion of kallikrein has been reported to be decreased in human and experimental forms of hypertension (31). There is experimental evidence linking the genesis of hypertension to a defect operating through kinin-prostaglandin interactions. In the first study, renal prostaglandin levels were shown to be dependent on the activity of the kallikrein-kinin system, as changes in renal kallikrein release were associated with corresponding changes in prostaglandin levels as reflected by excretion of prostaglandins (32). In the second study, cited previously, inhibition of prostaglandin synthesis by indomethacin caused a sustained elevation of blood pressure in the rabbit (15). Prostaglandin deficiency, secondary to decreased kallikrein release, therefore, could contribute to elevated blood pressure. Taken together, these studies urge consideration of the following working hypothesis: a deficiency in the renal kallikrein-kinin system contributes to the development of hypertension by decreasing the production of PGE_2 and, perhaps, PGI_2 which normally mediate an antihypertensive function (33).

Our understanding of the action of the converting enzyme inhibitor, captopril, must include a consideration of this vasodepressor system. Our work provides the basis for this extension (34,35). Captopril is thought to have antihypertensive effects related to preventing conversion of angiotensin I to angiotensin II (36); however, it also elevates the activity of the kallikrein-kinin and prostaglandin systems (37). Angiotensin converting enzyme, which is inhibited by captopril, is the same enzyme that degrades kinins (38). Thus, inhibition of converting enzyme increases the activity of the kallikrein-kinin system while depressing that of the renin-angiotensin system. A secondary effect of converting enzyme inhibition may be elevation of prostaglandin levels in tissues such as blood vessels and the tubules of the kidney. Therefore, the antihypertensive property of converting enzyme inhibitors may be related to augmentation of the activity of a major component of naturally occurring vasodepressor function, the kallikrein-kinin-prostaglandin system.

HYDRALAZINE

We have also obtained evidence that one of the antihypertensive
vasodilator agents, hydralazine, may act through enhanced release
of prostaglandins. In this study conducted in the anesthetized
dog, three doses of hydralazine, selected for their different
effects on renal blood flow, were infused into the renal artery
and changes in mean aortic blood pressure,renal blood flow and
concentration of PGE-like material in renal venous blood were
measured (Table 1). It is probable that the renal venous
concentration of PGE-like material referred to in Table 1 may
receive a substantial contribution from one or more products of
prostacyclin. This study shows a remarkable correlation between
the concentration of PGE-like material in renal venous blood, as
well as its rate of efflux from the kidney, and the renal
vasodilator response to hydralazine. Moreover, when high
concentrations of hydralazine were infused, causing decreased
renal blood flow, a marked reduction in the concentration and
efflux of PGE-like material occurred. Spokas and Wang have
reported that treatment of dogs with indomethacin prevents the
renal vasodilator action of hydralazine but not its dilator effects
in other regional vascular beds (39). These findings mandate that the
mechanism of action of vasodilator antihypertensive agents be re-
evaluated in terms of a possible prostaglandin mechanism.

CONCLUSIONS

Prostaglandins participate in the regulation of vascular
reactivity and blood pressure by opposing the vasoconstrictor and
antinatriuretic actions of pressor hormones, and by moderating
the release of norepinephrine from vasoconstrictor nerves. Blood
vessels synthesize prostaglandins intramurally, where their
local release influences vascular reactivity. PGI_2 and 6-keto-PGE_1,
unlike PGE_2, may be circulating hormones and may influence
vascular resistance of organs remote from sites of synthesis.
Prostaglandins not only attenuate the effects of vaso-constrictor
hormones but also amplify the effects of the kallikrein-kinin
system intrarenally and within the vasculature.

ACKNOWLEDGEMENT

This work was supported by the Heart, Lung and Blood Institute
of National Institutes of Health (grants HL-18845, HL-22075).

REFERENCES

1. J. C. McGiff, K. Crowshaw, N. A. Terragno and A. J. Lonigro:
    Renal Prostaglandins: Possible Regulators of the Renal Actions
    of Pressor Hormones. Nature, 227:1255-1257 (1970).

TABLE I

Hydralazine: Effects on Blood Pressure, Renal Blood Flow, Renovascular Resistance and Renal Venous PGE-like Material

	Control	Hydralazine Dose (intrarenally)		
		50 ug min^{-1}	500 ug min^{-1}	5000 ug min^{-1}
MABP (mm Hg)	95±3	93±3	88±5	94±4
RBF (ml min^{-1})	313±24	379±22	298±24	228±31
RVR (mm Hg ml^{-1}min^{-1})	0.31±0.03	0.25±0.01	0.30±0.02	0.44±0.05
"PGE" efflux (ng min^{-1})	36±11	60±16	46±9	9±5
"PGE" concentration (ng ml^{-1})	0.11±0.03	0.19±0.06	0.17±0.04	0.04±0.03

Hydralazine was infused into the renal artery of the anesthetized dog. Values are means ±SE.
MABP = mean aortic blood pressure; RBF = renal blood flow;
RVR = renal vascular resistance; "PGE" efflux = RBF x "PGE" concentration;
"PGE" concentration = determined in renal venous blood, measured as PGE$_2$ equivalents by bioassay.

2. J. C. McGiff, K. Crowshaw, N. A. Terragno and A. J. Lonigro:
    Release of a Prostaglandin-Like Substance into Renal Venous
    Blood in Response to Angiotensin II. Circ. Res., 26 and 27
    suppl.1:121-130 (1970).
3. J. C. McGiff, K. Crowshaw, N. A. Terragno, A. J. Lonigro, J. C.
    Strand, M. A. Williamson, J. B. Lee and K. K. F. Ng.:
    Prostaglandin-like Substances Appearing in Canine Renal Venous
    Blood During Renal Ischemia: Their Partial Characterization
    by Pharmacologic and Chromatographic Procedures. Circ. Res.,
    27:765-782 (1970).
4. J. C. McGiff, K. Crowshaw, N. A. Terragno, K. U. Malik and
    A. J. Lonigro: Differential Effect of Noradrenaline and
    Renal Nerve Stimulation on Vascular Resistance in the Dog
    Kidney and the Release of a Prostaglandin E-like Substance.
    Clin. Sci., 42:223-233 (1972).
5. E. W. Dunham and B. G. Zimmerman: Release of Prostaglandin-
    like Material from Dog Kidney during Renal Nerve Stimulation.
    Am. J. Physiol., 219:1279-1299 (1970).
6. S. Moncada, R. J. Gryglewski, S. Bunting an J. R. Vane: An
    Enzyme Isolated from Arteries Transforms Prostaglandin
    Endoperoxides to an Unstable Substance that Inhibits
    Platelet Aggregation. Nature, 263:663-666 (1976).
7. S. Moncada, R. Korbut, S. Bunting and J. R. Vane.: Prostacyclin
    is a Circulating Hormone. Nature, 273:767-768 (1978).
8. J. C. McGiff, N. A. Terragno, J. C. Strand, J. B. Lee, A. J.
    Lonigro and K. K. F. Ng.: Selective Passage of Prostaglandin
    Across the Lung. Nature, 223:742-745 (1969).
9. J. C. Frölich, B. J. Sweetman, K. Carr and J. A. Oates:
    Prostaglandin Synthesis in Rabbit Renal Medulla. Life Sci.,
    17:1105-1112 (1975).
10. N. A. Terragno, D. A. Terragno: Prostaglandin Metabolism in
    the Fetal and Maternal Vasculature, Fed. Proc., 38:75-77
    (1979).
11. A. G. Herman, T. J. Verbeuren, S. Moncada, J. R. Vane and P. M.
    Vanhoutte: Effect of Prostacyclin on Myogenic Activity and
    Adrenergic Neuroeffector Interaction in Isolated Canine Veins.
    Arch. Int. Pharmacodyn. Ther., 232:340-341 (1978).
12. A. E. Doyle and J. R. E. Fraser: Vascular Reactivity in
    Hypertension. Circ. Res., 9:755-761 (1961).
13. N. A. Terragno, D. A. Terragno and J. C. McGiff: Contribution
    of Prostaglandins to the Renal Circulation in Conscious,
    Anesthetized and Laparotomized Dogs. Circ. Res., 40,6:
    590-595 (1977).
14. A. J. Lonigro, H. D. Itskovitz, K. Crowshaw, and J. C. McGiff:
    Dependency of Renal Blood Flow on Prostaglandin Synthesis in
    the Dog. Circ. Res., 32:712-717 (1973).
15. J. Colina-Chourio, J. C. McGiff and A. Nasjletti: Effect of
    Indomethacin on Blood Pressure in the Normotensive
    Unanesthetized Rabbit: Possible Relation to Prostaglandin
    Synthesis Inhibition. Clin. Sci., 57:359-365 (1979).

16. D. A. Terragno, K. Crowshaw, N. A. Terragno and J. C. McGiff: Prostaglandin Synthesis by Bovine Mesenteric Arteries and Veins. Circ. Res., 36 and 37, suppl. 1:76-80 (1975).

17. S. Moncada, E. A. Higgs and J. R. Vane: Human Arterial and Venous Tissue Generate Prostacyclin (prostaglandin X), a Potent Inhibitor of Platelet aggregation. Lancet i:18-20 (1977).

18. N. A. Terragno, J. C. McGiff and D. A. Terragno: Synthesis of Prostaglandins by Vascular and Nonvascular Renal Tissues and the Presence of an Endogenous Prostaglandin Synthesis Inhibitor in the Cortex. In: Advances in Pharmacology and Therapeutics, Vol.4. Prostaglandins - Immunopharmacology, B. B. Vargaftig, ed., Pergamon Press, Oxford and New York (1979).

19. P. Y-K. Wong and J. C. McGiff: Detection of 15-hydroxy-prostaglandin dehydrogenase in Bovine Mesenteric Blood Vessels. Biochim. Biophys. Acta., 500:436-439 (1977).

20. P. Y-K. Wong, F. F. Sun and J. C. McGiff: Metabolism of Prostacyclin in Blood Vessels. J. Biol. Chem., 253, 16: 55-5557 (1978).

21. C. P. Quilley, J. C. McGiff, W. H. Lee, F.F. Sun and P. Y-K. Wong: 6-keto PGE_1, a Possible Metabolite of Prostacyclin: Cardiovascular and Platelet Anti-aggregatory Effects. Hypertension (In Press).

22. P. Y-K. Wong, J. C. McGiff, F. F. Sun and W. H. Lee: 6-keto Prostaglandin E_1 Inhibits the Aggregation of Human Platelets. Eur. J. Pharmacol. (In Press).

23. C. P. Quilley, P. Y-K. Wong and J. C. McGiff: Hypotensive and Renovascular Actions of 6-keto Prostaglandin E_1, a Metabolite of Prostacyclin. Eur. J. Pharmacol., 57:273-276 (1979).

24. K. U. Malik and J. C. McGiff: Modulation by Prostaglandin of Adrenergic Transmission in the Isolated Perfused Rabbit and Rat Kidney. Circ. Res., 36:599-609 (1975).

25. P. G. Baer and J. C. McGiff: Comparison of Effects of Prostaglandins E_2 and I_2 on Rat Renal Vascular Resistance. Eur. J. Pharmacol., 54:359-363 (1979).

26. P. B. Baer, M. L. Kauker and J. C. McGiff: Prostacyclin Effects on renal Hemodynamics and Excretory Functions in the Rat. J. Pharmacol. Exp. Therap., 208, 2:294-297 (1979).

27. J. M. Armstrong, G.J. Blackwell, R. J. Flower, J.C. McGiff, K. M. Mullane and J. R. Vane: Genetic Hypertension in Rats is Accompanied by a Defect in Renal Prostaglandin Catabolism. Nature, 260, 552:582-586 (1976).

28. P. Y-K. Wong, P. G. Baer and J. C. McGiff: Evidence for an Endogenous Inhibitor of 15-Hydroxyprostaglandin Dehydrogenase in New Zealand Genetically Hypertensive Rat Kidneys. Japanese Heart J., 20, suppl. 1:186-188 (1979).

29. J. C. McGiff, N. A. Terragno, K. U. Malik and A. J. Lonigro: Release of a Prostaglandin E-like Substance from Canine Kidney by Bradykinin. Circ. Res., 31:36-43 (1972).

30. J. C. McGiff and A. Nasjletti: Renal Prostaglandins and the
     Regulation of Blood Pressure. In: Prostaglandins and Cyclic
     AMP, Biologic Actions and Clinical Application, R. H. Kahn
     and W. E. M. Lands, eds., Academic Press Inc., New York and
     London (1973).

31. H. S. Margolius, R. Geller, W. de Jong, J. J. Pisano and
     A. Sjoerdsma: Urinary Kallikrein Excretion in Hypertension.
     Circ. Res., 31. suppl. 11: 125-131 (1972).

32. A.Nasjletti,J. C. McGiff and J. Colina-Chourio: Interrelations
     of the Renal Kallikrein-Kinin System and Renal Prostaglandins
     in the Conscious Rat. Circ. Res., 43, 5:799-807 (1978).

33. J. C. McGiff and A. Nasjletti: Kinins, Renal Function and
     Blood Pressure Regulation. Fed. Proc., 35:172-174 (1976).

34. A. Nasjletti, J. Colina-Chourio and J. C. McGiff: Disappearance
     of Bradykinin in the Renal Circulation of Dogs. Effects of
     Kininase Inhibition. Circ. Res., 37:59-65 (1975).

35. J. C. McGiff, H. D. Itskovitz and N. A. Terragno: The
     Actions of Bradykinin and Eledoisin in the Canine Isolated
     Kidney; Relationship to Prostaglandins. Clin. Sci. Mol.
     Med., 49:125-131 (1975).

36. M. A. Ondetti, B. Rubin and D. W. Cushman: Design of Specific
     Inhibitors of Angiotensin-Converting Enzyme: New Class of
     Orally Active Antihypertensive Agents. Science, 196:441-444
     (1977).

37. J. M. Vinci, D. Horwitz, R. M. Zusman, J. J. Pisano, K . J.
     Catt and H. R. Keiser: The Effect of Converting Enzyme
     Inhibition with SQ 20, 881 on Plasma and Urinary Kinins,
     Prostaglandin E, and Angiotensin II in Hypertensive Man.
     Hypertension, 1:416-426 (1979).

38. E. G. Erdös: The Kinins - A Status Report. Biochem.
     Pharmacol., 25:1563-1569 (1976).

39. E. G. Spokas and H. H. Wang: Regional Blood Flow and
     Cardiac Responses to Hydralazine. J. Pharmacol. Exp. Therap.
     (In Press),

PROSTAGLANDINS AND THE REGULATION OF RENIN RELEASE:

PROSTAGLANDINS AND THE REGULATION OF EXTRACELLULAR FLUID VOLUME

Peter C. Weber, Burkhard Scherer and Wolfgand Siess

Medizinische Klinik Innenstadt
University of Munich
Germany

Recent studies have brought about new insight in the inter-relationship between systemic and local hormones and the regulation of renal blood flow, glomerular filtration rate and the tubular handling of electrolytes. In discussing an interplay between two of these systems, namely the prostaglandin and the renin-angio-tensin systems, it is necessary to consider their respective local-izations within the kidney, factors causing their release and their intrarenal and systemic actions.

1. Formation of Prostaglandins in the Kidney

The kidney has a high capacity to synthesize prostaglandins. The formation of each of the different members of the prostaglandin (PG) family (PGE_2, PGD_2, $PGF_{2\alpha}$, PGI_2, TXA_2) has been demonstrated in the kidney, whereas PGA_2, previously thought to represent a circulating antihypertensive renal hormone arose artifactually from PGE_2 during analysis.

In the medulla and papilla there is a predominance of PG synthesis which is due mainly to the collecting ducts and to the interstitial cells. There is an appreciable rate of PG formation also in the kidney cortex (1) localized mainly in the vascular compartment. On the other hand, PG degradation and metabolism prevail in the kidney cortex. The main PG of the renal medulla and papilla is PGE_2, whereas 6-keto-$PGF_{1\alpha}$, the stable hydrolysis-product of PGI_2, predominates in the kidney cortex (2,3,4). In Table 1, the distribution of the different PG's in different zones of the normal rabbit kidney is shown.

In addition to the difference in the activity of the PG dehydrogenase between the kidney cortex (high activity) and the kidney medulla (low activity) (1) there is also a steep gradient for the enzyme PGE-9-ketoreductase which, in the rabbit kidney, shows highest activity in the kidney cortex (5). It seems, therefore, that the renal PG system is highly compartmentalized. As PG's act most probably as local hormones, this distribution of the PG system suggests different physiological functions of the cortical and medullary PG's.

In considering a connection between the renal PG's and renin within the cortex, it is important to point out that renal PG's could affect renal cortical function, by influencing renal vascular resistance and renin secretion. Due to the discovery of high PG formation in the renal medulla it was initially proposed that PG's, formed in the medulla, might be transported by several pathways such as tubular fluid or by lymphatics to the cortex where they could exert their actions. Although the renal cortex has a lower capacity than the medulla to produce PG's from arachidonic acid, recent studies make it more likely that PG production in the kidney cortex affects renal hemodynamics and renin secretion. In addition, whereas renal medullary PG's may operate mainly by modulating the effects of antidiuretic hormone and aldosterone in the distal tubule, thus acting in concert with the renin-angiotensin system to control sodium-, potassium-chloride and volume balance, renal cortical PG's may well affect distal tubular functions by their effects on renal blood flow.

2.   The Renin-Angiotensin System

2.1 The juxtaglomerular apparatus.

Renin is synthesized and stored in the epithelioid cells of the juxtaglomerular apparatus (JGA), a structure adjacent to the glomeruli, which are localized exclusively in the kidney cortex. The granular cells of the JGA are highly differentiated vascular smooth muscle cells within the media of the afferent arteriole as they contain both granules and myofibrils. They are in close proximity to the vascular endothelium and in intimate apposition to the macula densa (MD) cells. The latter are specialized cells of the distal tubule found at the juncture of the distal tubule with the afferent arteriole and the Goormaghtigh cells. Through these cells in the area formed by the MD and the afferent and the efferent arteriole the JG cells have anatomical connections to intraglomerular mesangial cells. There is also a dense network of adrenergic nerve endings around the JGA region

TABLE 1

Post mortem accumulation of prostaglandins (PG; µg/mg tissue) in different regions of the normal rabbit kidney. (Data from Larsson and Weber, 1978 and from Oliw, 1979). The measurements were performed with GC-MS.

	PGE_2	$PGF_{2\alpha}$	6-keto-$PGF_{1\alpha}$	TXB_2
Kidney cortex	0.4	0.4	1.4	not detectable
Kidney medulla	2.4	$3.7^{1)}$	2.1	0.2
Kidney papilla	4.2	0.4	3.5	0.2

1) outer medulla

2.2 The release of renin

The physiological consequences of release of the proteo-lytic enzyme renin from the granules within the JG cells result from a series of reactions. Renin cleaves from its substrate, angiotensinogen, the decapeptide-prohormone angiotensin I (A I) and its further reaction with the converting enzyme (or kininase II) which is concentrated in the vascular endothelium, generates the active octapeptide hormone angio-tensin II (A II). The major signals regulating synthesis and release of renin are extracellular volume, sympathetic nervous tone and the filling of the arterial tree. These signals operate through activation of one or more of three major mechanisms of renin release, the "baroreceptor", the adrenergic and the macula densa receptor.

3. Prostaglandins and the Regulation of Renin Release

Many of the experimental conditions known to be associated with an increase of renin secretion have also been shown to lead to the activation of renal PG formation. Thus, renal nerve stimulation and constriction of the renal artery have been shown to elicit a release of both, renin and PG's into the venous affluent.

Other factors which affect both, plasma renin activity (PRA) and renal venous or urinary PG's, are A II, bradykinin, catecholamines, potassium and loop diuretics. These observations can be taken as evidence of a connection between the PG and the renin angiotensin systems. It has been known since the studies of McGiff and coworkers (6) that angiotensin can release PGE-like compounds from the kidney, however, the converse, and effect of the renal PG system on renin secretion was not appreciated until the work of Larsson and coworkers (7), who demonstrated an increase of PRA following the infusion of the PG precursor, arachidonic acid, into the rabbit kidney.

Exogenous PG's as well as changes of intrarenal PG formation influence renin release, renal blood flow, sodium and volume excretion. Following arachidonic acid infusion, there is an increase of total renal blood flow, predominantly in the juxta-medullary cortex (8,9). Because of the complex interrelationship it is difficult to delineate the relative importance of PG's and renin in different functional states of the kidney. Whereas both hormonal systems seem to gain importance for the control of renal blood flow, glomerular filtration rate and systemic blood pressure with increasing deviation from control conditions, i.e. awake, undisturbed animal→sodium depletion→laparotomy, neither PG's nor the renin-angiotensin system seem to contribute to a major part to renal vascular resistance or renal blood flow autoregulation in the awake, salt replete animal (10). In unphysiological, or "stressed" conditions, blockade of PG formation will reduce and inhibition of the renin-angiotensin system will increase renal blood flow - with its consequences for sodium excretion - indicating the balancing influence of the two systems. It seems, therefore, that the kidney, by synthesizing PG's, increases renin secretion, but protects itself from the vasoconstrictor action of angiotensin, resulting from renin secretion in these conditions. These considerations and species differences in the renal effects of PG's (11) may explain some of the inconsistent results obtained following inhibition or stimulation of renal PG formation on renal blood flow and sodium-chloride excretion.

3.1 Exogenous PG's and renin release

Previous studies on the effects of exogenous PG's on renin secretion using systemic or intrarenal infusion of PGE_1, PGE_2, PGA_1 and PGA_2 gave inconsistent results (12 - 15). More recent studies by Yun et al. (16), Bolger et al. (17,18) and Gerber et al. (19) with intrarenal infusion of PGE_1, PGE_2, PGD_2, $PGF_{2\alpha}$ and PGI_2 also did not clarify which of the PG's and by which major mechanism that the PG's may be involved in renin secretion. All the PG's tested (with the exception of $PGF_{2\alpha}$) increased renin secretion from the kidney but showed different effects on renal plasma- or blood flow, glomerular filtration rate, sodium excretion and urinary volume. All together, these studies provide only information on the pharmacological effects of exogenous PG's on renin release. However, exogenous administration of one selected PG can not give relevant information on the physiological effects of endogenous PG's, and of the intermediary PG-endoperoxides formed and released within renal structures upon stimulation.

3.2   Stimulation of renal PG synthesis by arachidonic acid and renin release.

A more physiological way to study the consequences of increased intrarenal PG formation on kidney function and renin secretion is the infusion of the PG precursor arachidonic acid into the renal artery in doses which do not affect systemic hemodynamics or platelet aggregation. By this experimental design a spectrum of PG's and related compounds which is normally present will be produced at those sites in the kidney where the requisite enzymes and cofactors are available, i.e. at their physiological sites of action.

Intrarenal infusion of non-hypotensive doses of arachidonic acid in rabbits increased both PRA and urinary excretion of PG's (Figure 1). (7,8). Similar experiments were performed in rats where arachidonate increased PRA in both normally hydrated and volume-expanded rats (20). In the dog, Bolger et al. (21) found that arachidonic acid elevated PRA as well as sodium and water excretion. These studies have shown that activation of renal PG biosynthesis by using infusion of the PG precursor arachidonic acid elevates PRA. This interaction also occurs in the non-filtering kidney (22), indicating that renal tubular transport of PG's from the medulla to renal cortical sites is not a prerequisite for an effect of renal PG's on renin secretion.

3.3   Effects of PG's on renin release in vitro.

It was previously reported in a preliminary form that PGE_2 stimulates the release of renin from a suspension of rat renal cortical cells, while $PGF_{2\alpha}$ decreases renin release (23). In a later study, arachidonic acid, the natural PG endoperoxide PGG_2, and two synthetic, stable PG endoperoxide analogues stimulated the release of renin from rabbit renal cortical slices (24). PGE_2 had no effect, while $PGF_{2\alpha}$ inhibited renin release in a dose-dependent manner. Arachidonic acid was the most potent of the compounds studied, and increased renin

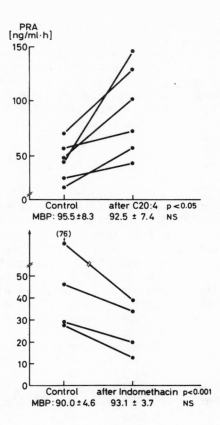

Fig. 1.   Effects of infusion of arachidonic acid (C20:4) (upper
          panel) into the renal artery and of indomethacin (lower
          panel) on plasma renin activity (PRA) in normal,
          anesthetized rabbits. Note, that there is no change of
          mean systemic blood pressure.

secretion about 4-fold. In all experiments in which there
was pretreatment with either indomethacin or eicosatetraynoic
acid (ETA), basal, as well as C20:4-stimulated renin release
was inhibited as compared to control (Figure 2). The results

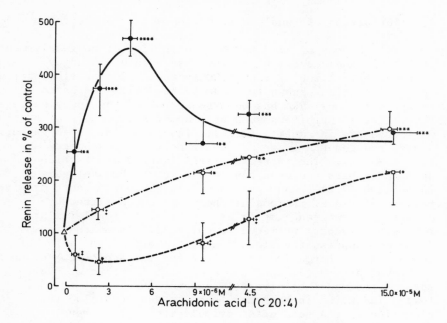

Fig. 2. Effects of various concentrations of arachidonic acid
alone (● ————— ●) and together with PG synthetase
inhibitors indomethacin (o–.–.–.o) and eicosa-5,8,11,
14-tetraynoic acid (ETA) (□----- □) on renin release in
per cent of control from slices of rabbit renal cortex.
Mean ± SE.

support the proposal that the increase of renin release seen
after stimulation of renal cortical PG synthesis is due to
the formation of PG endoperoxides from their precursor,
C20:4. The results further indicate that formation of $PGF_{2\alpha}$
inhibits renin secretion whereas the production of PGE_2
seems to have no direct effect on renin release in this in
vitro model. Because of the pronounced effect of C20:4 on
renin release in comparison to the very unstable natural PG
endoperoxides or the stable synthetic PG endoperoxide -
analogues a role of other PG endoperoxide-derived metabolites
on renin secretion, such as PGI_2 seems possible. Indeed,
recently it has been demonstrated that renal cortical formation
of PGI_2 may constitute one major pathway to increase renin
secretion (2,25). Taken together, these findings provide
strong evidence for an intrinsic role of the renal cortical
PG system in the mechanisms by which renin release is controlled.
Further support for the proposal connecting the PG and renin-
angiotensin systems comes from studies using PG synthesis
inhibitors.

3.4   Inhibition of renal PG formation and renin secretion.

In a number of studies the possibility of an involvement
of PG's in the secretion of renin has been explored by
pharmacological inhibition of PG synthesis in normal conditons
and in situations known to be associated with increased
renin secretion.   PRA has been found to be reduced by different
PG synthesis inhibitors such as indomethacin, aspirin and
meclofenamate in rabbits (7,26).   Indomethacin, in therapeutic
doses, reduced PRA in normal and hypertensive subjects
(27,28,29,30).   The increase of PRA induced by arachidonic
acid in rabbits and dogs can be blocked by PG synthesis
inhibition (7,21).   Another procedure, known to cause massive
release of renin, is renal ischemia produced either by
clamping of the renal arteries, or by acute renal failure
following glycerol or mercuric chloride.   Indomethacin was
found to suppress the elevation of PRA and accumulation of
intrarenal PG formation seen after the release of the clamp on
the renal artery (31) and to reduce the increase of PRA
seen in the model of glycerol-induced acute renal failure
(32).   Indomethacin has been found to suppress also the
elevation of PRA seen after stimulation of intrarenal
adrenergic receptors either in rabbits after bleeding or in
man after isoproterenol infusion or after orthostasis (33,
34) (Figure 3).

The involvement of different PG's with renin secretion
may be a direct one, due to direct stimulation of the
juxtaglomerular cells or, an indirect one due to an interaction of locally produced PG's with adrenergic transmission,
or the stretch or the tension of the wall of the afferent
arteriole.

4.   PG's and the Different Receptors for Renin Secretion

4.1   The adrenergic receptor.

An important receptor for renin release is the renal
adreno-receptor.   The sympathetic nervous system affects the
secretion of renin via the renal nerves and via circulating
catecholamines.   Sympathetic effects on renin secretion
appear to be mediated via both, β- and α-adrenergic receptors.
Stimulation of the β-receptor causes increased renin
secretion.   Renal vasoconstriction due to stimulation of
α-receptors (with a subsequent decrease of perfusion pressure
at the site of the afferent arteriole) could, indirectly,
increase renin secretion (consequent to the stimulation of
the baroreceptor- or the macula densa mechanisms); stimulation
of the α-receptor could also decrease renin secretion,
possibly by inhibiting the release of norepinephrine from

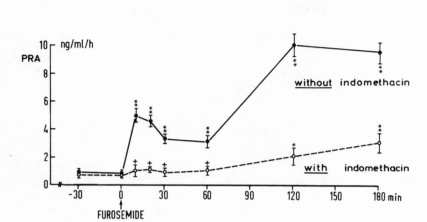

Fig. 3.   Time course of plasma renin activity (PRA) following 40
          mg furosemide i.v. at time zero in normal, male volunteers
          with (o ----- o) and without (●———●) pretreatment
          with indomethacin. Mean ± S.E. Note the complete
          suppression of the initial and the significant reduction
          of the later (at active orthostasis) increase of PRA by
          indomethacin.

renal sympathetic nerve endings and thereby decreasing β-
stimulation of renin secretion (for ref. 35). So far,
inhibition of PG synthesis has been shown to reduce the
increase of renin secretion following orthostasis or after
isoproterenol infusion, maneuvers assumed to increase renin
secretion via stimulation of renal adreno-receptors (33,34).
Since PG's are known to interfere with both, the release
of adrenergic neurotransmitters and with the vascular
response to catecholamines or nerve stimulation (36), it is
difficult, at present, to delineate the exact role of PG's
for this mechanism of renin secretion.

4.2   The baroreceptor mechanism.

     The receptor mechanism mediating renin release after
reduction of renal perfusion pressure is likely to be a
baroreceptor which signals to the juxtaglomerular granular
cells changes of stretch or tension of the wall of the
afferent arterioles (37). Reduction of perfusion pressure
or blood flow to the kidney is followed by the release of
both, renin and PG's. Recently, it was demonstrated in the

"non-filtering dog kidney" model, which included bilateral
adrenalectomy, renal denervation and continuous propranolol
infusion that a reduction of renal perfusion pressure
increased renal venous renin activity (22). Intrarenal
infusion of C20:4 increased and inhibition of PG synthesis
abolished both, the release of renin and the changes of
renal vascular resistance under these conditions, suggesting
an important contribution of renal cortical PG's on vascular
smooth muscle function (22,38). Since, in this model, there
is no transport of renomedullary PG's to the cortex and
since the macula densa- and the adrenergic mechansims for
renin release are interrupted, the results favour the concept
that PG's produced in cortical structures mediate renin
release following stimulation of the baroreceptor.

4.3   The interference of vascular and tubular mechanisms.

      Furosemide and similar loop diuretics cause a rapid
increase of renin release 10 to 15 minutes after i.v. injection
in animal or man. This is paralleled by a stimulation of renal
PG synthesis and by a decrease of renal vascular resistance
(39,40,26,34,41). Figure 3. PG synthesis inhibition abolishes
the elevation of renin secretion and the hemodynamic changes,
whereas sodium and water excretion are affected to a lesser
degree, or not at all (42,34). The concordance between the
increase of PRA, renal blood flow and urinary PG excretion
(Fig. 4) reflects most probably an increased synthesis of
PG's (34,41). The primary stimulus for the increase of PG
formation may be either furosemide-induced inhibition of
chloride transprot across the distal tubular cells at the site
of the macula densa, or a direct effect of furosemide on
vacular PG formation.

      Acute unilateral ureteral obstruction is associated with
an ipsilateral increase of renal blood flow and renin
secretion (43,44). The excretion of PG's in the obstructed
kidney is stimulated (45). PG synthesis inhbition prevents
the hyperemic response and the increased PG excretion in the
obstructed kidney and abolishes the elevation of PRA and
blood pressure all following ureteral obstruction. It is
assumed that, in this model, either changes in the pressure
gradients across vascular/tubular structures, or a diminished
electrolyte delivery in the distal tubule at the site of the
macula densa triggers renal PG formation with its consequences
for renal vascular resistance and renin secretion (46,47,3).

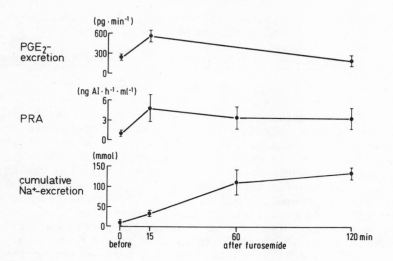

Fig. 4. Concordance between PGE_2 excretion and PRA after furosemide i.v. in man (Mean ± SE, n = 15). The subjects
remained in the supine position throughout the study.
Except for PRA at 60 and 120 min the values of each
parameter are significantly (p<0.05) different from the
preceeding one. Note that PRA and PGE_2 excretion have
declined again at 120 min after furosemide when cumulative
sodium excretion is still increasing.

Glomerular filtration rate is assumed to be partly controlled
by a feed-back system in which changes of (sodium)-chloride
concentration, -load or -uptake across the macula densa segment
of the distal tubule is processed in the juxtaglomerular
apparatus causing a change of glomerular arteriolar vasomotor
tone. As a result, glomerular filtration rate changes
inversely with loop of Henle flow rate. In micropuncture
experiments, inhibition of PG synthesis to about 10% of
control attenuates the feed-back response observed after
changes of loop of Henle flow rate (48). This diminution of
feed-back response can be restored by infusion of PGI_2 into
renal artery (49). The results suggest that PG's, possibly
PGI_2, may modify the juxtaglomerular feed-back system, either
directly or by mediating renin secretion, thereby participating
in the regulation of glomerular filtration rate.

Another possibility for renal PG's to influence
glomerular filtration rate might be an effect of the filtration
coefficient, either by affecting the filtration area of the
intraglomerular capillaries or by changing the permeability of
the filtration barriers (50). Such a mechanism seems

attractive since, very recently, the production of PG's
has been found in isolated glomeruli (51).

5.   Prostaglandins and the Regulation of Extracellular Volume

5.1 Sodium and potassium chloride balance.

The predominant role of the renin-angiotensin system is
to protect the body against losses of sodium-chloride and
water. Sodium-chloride depletion as well as low potassium-
chloride intake increases renin secretion and, thereby, the
formation of angiotensin. Angiotensin, and also a high
potassium-chloride intake exert a stimulatory effect on
aldosterone secretion which, by itself, stimulates sodium
retention and facilitates potassium excretion. An increasing
extracellular volume, as well as a high potassium intake
reduces renin secretion. It is therefore evident that, physio-
logically, a delicate balance exists between the mechanisms
which are involved in regulating sodium- and potassium-chloride
balance, and in controlling renin secretion and aldosterone
production.

The role of PG's in the regulation of sodium-chloride
excretion is a matter of controversy. A number of studies
indicate that renal PG's could have a natriuretic action
(52,53,21). Renal hemodynamic effects of PG's could reduce
tubular reabsorption and increase urinary excretion of
sodium. Other studies have indicated, however, an antinatriuretic role for the renal PG's (54,55).

In awake rabbits, a chronic increase of dietary NaCl
intake with free access to water induced a decrease of
urinary PG excretion (56,57,58)   (Table 2). In addition, the
pattern of PG excretion was altered: a marked reduction of
PGE_2 excretion was associated with either no decrease or a
minor decrease of $PGF_{2\alpha}$ excretion. The reduction of total
PG production in combination with a shift in the ratio of
PGE_2 to $PGF_{2\alpha}$ with a relative preponderance of $PGF_{2\alpha}$ at high
salt intake was proposed to be the result of a decrease of
PG synthesis in association with an increase of PGE_2-9-
ketoreductase activity in the kidney induced by high NaCl
intake (56)

Both, a reduction of PG synthesis as well as a relative
increase of $PGF_{2\alpha}$ formation have the potential to reduce
renin secretion. The reverse was found after low sodium-
chloride intake, e.g. an enhanced renal PG synthesis with a
predominant increase of PGE_2 excretion. These findings are
in accordance with the observation that restriction of sodium
intake leads to a relative increase of juxtamedullary blood

TABLE 2

Effect of chronic NaCl loading in rabbits on urinary
prostaglandin excretion (µg/day) (MEAN ± S.E.)

	Low NaCl	High NaCl	
PGE_2	1.9 ± 0.1	0.53 ± 0.17	Weber et al., 1977a
	1.5 ± 0.3	0.1 ± 0.04	Davila et al., 1978
$PGF_{2\alpha}$	2.1 ± 0.2	2.4 ± 0.3	Weber et al., 1977a
	3.4 ± 0.4	2.0 ± 0.5	Davila et al., 1978

flow (59), consistent with an increased renal PGE synthesis.
In addition, such salt intake-related changes in the formation
and metabolism of renal PG's, whether direct or subject
to the control by aldosterone, might be involved in modulating
the action of antidiuretic hormone at the distal tubule in
response to variations of NaCl intake.

In rats on their normal potassium and normal sodium
diet, PGE_2 excretion was found to be significantly higher
than $PGF_{2\alpha}$ excretion (60). High potassium-chloride intake
decreased the excretion of PGE_2 and increased that of $PGF_{2\alpha}$
and, by these effects, reversed the $PGE_2:PGF_{2\alpha}$ ratio.
Table 3.

The above mentioned findings together with results of
others obtained in hypokalemic man (61), or in dogs (62) are
evidence for the assumption that both, sodium-chloride as well
as potassium-chloride balance play a role in the renal
production of PG's. It seems that in conditions with a
high sodium-chloride intake the formation of PG's, predominantly
that of PGE_2 is decreased. In contrast, both, hypokalemia as
well as a low dietary sodium-chloride intake seem to stimulate
PG formation.

In addition, the demonstration of PG synthesis and of PGE
9-ketoreductase activity in vascular walls (63,64,65) opens
the possibility that such sodium-chloride or potassium-chloride
intake-related effects on PG production, if operating in

TABLE 3

Influence of Potassium Chloride Loading on Urinary
Prostaglandins in Rats (Mean ± SD)

	KCl NaCl (gm/100 gm food)		PGE_2 $PGF_{2\alpha}$ (ng/KG b.w./day)		ratio $\frac{PGE_2}{PGF_{2\alpha}}$
(n=7)	0.23	0.35	270 ± 65	180 ± 30	1:0.6
(n=7)	1.10	0.35	100 ± 35*	300 ± 45*	1:3.0*

*p<0.01 vs low KCl (0.23) intake

vascular smooth muscle cells,could explain, in part, the
dependence of vascular reactivity to pressor hormones like A
II or norepinephrine upon changes in sodium-chloride or
potassium-chloride balance (66,62,67).

5.2 PG-aldosterone interactions.

A II is an important stimulus for aldosterone production
in high renin states. A II stimulates also PG synthesis in
a variety of tissues. Therefore, an interaction of PG's with
the release and action of aldosterone may have physiological
importance. The involvement of PG's in the biosynthesis and
release of adrenocortical hormones has been studied by
several authors, but the results are contradictory. PGE
compounds have been found both to inhibit and to stimulate
aldosterone production from adrenals in vitro (68,69).
Basal aldosterone output in vitro was inhibited by the addition
of PG synthesis inhibitors.

Early observations in animals and in man demonstrated that
the natriuretic effects of the aldosterone antagonists,
spironolactone, was markedly antagonized by the concurrent
administration of aspirin (70,71). The effect of aspirin in
inhibiting the PG-cyclooxygenase was not known at that time.
It is, however, difficult to link this finding to the PG's in
a logical way at the present state of knowledge. Sodium
deprivation with high renin-angiotensin and aldosterone secretion
is associated with an enhancement in the urinary excretion of PG's
(56,58). This would suggest the possibility of an involvement
of PG's in the sodium conserving action of aldosterone.
This could explain that an aldosterone antagonist inhibits PG

formation. The antagonizing effect of aspirin on the
natriuretic effect of spironolactone could, however, be due
also to inhibition of the tubular secretion of spironolactone
rather than PG synthesis inhibition (72). Besides, many
non-steroidal anti-inflammatory drugs also have a substantial
mineral-ocorticoid activity, as shown in aldosterone receptor
assay (73).

The difficulty in establishing a clear concept about
the position and function of the PG system for the renin-
angiotensin-aldosterone-related control of sodium-chloride
balance and extra-cellular volume is further illustrated by
two recent studies in which indirect evidence is presented
for both, an inhibitory as well as a stimulatory effect of
aldosterone on the activity of phospholipase A, and hence PG
production (74,75).

6.   PG's and Renin in Essential Hypertension

In a number of patients with stable, uncomplicated essential
hypertension, PRA is suppressed (for ref. see 76). In addition, by
using maneuvers which normally either increase or decrease renin
secretion, a general unresponsiveness of renin release has been
documented in the majority of patients with essential hypertension
(77,78,79). Another common feature of patients with essential
hypertension is that an increase of renal vascular resistance
seems to correlate with a decrease of renin secretion (80.81).

The demonstration of a primary role of renal cortical PG's
in the release of renin, the finding of the pronounced vasoactive
properties of these compounds, and the possible involvement of
PG cyclo-oxygenase-derived products on the function of the
baroreceptor at the site of the juxtaglomerular apparatus points
to a defect in the synthesis and/or metabolism of locally produced
PG's as a possible denominator of both, the decrease in renin
secretion and the increase of renal vascular resistance in essential
hypertension (82). Furthermore, renin release, if studied under
defined conditions may be used as a marker of the intrinsic, PG-
related vasodilating capacity of the vasculature in the kidney
cortex (34,41). After furosemide, the initial increase of PRA and
of PGE_2 is significantly reduced in patients with essential hypertension as compared to controls,whereas $PGF_{2\alpha}$ formation is not different
(82,83) (Figure 5). Similar findings have been reported in two
other studies. Abe et al. (84) observed a reduced increase of PGE_2
excretion after furosemide in essential hypertensive patients, and
Tan et al. (85) found a reduction of 24-h-urinary PGE_2 excretion
in essential hypertensive patients, the reduction being most
pronounced in females with low-renin essential hypertension.

The results suggest that the reduced increase of renin release observed in essential hypertensive patients initially after furosemide is the result of reduced PG production at the site of, or near the renin producing structures. Although one cannot identify PGE_2 as the main responsible compound of the PG system which mediates renin secretion, it seems safe to conclude, that the reduction in its urinary excretion associated with unchanged $PGF_{2\alpha}$ formation immediately after furosemide reflects an impairment of renal PG formation. The defect in renal PG-synthesis and/or metabolism in patients with essential hypertension may include an alteration in the availability of the PG precursor arachidonic acid, a reduced formation of PG-endoperoxides or of PG-endoperoxide-derived compounds with renin stimulating (and vascular smooth muscle tone-reducing) activity or inadequate $PGF_{2\alpha}$ formation at reduced total PG production. Such alterations in the synthesis or metabolism of renal PG's are capable of diminishing renin secretion. In addition, such defects in PG formation will increase renal vascular resistance and decrease renal blood flow.

It could be that the reduction of PG formation and of renin secretion found in essential hypertensive patients reflects an impairment of kidney function, induced by chronically elevated blood pressure. However, observations in man and in genetically hypertensive (or hypertension-prone) rats strengthen the concept that impaired renal PG production and the unresponsiveness of renin secretion may occur in parallel at an early stage in the development of essential hypertension: (1) Suppression of PRA is observed in most strains of genetically hypertensive rats at a very early (some times prehypertensive) stage of the disease (86,87); (2) suppression of renin responsiveness has been documented in a number of normotensive (some years later hypertensive) offspring of hypertensive parents after a definite stimulus which normally increases renin secretion (88); (3) Ahnfelt-Rønne and Arrigoni-Martelli (89) have found an increased renal production of $PGF_{2\alpha}$ in young, genetically hypertensive rats; and (4) we have found in human neonates a positive correlation between urinary $PGF_{2\alpha}$ excretion and blood pressure (90).

In any case, if intact PG synthesis in the kidney cortex is an essential step for the renin release mechanism, a low, or an unresponsive PRA (whether due to genetic or to environmental factors, e.g. high NaCl-intake) in turn, should reflect a reduction of PG formation. The beneficial effects of diuretics for blood pressure control in patients with low-renin essential hypertension, may depend on their potency to increase the production of PG's either directly, or secondarily to the decrease of extracellular volume. Finally, a primary prevention of essential hypertension by a reduction of sodium-chloride intake may well operate, in part, through a PG-related mechanism, in the kidney as well as in the blood vessel wall.

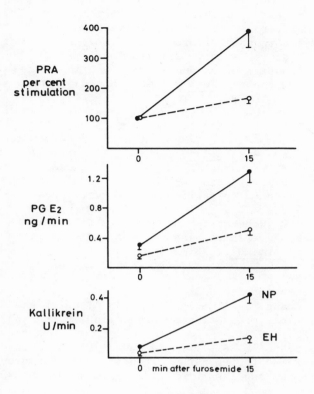

Fig. 5.   Reduced increase of plasma renin activity (PRA)
(upper panel), of urinary PGE_2 (middle panel) and of
kallikrein excretion (lower panel) after furosemide in
essential hypertensive patients (EH; (o ----- o);
n = 35, Mean ± S.E.) as compared to normotensive
controls (NP; (●——— ●); n = 22).

Acknowledgement

This study was supported by the Deutsche Forschungsgemeinschaft
We 681/4.   S. Havenstein helped in preparing the manuscript.

REFERENCES

1.   C. Larsson and E. Änggard, Regional differences in the
formation and metabolism of prostaglandins in the rabbit
kidney, Europ. J. Pharmacol., 21: 30-36 (1973).

2. A. R. Whorton, M. Smigel, J. A. Oates and J. C. Frölich,
    Regional differences in prostacyclin formation by the kidney:
    Prostacyclin is a major prostaglandin of renal cortex,
    Biochim. Biophys. Acta., 529: 176-180 (1978).
3. E. Oliw, Prostaglandins and kidney function. An experimental
    study in the rabbit, Acta Physiol. Scand., Suppl. 461: 7-55
    (1979).
4. C. Larsson and P. C. Weber, Renal prostaglandins an renin
    release, Acta Biol. Med. Germ., 37: 857-862 (1978).
5. K. J. Stone and M. Hart, Prostaglandin-E$_2$-9-ketoreductase in
    rabbit kidney, Prostaglandins, 10: 273-288 (1975).
6. J. McGiff, K. Crowshaw, N. A. Terragno and A. J. Lonigro,
    Release of a prostaglandin-like substance into renal venous
    blood in response to angiotensin II, Circ. Res., 27, Suppl. I:
    121-131 (1970).
7. C. Larsson, P. Weber and E. Änggård, Arachidonic increases and
    indomethacin decreases plasma renin activity in the rabbit,
    Europ. J. Pharmacol., 28: 391-394 (1974).
8. C. Larsson and E. Änggård, Increased juxtamedullary blood flow
    on stimulation of intrarenal prostaglandin biosynthesis,
    Europ. J. Pharmacol., 25: 326-334 (1974).
9. L. C. T. Chang, J. A. Splawinski, J. A. Oates and A. S. Nies,
    Enhanced renal prostaglandin production in the dog, Circ. Res.,
    36: 204-207 (1975).
10. N. A. Terragno, D. A. Terragno and J. McGiff, Contribution of
    prostaglandins to the renal circulation in conscious,
    anesthetized, and laparotomized dogs, Circ. Res., 40: 590-595
    (1977).
11. K. U. Malik, Prostaglandins - modulation of adrenergic nervous
    system, Fed. Proc., 37: 203-207 (1978).
12. A. J. Vander, Direct effects of prostaglandin on renal function
    and renin release in anesthetized dog, Am. J. Physiol., 214:
    218-221 (1968).
13. C. Werning, W. Vetter, P. Weidmann, H. U. Schweikert, D.
    Stiel and W. Siegenthaler, Effect of prostaglandin E$_1$ on
    renin in the dog, Am. J. Physiol., 220: 852-856 (1971).
14. M. P. Fichman, G. Littenburg, G. Brooker and R. Horton,
    Effect of prostaglandin A$_1$ on renal and adrenal function in
    man, Circ. Res., 30-31, Suppl. II: 19-35 (1972).
15. A. Hornych, N. Safar, N. Papanicolaou, P. Meyer and P.
    Milliez, Renal and cardiovascular effects of prostaglandin A$_2$
    in hypertensive patients, Europ. J. Clin. Invest., 3: 391-398
16. J. C. H. Yun, G. D. Kelly, F. C. Bartter and G. W. Smith II,
    Role of prostaglandins in the control of renin secretion in the
    dog (II), Life Sciences, 23: 945-952.
17. P. M. Bolger, G. M. Eisner, P. W. Ramwell and L. M. Slotkoff,
    Renal actions of prostacyclin, Nature, 271: 467-469 (1978).

18. P. M. Bolger, G. M. Eisner, P. Terez Shea, P. W. Ramwell and
L. M. Slotkoff, Effects of PGD_2 on canine renal functions,
Nature, 267:628-630 (1977).

19. J. G. Gerber, A. S. Nies, G. C. Friesinger, J. F. Gerkens,
R. A. Branch, and J. A. Oates, The effect of PGI_2 on canine
renal function and hemodynamics, Prostaglandins, 16: 519-528
(1978).

20. P. Weber, H. Holzgreve, R. Stephan, and R. Herbst, Plasma
renin activity and renal sodium and water excretion following
infusion of arachidonic acid in rats, Europ. J. Pharmacol.,
34: 299-304 (1975).

21. P. M. Bolger, G. M. Eisner, P. W. Ramwell and L. M. Slotkoff,
Effect of prostaglandin synthesis on renal function and renin
in the dog, Nature, 259: 244-245 (1976).

22. J. L. Data, J. G. Gerber, W. J. Crump, J. C. Frölich, J. W.
Hollifield and A. S. Nies, The prostaglandin system. A
role in canine baroreceptor control of renin release. Circ. Res.,
42: 454-458 (1978).

23. M. E. Dew and A. M. Michelakis, Effect of prostaglandins on
renin release in vitro, Pharmacologist, 16: 198A (1974).

24. P. C. Weber, C. Larsson, E.Änggard, M. Hamberg, E. J. Corey,
K. C. Nicolaou and B. Samuelsson, Stimulation of renin release
from rabbit renal cortex by arachidonic acid and prostaglandin
endoperoxides, Circ. Res., 39: 868-874 (1976).

25. A. R. Whorton, K. Misono, J. Hollifield, J. C. Frölich, T.
Inagani and J. A. Oates, Prostaglandins and renin release:
I. Stimulation of renin release from rabbit renal cortical
slices by PGI_2, Prostaglandins, 14: 1095-1104 (1977).

26. J. C. Romero, C. L. Dunlap and C. G. Strong, The effect of
indomethacin and other anti-inflammatory drugs on the renin-
angiotensin system, J. Clin. Invest., 58: 282-288 (1976).

27. K. W. Rumpf, S. Frenzel, H. D. Lowitz and F. Scheler, The
effect of indomethacin on plasma renin activity in man under
normal conditions and after stimulation of the renin-
angiotensin system, Prostaglandins, 10: 641-647 (1975).

28. R. V. Patak, B. K. Mookerje, C. J. Bentzel, P. E. Hysert,
M. Babej ,and J. B. Lee, Antagonism of the effects of furosemide
by indomethacin in normal and hypertensive man, Prostaglandins,
10: 649-659 (1975).

29. A. J. M. Donker, L. Arisz, J. R. H. Brentjens, G. K. van der
Hem and H. J. G. Hollemans, The effect of indomethacin on
kidney function and plasma renin activity in man, Nephron.,
17: 288-296 (1976).

30. J. C. Frölich, J. W. Hollifield, J. C. Dormois, B. L. Frölich,
H. Seyberth, A. M. Michelakis, J. A. Oates, Suppression of
plasma renin activity by indomethacin in man, Circ. Res.,
39: 447-452 (1976).

31. C. Larsson, P. Weber and E. Änggard, Stimulation and inhibition of renal PG biosynthesis: Effects on renal blood flow and on plasma renin activity, Acta. Biol. Med. Germ., 35: 1195-1200 (1976).

32. V. E. Torres, C. G. Strong, J. C. Romero and D. M. Wilson, Indomethacin enhancement of glycerol-induced acute renal failure in rabbits, Kidney International, 7: 170-178 (1975).

33. J. C. Frölich, J. W. Hollifield and J. A. Oates, Effect of indomethacin on isoproterenol induced renin release, Clin. Res., 24: 9 A (1976).

34. P. C. Weber, B. Scherer and C. Larsson, Increase of free arachidonic acid by furosemide in man as the cause of prostaglandin and renin release, Europ. J. Pharmacol., 41: 329-332 (1977).

35. A. Reid, B. J. Morris and W. F. Ganong, The renin-angiotensin system, Ann. Rev. Physiol., 40: 377-410 (1978).

36. P. Hedquist, Prostaglandin action on transmitter release at adrenergic neuroeffector junctions, In: "Advances in Prostaglandin and Thromboxane Research", Vol. I: 357-363, Raven Press, New York (1976).

37. L. Tobian, A. Tomboulian and J. Janecek, Effect of high perfusion pressures on the granulation of juxtaglomerular cells in an isolated kidney, J. Clin. Invest., 3ß: 605-610 (1959).

38. J. G. Gerber, J. L. Data and A. S. Nies, Enhanced renal prostaglandin production in the dog. The effect of sodium arachidonate in nonfiltering kidney, Circ. Res., 42: 43-45 (1978).

39. H. E. Williamson, W. A. Bourland, G. R. Marchand, D. B. Farley and D. E. van Orden, Furosemide induced release of prostaglandin E to increase renal blood flow, Proc. Soc. Exptl. Biol. Med., 150: 104-106 (1975).

40. U. B. Olsen and I. Ahnfelt-Rønne, Bumetanide induced increase of renal blood flow in conscious dogs and its relation to local renal hormones (PGE, kallikrein and renin), Acta Pharmacol. et Toxicol., 38: 219-228 (1976).

41. B. Scherer and P. C. Weber, Time-dependent changes in prostaglandin excretion in response to frusemide in man, Clin. Sci., 56: 77-81 (1979).

42. M. D. Bailie, J. A. Barbour and J. B. Hook, Effect of indomethacin on furosemide-induced changes in renal blood flow, Proc. Soc. Exptl. Biol. Med., 148: 1173-1176 (1975).

43. A. J. Vander and R. Miller, Control of renin secretion in the anesthetized dog, Am. J. Physiol., 207: 537-546 (1964).

44. E. D. Vaughan Jr., J. H. Shenasky II and J. Y. Gillenwater, Mechanism of acute hemodynamic response to ureteral occlusion, Inv. Urol., 9: 109-114 (1971).

45. P. Cadnapaphornchai, G. Aisenbrey, K. M. McDonald, T. J.
     Burke and R. W. Schrier, Prostaglandin-mediated hyperemia and
     renin-dediated hypertension during acute ureteral obstruction,
     Prostaglandins, 16: 965-971 (1978).
46. I. Eide, E. Løyning, Ø. Langard and F. Kiil, Mechanism of
     renin release during acute ureteral constriction in dogs,
     Circ. Res., 40: 293-299 (1977).
47. U. B. Olsen, The effect of ureteral occlusion and renal venous
     constriction on kidney kallikrein-kinin and prostaglandin
     systems in dogs, Acta Physiol. Scand., 104: 443-452 (1978).
48. J. Schnermann, G. Schubert, M. Hermle, R. Herbst, N. T. Stowe,
     S. Yarimizu and P. C. Weber, The effect of inhibition of
     prostaglandin synthesis on tubuloglomerular feedback in the
     rat kidney, Pflügers Archiv., 379: 269-279 (1979).
49. J. Schnermann and P. C. Weber, A role of renal cortical prosta-
     glandins in the control of glomerular filtration rate
     in rat kidneys, International Conference on Prostaglandins,
     Washington, D.C. In: Advances in Prostaglandin and Thromboxane
     Research", Vol. 7:1047-1052, Raven Press, New York (1980).
50. Ch. Baylis and B. M. Brenner, Modulation by prostaglandin
     synthesis inhibitors of the action of exogenous angiotensin
     II on glomerular ultrafiltration in the rat, Circ. Res.,
     43: 889-898 (1978).
51. V. W. Folkert and D. Schlöndorff, Prostaglandin synthesis in
     isolated glomeruli, Prostaglandins, 17: 79-86 (1979).
52. J. B. Lee, R. V. Patak and B. K. Mookerje, Renal prostaglandins
     and the regulation of blood pressure and sodium and water
     homeostasis, Am. J. Med., 60: 798-816 (1976).
53. J. Tannenbaum, J. A. Splawinski, J. A. Oates and A. S. Nies,
     Enhanced renal prostaglandin production in the dog, I.
     Effects on renal function, Circ. Res., 36: 197-203 (1975).
54. L. Tobian, M. O'Donnel and P. Smith, Intrarenal prostaglandin
     levels during normal and high sodium intake, Circ. Res., Suppl.
     1: 34/35: 83-89 (1974).
55. M. A. Kirschenbaum and J. H. Stein, The effect of inhibition
     of prostaglandin synthesis on urinary sodium excretion in the
     conscious dog, J. Clin. Invest., 57: 517-521 (1976).
56. P. C. Weber, C. Larsson and B. Scherer, Prostaglandin E_2-9-
     ketoreductase as a mediator of salt intake-related prosta-
     glandin-renin interaction, Nature, 266: 65-66 (1977).
57. B. Scherer, W. Siess and P. C. Weber, Radioimmunological and
     biological measurement of prostaglandins in rabbit urine:
     Decrease of PGE_2 excretion at high NaCl intake, Prostaglandins,
     13: 1127-1139 (1977).
58. D. Davila, T. Davila, E. Oliw and E. Änggard, The influence of
     dietary sodium on urinary prostaglandin excretion, Acta.
     Physiol. Scand., 103: 100-106 (1978).

59. N. K. Hollenberg, M. Epstein, R. D. Guttmann, M. Conroy,
     R. I. Basch and J. P. Merrill, Effect of sodium balance on
     intrarenal distribution of blood flow in normal man, J. Appl.
     Physiol., 28: 312-317 (1970).
60. P. C. Weber, B. Scherer and J. Schnermann, Effect of sodium and
     potassium chloride loading on urinary prostaglandin excretion
     in the rat, Clin. Res., 26: 478 A (1978).
61. J. R. Gill, J. C. Frölich, R. E. Bowden, A. A. Taylor, H. R.
     Keiser, H. W. Seyberth, J. A. Oates and F. C. Bartter,
     Bartter's syndrome: A disorder characterized by high urinary
     prostaglandins and a dependence of hyperreninemia on
     prostaglandin synthesis. Am. J. Med., 161: 43-51 (1976).
62. O. G. Galvez, W. H. Bay, B. W. Roberts and T. F. Ferris,
     The hemodynamic effects of potassium deficiency in the dog,
     Circ. Res., 40 (Suppl. 2): 11-16 (1977).
63. M. A. Gimbrone Jr. and R. W. Alexander, Angiotensin II
     stimulation of prostaglandin production in cultured human
     vascular endothelium, Science, 189: 219-220 (1975).
64. P. Y.-K. Wong, D. A. Terragno, N. A. Terragno and J. C. McGiff,
     Dual effects of bradykinin on prostaglandin metabolism:
     Relationship to the dissimilar vascular actions of kinins,
     Prostaglandins, 13: 1113-1125 (1977).
65. C. L. Limas, Selective stimulation of venous prostaglandin
     E-9-ketoreductase by bradykinin, Biochim. Biophys. Acta.,
     498: 306-315 (1977).
66. G. J. Strewler, K. J. Hinrichs, L. R. Guiod and N. K. Hollenberg,
     Sodium intake and vascular smooth muscle responsiveness to
     norepinephrine and angiotensin in the rabbit, Circ. Res.,
     31: 758-765 (1972).
67. A. B. Silverberg, P. A. Mennes and P. E. Cryer, Resistance to
     endogenous norepinephrine in Bartter's syndrome, Am. J. Med.,
     64: 231-235 (1978).
68. K. V. Honn and W. Chavin, Role of prostaglandins in aldosterone
     production by the human adrenal, Biochem. Biophys. Res. Comm.,
     72: 1319-1326 (1976).
69. T. Saruta and N. M. Kaplan, Adrenocortical steroidogenesis:
     The effect of prostaglandins, J. Clin. Invest., 51:
     2246-2251 (1972).
70. H. C. Elliot, Reduced adrenocortical steroid excretion rates
     in man following aspirin administration, Metabolism, 11:
     1015-1018 (1962).
71. M. G. Tweeddale and R. J. Ogilvic, Antagonism of spironolactone-
     induced natriuresis by aspirin in man, New Engl. J. Med.,
     26: 198-200 (1973).
72. L. E. Ramsey, I. R. Harrison, J. R. Shelton and C. W. Vose,
     Influence of acetylsalycic acid on the renal handling of
     spironolactone metabolite in healthy subjects, Europ. J. Clin.
     Pharmacol., 10: 43-48 (1976).

73. D. Feldman and C. Couropmitree, Intrinsic mineralocorticoid agonist activity of some non-steroidal anti-inflammatory drugs, J. Clin. Invest., 57: 1-7 (1976).

74. R. M. Zusman, H. R. Keiser and J. S. Handler, Effect of adrenal steroids on vasopressin-stimulated PGE synthesis and water flow, Am. J. Physiol., 234(6), F 532-F 540 (1978).

75. T. Yorio and P. J. Bentley, Phospholipase A and the mechanism of action of aldosterone, Nature, 271: 79-81 (1978).

76. M. J. Dunn and R. L. Tannen, Low-renin hypertension, Kidney International, 5: 317-325 (1974).

77. P. L. Padfield, M. E. M. Allison, J. J. Brown, A. F. Lever, R. G. Luke, C. C. Robertson, J. I. S. Robertson and M. Tree, Effect of intravenous frusemide on plasma renin concentration: Suppression of response in hypertension, Clin. Sci. Mol. Med., 49: 353-358 (1975).

78. G. W. Thomas, J. G. G. Ledingham, L. J. Beilin, A. N. Stott and K. M. Yeates, Reduced renin activity in essential hypertension: A reappraisal, Kidney International, 13: 513-518 (1978).

79. M. L. Tuck, G. H. Williams, R. G. Dluhy, M. Greenfield and T. J. Moore, A delayed suppression of the renin-aldosterone axis following saline infusion in human hypertension. Circ. Res., 39: 711-717 (1976).

80. M. A. D. H. Schalekamp, M. P. A. Schalekamp-Kuyken and W. H. Birkenhäger, Abnormal renal haemodynamics and renin suppression in hypertensive patients, Clin. Sci., 38: 101-110 (1970).

81. D. B. Case, W. J. Casarella, J. H. Laragh, D. L. Fowler and P. M. Cannon, Renal cortical blood flow and angiography in low- and normal-renin essential hypertension, Kidney International, 13: 236-244 (1978).

82. P. C. Weber, B. Scherer, H.-H. Lange, E. Held and J. Schnermann, Renal prostaglandins and renin release: Relationship to regulation of electrolyte excretion and blood pressure, Proc. VIIth Intern. Congr. of Nephrology, Montreal, pp.99-106, Karger, Basel (1978).

83. P. C. Weber, B. Scherer, E. Held and W. Siess, Reduction of renal prostaglandin formation in essential hypertension, International Conference on Prostaglandins, Washington, D.C., In: "Advances in Prostaglandin and Thromboxane Research", Vol. 7: 1145-1148, Raven Press, New York (1980).

84. K. Abe, M. Yasujima, S. Chiba, N. Irokawa, T. Ito and K. Yoshinaga, Effect of furosemide on urinary excretion of prostaglandin E in normal volunteers and patients with essential hypertension, Prostaglandins, 14: 513-521 (1977).

85. S. Y. Tan, P. Sweet and P. J. Mulrow, Impaired renal production of prostaglandin E_2: A newly identified lesion in human essential hypertension, Prostaglandins, 15: 139-149 (1978).

86. J. Iwai, L. K. Dahl and K. D. Knudsen, Genetic influence on the renin-angiotensin system, Circ. Res., 32: 678-684 (1973).

87. G. Bianchi, P. G. Baer, U. Fox, L. Duzzi, D. Pagetti and
     A. M. Giovannetti, Changes in renin, water balance, and sodium
     balance during development of high blood pressure in genetically
     hypertensive rats, Circ. Res., 36-37: Suppl. 1, 153-161
     (1975).
88. A. F. Fasola, B. L. Martz and O. M. Helmer, Plasma renin
     activity during supine exercise in offspring of hypertensive
     parents, J. Appl. Physiol., 25: 410-415 (1968).
89. I. Ahnfelt-Rønne and E. Arrigoni-Martelli, Increased $PGF_{2\alpha}$
     synthesis in renal papilla of spontaneously hypertensive
     rats, Biochem. Pharmacol., 27: 2363-2367 (1978).
90. B. Scherer and P. C. Weber, Urinary prostaglandins (PG)
     in the newborn: Relationship to U_{osm}, U_{K^+} and blood pressure,
     International Conference on Prostaglandins, Washington, D.C.
     In: "Advances in Prostaglandin and Thromboxane Research",
     Vols. 6, 7 (1980) Raven Press, in press.

GENDER DIFFERENCES IN THE EFFECT OF ARACHIDONATE METABOLITES

P. W. Ramwell, J. W. Karanian, F. Maggi and E. R. Ramey

Department of Physiology and Biophysics
Georgetown University Medical Center
Washington, DC 20007

INTRODUCTION

The arachidonate metabolites not only constitute a large class of endogenous substances of high biological activity but they also possess powerful thrombogenic and anti-thrombogenic properties. The greater morbidity and mortality from cardiovascular disease of men as compared to women is well established. Thus, sex differences may be related to gender differentiation among the arachidonate metabolites (1). In this paper we briefly review the current situation.

TISSUE SOURCES

The free arachidonate concentration in the human is low (3 µg/ml) and independent of the total FFA level (2). The feeding of ethyl arachidonate to men for 2 to 3 weeks increased the percentage of arachidonate in the triglycerides, phospholipids, and cholesterol esters but not the plasma-free arachidonate. In humans at rest the fractional turnover rate of arachidonate is higher (50%) than that of oleate, but during exercise the arterial concentration and turnover rate of arachidonate did not change while the arterial concentration of oleate decreased 10% and the fractional turnover rate increased 90%. No significant net transport of arachidonate could be detected between muscle tissue, lungs, the kidney and the liver (3). Interestingly, the fractional turnover rate on a weight basis (4) was higher (40%) for women although the arterial concentrations of arachidonate were not significantly different in contrast to animals where the female plasma arachidonate is significantly higher than the male. Probably little arachidonic acid is metabolized by β oxidation, chain elongation

271

or autoxidation.   Incorporation into the phospholipid, triglyceride and cholesterol esters occurs but the main catabolic route may be via peroxidation and endoperoxidation.

Significance of Arachidonic Acid

The question arises as to the initiating role of arachidonic acid in pathophysiology. Prostaglandins do not appear to be stored. Increased prostaglandin release which occurs in many situations, is a reflection of prior arachidonic acid release. However, although prostaglandins have been measured in many of these circumstances, the same cannot be said for arachidonic acid. The occurrence of this acid in the plasma as a free acid, as an ester of cholesterol or in its key location in the 2 position of phospholipids is well known. What is not generally known is that arachidonic acid is unique in that it has a high turnover rate in human plasma and it appears to be regulated in a completely different manner from the other fatty acids which respond in concert to feeding, starvation and to nicotinic acid.

Dietary Sources

Diets deficient in arachidonic acid, or its precursor, linoleic acid, are well known to cause poor growth, skin disorders and decreased fertility in animals. Carnivores, such as cats, cannot convert linoleic acid to arachidonic acid by chain elongation and desaturation, and therefore require arachidonate to be present in their diet. Estradiol but not testosterone is well known to increase both free and esterified arachidonate in plasma (5,6). The sex differences in plasma arachidonate incorporation by rat platelets is abolished by fasting (7). Deficiency syndromes are observed in male trauma patients and patients with extensive intestinal resection. Children who have diets lacking these two fatty acids are especially susceptible. The diet has to be substantially deficient since the characteristic infant eczema is easily eliminated if linoleate is added to the diet in sufficient quantities to make up 1% of the total calories consumed.

Arachidonate Lipoxygenases

No data are available on sex differences in the activity of the 5 and 12 lipoxygenases. Aspirin sensitive asthma is more frequent in females. This suggests that the 5 lipoxygenase pathway which leads to SRS formation may be enhanced by estradiol (8).

Cyclo-Oxygenase

No data are available on sex differences in the activity of

this enzyme. However, sex differences have been observed following
intravenous administration of free arachidonate in mice. This
procedure produces pulmonary platelet aggregation followed by
hypoxia, at which time the animals lose their righting reflex.
Fig. 1 shows that males are more responsive to arachidonate than
the female. The protective effect of aspirin is seen in Fig. 2.
The next Figures (3 and 4) show the sensitizing effects of
pretreatment with testosterone in male and female mice respectively
(9). These data have been confirmed using a slightly different
model in which mortality rate is used as the end point following
intravenous administration of arachidonate to anesthetized mice
(10 . In this series of experiments the death rate was reduced
not only by the cyclo-oxygenase inhibitor indomethacin, but also
by pretreatment with cortisone (Fig. 5).

These data indicate that there may be a sex difference in (i)
cyclo-oxygenase activity, (ii) thromboxane and prostacyclin
synthetase, (iii) platelet aggregation and (iv) contributing
factors such as pulmonary vasoconstriction.

Platelet Aggregation

In rats and guinea pigs, platelet aggregation is sex
dependent. Male platelets react to many agents more readily than
do platelets from females. Again, the evidence is that this sex
difference is due to testosterone rather than estradiol (11).

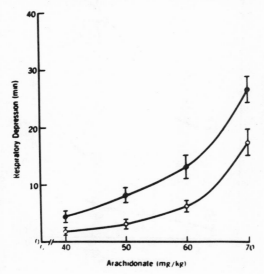

Fig. 1. Gender differences in respiratory depression to sodium
         arachidonate (i.v.) in mice. Each point on this figure
         and figure 2 to 5 represents the mean of 30-35 animals
         ±SE.•-• Male;o-o Female.

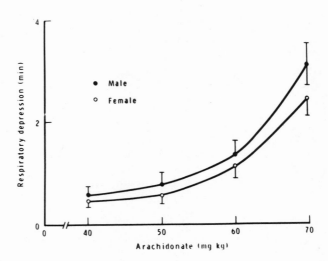

Fig. 2.   Effect of aspirin (40 mg/kg) two hours prior to arachidonate administration.   No significant gender differences were apparent.

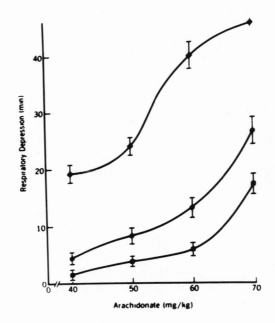

Fig. 3.   The potentiating effect of testosterone treatment and the inhibitory effect of estradiol on pulonary depression in male mice.   •-• Control; ▲-▲ Testosterone; ■-■ Estradiol.

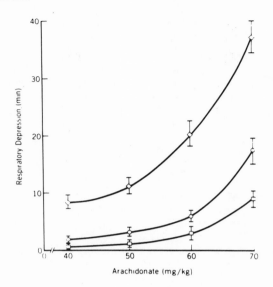

Fig. 4.   Effect of testosterone and estradiol on the responsiveness
of female mice to arachidonate. o-o Control;Δ-Δ
Testosterone;□ -□ Estradiol.

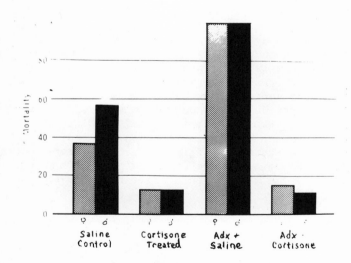

Fig. 5.   Mortality (%) following arachidonate (50 mg/kg i.v.) in
intact and adrenolectomized (Adx) mice untreated or
treated with cortisone (10 mg/kg/day s.c.) for four
days.

In humans the situation is reversed, i.e. platelets from females aggregate more readily than males. However, aspirin inhibits the aggregation of platelets from males more than from females (unpublished). Whether these sex differences are related cyclo-oxygenase activity and thromboxane synthetase activity remains to be determined. These gender differences may be due to differences in arachidonate release rather than to differences in arachidonate catabolism.

Thrombus Formation

The sex differences seen in thromboembolic diseases in humans can be initiated in animal models by the insertion of a plastic loop into the abdominal aorta. The thrombus formed in the externalized loop can be weighed and the overall effect on the animals observed. The results indicate that testosterone exacerbates the thrombotic process and both thrombus weight and mortality rates are greater in males than in females. Further, administration of testosterone to either male or female exaggerates the damaging effects of the procedure. Pretreatment with aspirin significantly protects against the damaging androgen effects (12). This protection is greater in the male animals and is consistent with recent reports of protection with cyclo-oxygenase inhibitors in humans (see below). In the animal studies it was possible to study the effect of anti-androgens. The non-steroidal anti-androgen, Flutamide (Schering) had a protective effect (Fig. 6).

Sex Differences in the Clinical Use of Cyclo-Oxygenase Inhibitors

Three studies have been reported in which men appear to be protected more than women by this class of drugs; first, in protecting against a second myocardial infarct (13); second in protecting against trasient cerebral ischemia (14) and third in protecting against venous thrombosis following hip replacement surgery (15). These data are consistent with our animal studies described earlier in which aspirin inhibited platelet aggregation and thrombus formation more in males than females. Other workers (16) find that the accretion of fibrinogen to thrombi was the same in rabbits of both sexes. However, treatment with aspirin significantly reduced fibrinogen accretion in the male and not the female.

Vascular Contractility

Isolated aortic strips like all smooth muscle contract in response to a superfusion of the stable prostaglandin endoperoxide analogue U46619. The male aortic strip of both rats and rabbits (17) is more responsive than the female (Fig. 7). These data suggest that there may be sex differences in the receptors for the drug or the excitation - contraction coupling mechanism.

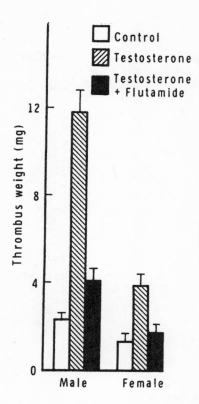

Fig. 6. The effect of the non-steroidal anti-androgen flutamide on arterial thrombi formation in an artificial aorta loop of male and female rats before and after treatment with testosterone.

No gender differences were observed in aorta dry weight. In the rat, the male aorta response was inhibited significantly more by aspirin and by indomethacin than the response in the female (Fig. 8).

Blood Pressure Responses

In the anesthetized rat the vasodepressor response to arachidonate is smaller in the male or androgen treated animal than in the female (18). However, no sex differences were observed in blood pressure responses to PGI_2 which with PGE_2 may be the primary metabolic products responsible for the net pressure response to intravenous arachidonate. Indomethacin was found to potentiate the pressor response to intravenous norepinephrine more in females than in males.

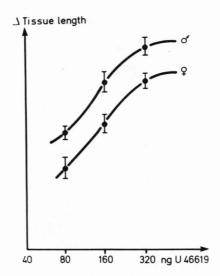

Fig. 7. Gender differences in contractility of the superfused
rat aorta preparation to the stable endoperoxide analogue,
Upjohn 46619.

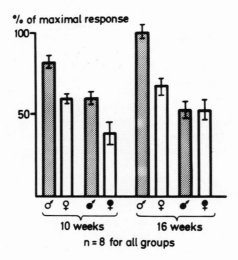

Fig. 8. Differences (♂ ♀) in contractility of the rat aorta
during development (10-16 weeks) and after superfusing
with indomethacin, 4 ug/ml (♂ ♀).

DISCUSSION

These data show there are sex differences in the magnitude of physiologic responses to prostaglandin metabolites. These substances probably play a major role in the maintenance of cardiovascular homeostasis. It is here that the sex differences observed in morbidity and mortality from cardiovascular disease may be clarified and manipulated.

Sex differences occur in the synthesis and turnover of arachidonate. It is conjectural whether sex differences exist in the 5 and 12 lipoxygenase and cyclo-oxygenase enzymes or in the individual pathways leading to SRS, or to prostaglandins and thromboxane. However, gender differences have been shown to occur in the response of isolated vascular tissue and in overall blood pressure changes.

Finally, it is known that the activity of the primary metabolizing enzyme, prostaglandin 15-degydroxygenase, is increased in the lung during pregnancy, or following progesterone treatment in the rabbit (19). The lungs are rich in this enzyme. Except for prostacyclin most prostaglandins are largely removed in a single transit of this organ (20). Preliminary studies of the effect of testosterone and estradiol treatment in the dog, indicate that these steroids may also affect pulmonary transit or the sylmstemic pressure responses of arachidonate and PGE_2 (21).

Our working hypothesis was that during the life span process, males generate more endoperoxide than do females. The products formed from the endoperoxide depend upon the tissue. If this is the case,one might expect males to produce more prostacyclin from the endothelium and more thromboxane from the platelets than do females. In the lung vasculature (Fig. 8) and aorta at least, this seems to be the case for prostacyclin (22). Whether there is a gender difference in prostaglandin receptors is an interesting question. Our data from the isolated rat aorta preparation indicate that this may be the case (Fig. 9).

Most investigators use males in order to minimize possible variances due to female estrous. However, it is clear from the above review that in addition to estrous related variances, the sex differences per se in pathophysiological processes are significant. If these differences are indded related to the arachidonate cascade, then the clarification of the humoral regulation of these pathways and receptors in cardiovascular tissues will provide a rational basis for therapeutic intervention for these male related diseases.

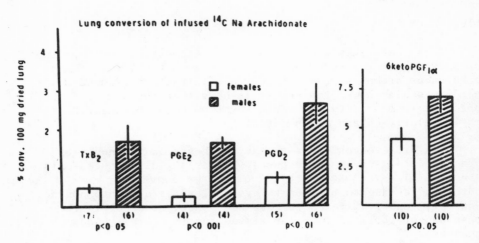

Fig. 9.   Gender differences in the conversion of ^{14}C-arachidonate
by the perfused rat lung.

ACKNOWLEDGEMENT

        This work was supported by

             Grant HL 18718
                   HL 17516

REFERENCES

1. P. W. Ramwell, E. M. K. Loevey and A. L. Sintetos, Biol. of
    Reprod., 16: 70-87 (1977).
2. L. Hagenfeldt, Ark. Keni., 29:57 (1968).
3. I. Hagenfeldt and J. Wahren, Metabolism, 24:799 (1975).
4. L. Hagenfeldt, K. Hagenfeldt and A. Wennmalin, Horm. Metab. Res.,
    7:467 (1975).
5. R. L. Lyman, Prog. Chem. Fats Other Lipids, 9:195 (1968).
6. E. M. K. Loevey, Advances in Prost. and Thromb. Res. Vol.
    6-8 (1980).
7. E. M. K. Loevey, Advances in Prost. and Thromb.Res. Vol.
    6-8 (1980).
8. M. Foegh, Nature, 281:14 (1979).
9. A. D. Uzunova, E. R. Ramey and P. W. Ramwell, Prostaglandins,
    13:995 (1977).
10. J. C. Penhos, M. Montalbert-Smith, F. Rabbani, E. R. Ramey and
    P. W. Ramwell, Prostaglandins, 18 (1979).

11. M. Johnson, E. R. Ramey and P. W. Ramwell, Am. J. Physiol., 232:H381 (1977).
12. A. D. Uzanova, E. R. Ramey and P. W. Ramwell, Am. J. Physiol., 234: H454-459 (1978).
13. S. Sherry, N. Engl. J. Med., 298:289 (1968).
14. Barnett, N. Engl. J. Med., 299:53 (1978).
15. M. M. Harris, E. W. Salzman, C. A. Athanacoulis, A. C. Waltman and R. W. DeSanctis, N. Engl. J. Med., 297:1246 (1977).
16. J. G. Kelton, J. Hirsh, C. J. Carter and M. R. Buchanan, Blood, 52:1073 (1978).
17. A. L. Sintetos, P. W. Ramwell and E. R. Ramey, Fed. Proc., 37:731 (1978).
18. P. J. Baker, E. R. Ramey and P. W. Ramwell, Am. J. Physiol., 235:242 (1978).
19. J. R. Bedwani and P. B. Marley, Brit. J. Pharmacol., 50:459 (1974).
20. H. M. Waldman, I. Alter, P. A. Kot, J. C. Rose and P. W. Ramwell, J. Pharmacol. Exp. Therap., 206:289 (1978).
21. H. M. Waldman, I. Alter, P. A. Kot, J. C. Rose, E. R. Ramey and P. W. Ramwell, Proc. Soc. Exp. Biol., 158:442 (1978).
22. R. H. Harris, Y. Maddox, E. R. Ramey and P. W. Ramwell, Proc. IV Internat. Prostaglandins Conf., 46 (1979).

PROSTAGLANDIN ANALOGS THAT ANTAGONIZE THE VASCULAR RESPONSES

TO PARTICULAR PROSTAGLANDINS

Thomas M. Fitzpatrick, Robert B. Stinger
Peter W. Ramwell and Peter A. Kot

Department of Physiology and Biophysics
Georgetown University Medical Center
Washington, D.C. 20007

In the current literature, there are numerous reports of the biological activity of exogenously administered prostaglandins and variations in the endogenous production of prostaglandins under varie physiologic conditions. However, no method has been developed that clearly differentiates the in vivo actions of each biologically active product of arachidonic acid metabolism. Thus, the true physiologic and pathophysiologic significance of these compounds remains somewhat theoretical.

In the past, the development of specific antagonists that compete with various vasoactive compounds such as histamine (7) and the catecholamines (18) has furthered our awareness of the pharmacologic actions of these substances. To date there have been no consistant attempts to systematically develop antagonists that are specific for the known vasoactive prostaglandins.

Ideally, an effective antagonist should bind competitively to particular prostaglandin receptors and displace the active compound (8). Following this rationale, Fried et al. (10) synthesized a series of 7-oxa-prostaglandin analogs in which oxygen replaced the methylene group at the 7-position (23). Several of these compounds antagonized PGE_1 induced contractions of the isolated gerbil colon (9). However, they have also demonstrated weak agonist effects on some gastrointestinal (2) and vascular tissues (20,19). Likewise, the 7-oxa-prostaglandins are not effective antagonists to the vascular actions of prostaglandins in the rat (9) and dog (16).

Several non-prostanoic compounds have also been noted to attenuate responses to various prostaglandins. For instance, a dibenzoxazepine derivative (SC-19220), which was initially tested

as an anticonvulsant and analgesic agent (6), specifically inhibits
prostaglandin induced contractions of the isolated guinea pig
ileum at low concentrations (21,2). Yet it does not affect the
relaxation of circular gastrointestinal muscle produced by the
E prostaglandins (1).   SC-19220 is less specific and less effective
on vascular tissues. It antagonizes the contractile responses to
both PGE_2 and 5-hydroxytryptamine on isolated human umbilical
arteries (20), and does not affect prostaglandin responses on
isolated pulmonary veins (4). The in vivo cardiovascular actions
of the various prostaglandins are also unaffected by SC-19220 (21).

Polyphloretin phosphate (PPP) is a mixture of polyester
polymers that affects the activity of many enzymes, including
hyaluronidase, alkaline phosphatase, and urease (8). Intra-arterial
administration of PPP blocks changes in ocular membrane permeability
(3), that have been associated with a mixture of prostaglandins
(8). In vitro, PPP produces selective and reversible inhibition of
the contractile action of both E and F prostaglandins on most
gastrointestinal smooth muscle preparations (23). Low concentrations
of PPP selectively antagonize the contractile response to PGE_2 on
strips of human umbilical artery. (Concentrations above 100 ug/ml
also inhibit the response to 5-hydroxytryptamine (20)).

Unlike SC-19220 and 7-oxa-prostaglandin, PPP (200 mg/kg)
does block the cardiovascular actions of $PGF_{2\alpha}$ (25,15), yet is
ineffective in inhibiting the vasodepressor actions of PGE_1 and
PGE_2 (17). Such high doses of PPP significantly decrease systemic
arterial pressure (15) and may in fact exert its inhibitory action
at sites other than the prostaglandin receptor, such as the
adenylate cyclase level (13,12).

Although each antagonist appears to competitively block the
response to prostaglandins in certain tissues (1), there has been
only limited success in the in vivo inhibition of prostaglandin
activity (8). Only the 7-oxa-prostaglandins appear to act at the
prostaglandin receptor. Thus, continued efforts should be made to
systematically screen new prostaglandin analogs in an attempt to
find more selective and effective antagonists (1). With this in
mind, we have tested two series of new prostaglandin analogs in
hopes of finding antagonists that are specific for the hemodynamic actions of individual prostaglandins.

A series of $PGF_{1\alpha}$ and $PGF_{2\alpha}$ analogs, synthesized by Corey,
were evaluated as prostaglandin antagonists in our laboratory.
Two of these compounds, N-dimethylamine and N-dimethylamide $PGF_{2\alpha}$
differ from $PGF_{2\alpha}$ only by substitution of the respective dimethyl-
amine groups on carbon 1 as shown if Figure 1. Each of the
analogs was a potent antagonist of PGE_2 and $PGF_{2\alpha}$ responses on
the gerbil colon preparation and did not block similar effects of
acetylcholine or bradykinin. Neither exhibited any agonist

activity in this preparation (14). Subsequently, the antagonism of both analogs was tested against the pulmonary pressor action of $PGF_{2\alpha}$ and arachidonic acid in the isolated canine lung lobe.

In this in situ preparation the lower left lung lobe is isolated from the remainder of the pulmonary circulation by cannulating the lobar artery and vein. The bronchus is left intact to maintain ventilation to the lobe. Autologous citrated blood was collected in a 200 ml siliconized reservoir, maintained at 37°C and perfused through the isolated lung lobe via the lobar artery. Mean perfusion pressure was monitored at the inflow catheter and maintained at 12-16 mm Hg. Venous blood drained passively into the reservoir and recirculated through the lobe. Since flow was maintained at a constant rate with a peristaltic pump, changes in perfusion pressure were indicative of changes in pulmonary vascular tone.

Each analog was infused into the inflow catheter at a constant rate (160 ng/min) and produced no change in perfusion pressure. $PGF_{2\alpha}$ (1 ug/kg) was administered by bolus injection before, during, and after infusion of the analog. Arachidonic acid (100 ug/kg), which is also a pulmonary vasoconstrictor in this preparation (26), was administered by bolus injection before and after the infusion.

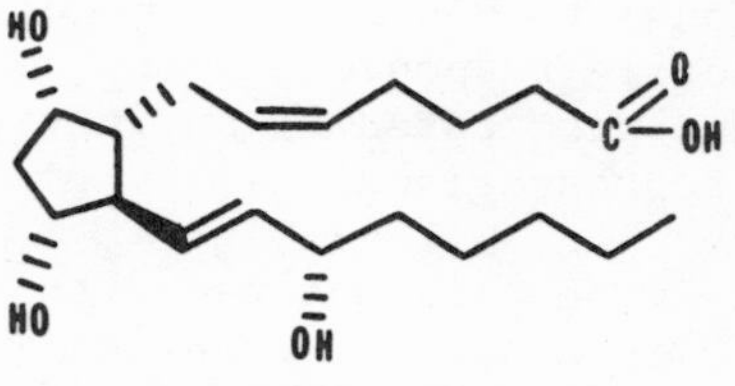

$PGF_{2\alpha}$

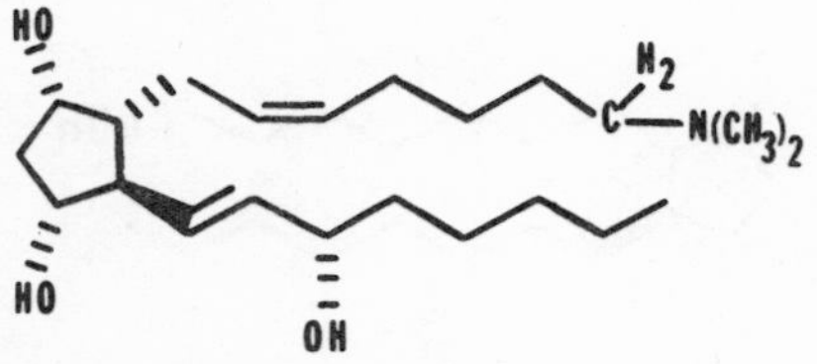

N-dimethylamine

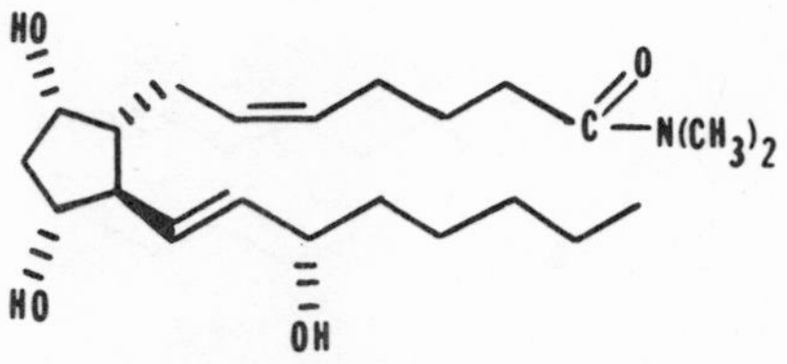

N-dimethylamide

Fig. 1. Structural differences between $PGF_{2\alpha}$ and N-dimethylamino analogs.

During the control period, both $PGF_{2\alpha}$ and arachidonic acid increased lobar arterial pressure 53.9 ± 4.4 and 82.8 ±9.6% (mean ± S.E.), respectively. After infusion of either analog, the response to $PGF_{2\alpha}$ was markedly attenuated. N-dimethylamine $PGF_{2\alpha}$, at a concentration of 3.2 ug/ml reduced the $PGF_{2\alpha}$ response to 14.1 ± 2.3%, representing an approximate 75% decrease from the control response. The N-dimethylamide analog, less potent of the two analogs, required 8.0 ug/ml to produce a similar reduction (14.0 ± 3.9%).

In contrast, after infusion of either the N-dimethylamine or the N-dimethylamide analogs, arachidonic acid still produced increases of 82.4 ± 6.5 and 95.2 ± 15.2%, respectively. Thus, both analogs selectively antagonize the pulmonary pressor actions of $PGF_{2\alpha}$.

These data further suggest the usefulness of these analogs in differentiating active components of arachidonic acid metabolism. For instance, the pumonary pressor response to arachidonic acid is due not to significant production of $PGF_{2\alpha}$ but more likely the production of endoperoxides and/or thromboxanes.

Fried et al. (11) have suggested that selective removal of the hydroxyl groups from carbons of natural prostaglandins reduces the agonist property of that analog. As depicted in Figure 2, 11-15-bisdeoxy PGE_1 differs from the natural PGE_1 by removal of hydroxyl groups from both carbon 11 and carbon 15. On the isolated gerbil colon preparation, this analog is a specific antagonist of the contractile response to PGE_1, and had no agonist activity or affect on the contractile response to $PGF_{2\alpha}$ or acetylcholine (24). This bisdeoxy compound was tested as an in vivo antagonist to several vasodepressor prostaglandins.

Male Wistar rats were anesthetized with sodium pentobarbital (50 mg/kg IP). The common carotid arteries were cannulated for recording systemic arterial pressure and infusion of the analog. The external jugular vein was cannulated for injections of the prostaglandins.

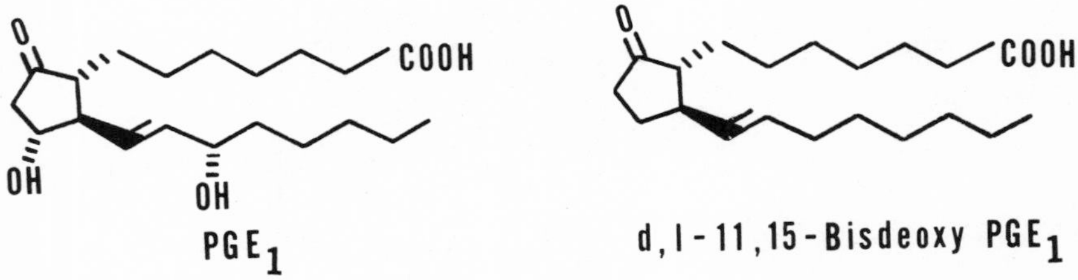

Fig. 2.   Variations between PGE_1 and d,1-11,15 Bisdeoxy PGE_1.

Prostacyclin (PGI_2; 0.3 ug/kg), PGE_1 (3.0 ug/kg) and PGE_2 (3.0 ug/kg) were administered at five minute intervals before, during and after infusion of the analog. The bisdeoxy PGE_1 was infused at a rate of 200 ug/kg/min and produced no changes in systemic arterial pressure. Control doses of the prostaglandins were approximately equidepressor with PGI_2, PGE_1 and PGE_2 producing decreases in systemic arterial pressure of 37.9 ± 2.4, 41.2 ± 1.8 and 38.7 ± 2.8%, respectively. Following a fifty minute infusion period the response to PGE_1 was reduced to a 20.2 ± 2.6% decrease, which represents a 50% reduction in activity of PGE_1. Responses to PGE_2 (43.9 ± 6.0%) and PGI_2 (35.8 ± 4.0) were virtually unchanged. Twenty minutes after the infusion was terminated, PGE_1 again produced a 36.8 ± 2.9% decrease in systemic arterial pressure which was not significantly different from the control value.

Therefore, this analog appears to be specific for the PGE_1 receptor and may in fact be a useful pharmacologic tool that differentiates the actions of the PGE_1 and PGE_2 on vascular tissue.

Although these are preliminary studies, the data strongly suggest that specific prostaglandin antagonists can be developed that are effective on systemic preparations as well as on isolated bioassay tissues. In addition, they have already been useful in differentiating the vascular actions of prostaglandin-like substances and may lead to the development of new therapeutic agents.

REFERENCES

1. A. Bennett, Prostaglandin antagonists, p.83, in: "Advances in Drug Research", N. J. Harper and A. B. Simmonds, eds., Academic Press, New York (1974).
2. A. Bennett and J. Posner, Studies on prostaglandin antagonists, Br. J. Pharmacol., 42:584 (1971).
3. B. R. Beitch and K. E. Eakins, The effects of prostaglandins on the intraocular pressure of the rabbit, Br. J. Pharmacol., 37:158 (1969).
4. J. F. Burka and P. Eyre, Studies of prostaglandins and prostaglandin antagonists on bovine pulmonary vein in vitro, Prostaglandins, 6:333 (1974).
5. N. Chand and P. Eyre, Effects of prostaglandin E_1, E_2 and $F_{2\alpha}$ and polyphloretin phosphate on carotid blood pressure of domestic fowl, Arch. Int. Pharm. Ther., 221:261 (1976).
6. W. E. Coyne and J. W. Cusic, Anticonvulsant semicarbazides, J. Med. Chem., 11:1158 (1968).
7. W. W. Douglas, Histamine and antihistamines; 5-hydroxytryptamine and antagonists, p.621, in: "The Pharmacological Basis of Therapeutics", L. S. Goodman and A. Gilman, eds., The Macmillan Company, New York (1970).

8.   K. E. Eakins and J. H. Sanner, Prostaglandin antagonists, p.261,,
     in: "The Prostaglandins, Progress in Research", S. M. M. Karim,
     ed., Medical and Technical Pub. Co. Ltd., London (1972).

9.   J. D. Flack, Biological significance of the prostaglandins,
     p.174, in: "Recent Progress in Hormone Research", P. W. Ramwell
     and J. E. Shaw, eds., Academic Press, New York (1970).

10. J. Fried, S. Heim, S. J. Etheredge, P. Sunder-Plassman,
     T. S. Santhanakrishan and J. Himizu, Synthesis of 15-
     desoxy-7-oxaprostaglandin $F_{1\alpha}$ and related substances, in:
     "Prostaglandin Symposium of the Worcester Foundation for
     Experimental Biology", P. W. Ramwell and J. E. Shaw, eds.,
     John Wiley and Sons, New York (1968).

11. J. Fried, T. S. Santhanakrishnan, J. Himizu, C. H. Lin, S. H.
     Ford, B. Rubin and E. O. Grigas, Prostaglandin antagonists:
     synthesis and smooth muscle activity, Nature, 223:208 (1969).

12. S. Hynie, J. Cepelik, M. Cernohorsky, V. Klenerova, J.
     Skrivanova and M. Wenke, 7-oxa-13 prostanoic acid and poly-
     phloretin phosphate as non-specific antagonist of the stimulatory
     effects of different agents on adenylate cyclase from various
     tissues, Prostaglandins, 10:971 (1975).

13. F. A. Keuhl and J. L. Humes, Direct evidence for a prostaglandin
     receptor and its application to prostaglandin measurement,
     Proc. Nat. Acad. Sci. U.S.A., 69:480 (1972).

14. Y. T. Maddox, P. W. Ramwell, C. S. Shiner and E. J. Corey, Amide
     and 1-amino derivatives of F prostaglandins as prostaglandin
     antagonists, Nature, 273:549 (1978).

15. A. A. Mathe, K. Strandberg and B. Fredholm, Antagonism of
     prostaglandin $F_{2\alpha}$ induced bronchoconstriction and blood pressure
     changes by polyphloretin phosphate in the guinea pig and cat,
     J. Pharm. Pharmac., 24:378 (1972).

16. J. Nakano, Relationship between the chemical structure of
     prostaglandins and their vasoactivities in dogs, Br. J. Pharmacol.
     44:63 (1972).

17. J. Nakano, A. V. Prancan and S. Moore, Effect of the
     prostaglandin antagonists in the vasoactivities of prosta-
     glandin E_1 (PGE_1), E_2 (PGE_2), A_1 (PGA_1) and $F_{2\alpha}$ ($PGF_{2\alpha}$),
     Clin. Res., 19:712 (1971).

18. M. Nickerson, Drugs inhibiting adrenergic nerves and structures
     innervated by them, p.549, in: "The Pharmacological Basis of
     Therapeutics", L. S. Goodman and A. Gilman, eds., The
     Macmillan Company, New York (1970).

19. N. Ozaki, J. D. Kohli, L. I. Goldberg and J. Fried, Vascular
     smooth vuscle activity of 7-oxa-13-prostanoic acid, Blood
     Vessels, 16:52 (1979).

20. M. K. Park and D. C. Dyer, Effect of polyphloretin phosphate
     and 7-oxa-13-prostanoic acid on vasoactive actions of prosta-
     glandin E_2 and 5-hydroxytryptamine on isolated human umbilical
     arteries, Prostaglandins, 3:913 (1973).

21. J. H. Sanner, Antagonism of prostaglandin E_2 by 1-acetyl-2-
     (8-chloro-10,11-dihydrodibenz b,f 1,4 oxazepine-10-carbonyl)
     hydrazine (SC-19220), Arch. Int. Pharmacodyn, Ther., 180:46(1969).

22. J. Sanner, Prostaglandin inhibition with a dibenzoxazepine
     hydrazide derivative and morphine, Ann. N.Y. Acad. Sci., 180:
     396 (1971).

23. J. Sanner and K. E. Eakins, Prostaglandin antagonists, p.139,
     in: "Prostaglandins: Chemical and Biological Agents
     S. M. M. Karim, ed., University Park Press, Baltimore (1976).

24   E. L. Tolman, R. Partridge and E. T. Barris, Prostaglandin
     E antagonists activity of 11,15-bisdeoxy prostaglandin E_1 and
     congeners, Prostaglandins, 14:11 (1977).

25. R. Villanueva, L. Hinds, R. L. Katz and K. E. Eakins, The
     effect of polyphloretin phosphate on some smooth muscle
     actions of prostaglandins in the cat, J. Pharm. and Exp. Ther.,
     180:78 (1972).

26. T. C. Wicks, J. C. Rose, M. Johnson, P. W.Ramwell and P. A. Kot,
     Vascular responses to arachidonic acid in the perfused canine
     lung, Cir. Res., 38:167 (1976).

PROSTAGLANDINS AND THE UTERINE CIRCULATION

Norberto A. Terragno and Alicia Terragno

Department of Pharmacology
New York Medical College
Valhalla, NY 10595, U.S.A.

By late pregnancy, uterine blood flow is 30 to 40 times that of the non-pregnant state (1). The great capacity of the uterine vasculature to adapt itself to the enormous increase in the physiological demands imposed by gestation might be caused by either the appearance of new or increased production of pre-existing compounds which influence uterine vascular resistance. The mechanism which regulates blood flow to the pregnant uterus is not well defined; the proposal that it involves uterine prostaglandins is supported by our studies.

The uterine vascular bed of late pregnancy has the following distinguishing characteristics: 1) it appears to be in a state of nearly complete vasodilatation as it does not respond with reactive hyperemia to an ischemic stimulus (2,3); 2) it does not autoregulate (4); 3) local vasoconstrictor actions of pressor hormones and adrenergic nerve stimulation are markedly depressed as are reflex vasoconstrictor responses (5-7). Although these observations were made in experimental animals, diminished vascular reactivity in man is also implied by the successively reduced pressor effect of intravenously administered angiotensin II during the progression of pregnancy when compared to the effect of the octapeptide in the non-pregnant state (8).

Local production of prostaglandins contributes to the regulation of regional blood flows and modulates vascular responses to vasoactive hormones (9,10). Augmented prostaglandin (PG) synthesis in an organ has been shown when blood flow to the organ is affected by an ischemic stimulus (11,12). For the renal circulation, a prostaglandin mechanism protects the renal circulation from possible deleterious effects of pressor hormones. The evidence just cited

is the basis of the hypothesis that a vasodilator compound which
supports the uterine circulation and opposes the vasoconstrictor
action of pressor stimuli is released from the uterus during
pregnancy. Vasodilator prostaglandins are ideal candidates to
mediate these effects. This hypothesis is also partially based on
the demonstrated large capacity of the uterus to release prostaglandins in response to various stimuli, such as estrogen treatment
(13) and uterine distention (14). Further, the synthesis and
release of prostaglandins from the gravid uterus may contribute to
some of the hemodynamic changes which occur at birth (15) and
could contribute to the antihypertensive function of the uteroplacental complex. The latter is invoked to account for the
amelioration of hypertension during gestation in both human and
experimental forms of hypertension.

    To investigate the possible participation of prostaglandins
in the regulation of blood flow to the uterus, we determined
the capacity of the pregnant uterus to release prostaglandins
into the venous effluent in response to vasoactive hormones.
We also studied, during pregnancy and in the non-pregnant state,
the capacity of different vascular elements of the uteroplacental
complex to synthesize prostaglandins as well as their responses
when stimulated by vasoactive substance. The participation of
vasodilator prostaglandins in the control of uterine vascular
reactivity in pregnancy was shown in experiments performed on
morphine-chloralose anesthetized dogs in late pregnancy. Intravenous administration of angiotension II (10-37 ng/kg/min) did not
constrict the uterine vascular bed under these experimental
conditions. Rather, in later pregnancy, angiotensin unexpectedly
increased uterine blood flow, although it still decreased renal
blood flow and increased systemic blood pressure (16). As we had
previously demonstrated that attenuation of the renal vasoconstrictor action of angiotensin was dependent on a prostaglandin
mechanism, we measured the concentration of PGF- and PGE-like
material in uterine venous blood, before and during angiotensin
administration. Simultaneous with the increase in uterine blood
flow induced by the peptide, the concentration of a PGE-like
substance in the venous effluent increased twofold (Fig. 1). After
blockade of prostaglandin synthesis with indomethacin, the same
dose of angiotensin II did not increase uterine blood flow; the
concentration of a PGE-like substance in uterine venous blood was
much lower during the control period and did not change when angiotensin was infused (Fig. 1). Uterine blood flow, whether measured
at rest or during infusion of angiotensin, and either in the presence
or absence of indomethacin, was highly correlated with the uterine
venous concentration of PGE-like material but not a PGF compound.
The participation of prostaglandins in the regulation of regional
blood flows and blood pressure was further suggested when we
reporduced, by blockade of prostaglandin synthesis, three of the
major hemodynamic changes occurring during toxemia of prognancy

(16,17) viz., increased uterine and renal vascular resistances and elevated systemic blood pressure. The uterine hyperemic action of angiotensin II was not seen in early pregnancy or in the non-pregnant state; rather angiotensin II decreased uterine blood flow and did not stimulate prostaglandin release (Fig. 2). However, at these times, the basal concentration of a PGE-like substance in uterine venous blood was either low or not detectable. This differential sensitivity of the uterine vasculature to angio-tensin, determined by the duration of gestation, appears to be related to the high prostaglandin biosynthetic capacity of the gravid uterus of late pregnancy, which can be further stimulated by antiotensin II.

There is an important finding in late pregnancy relative to uterine prostaglandin synthesis; namely, the resistance of cyclo-oxygenase to the inhibitory action of non-steroidal anti-inflammatory agents. A dose of indomethacin tenfold higher than that which markedly suppresses prostaglandin production in adult non-pregnant dogs, was required before any effects on uterine prostaglandin production could be demonstrated in late pregnancy (16,17). This relative refractoriness to prostaglandin synthesis inhibition of late pregnancy is not unique to the uterine circulation as it can be shown in other vascular territories. A dose of 2 mg/kg of indomethacin given intravenously to the non-pregnant dog reduced renal blood flow by 42%, whereas in late pregnancy a dose tenfold greater induced a decrease of renal blood flow of only 18% (Fig. 3). Lower doses were usually without effect on the renal circulation in late pregnancy. These observations recall our previous studies on the renal circulation: 1) continuous production of a PGE compound, under acute experimental conditions, contributed to the maintenance of resting renal blood flow (9); and 2) angio-tensin II, as well as norephinephrine, could increase renal synthesis of prostaglandins above basal levels (12).

Recent studies in our laboratory indicate that most of the PGE-like material which appears in the uterine venous blood in late pregnancy is 6 keto-$PGF_{1\alpha}$, the stable hydrolysis product of prostacyclin (PGI_2) (18). The identity of this compound was pre-viously masked since it has the same effects on the solvent system conventionally used to separate prostaglandins. The separation of PGE from 6 keto-$PGF_{1\alpha}$ can be accomplished by rechromatographing the PGE, 6 keto-$PGF_{1\alpha}$ zone in a second solvent system (19).

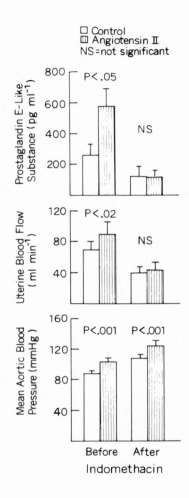

Fig. 1.   Effect of intravenous infusion of angiotensin II
          (10-37 ng/kg/min) on concentration of prostaglandin
          E-like substance in the uterine venous blood, uterine
          blood flow (of one horn) and mean aortic blood pressure,
          before and after the administration of indomethacin
          (10-25 mg/kg intravenously) in late pregnant dogs.
          Columns represent mean values and vertical bars standard
          error of the mean.

Several years ago we reported that blood vessels have the ability to synthesize prostaglandins;this ability can be inhibited by either indomethacin or meclofenamate and can be stimulated by various vasoactive hormones such as angiotensin II and bradykinin (20). The discovery that two additional arachidonic derivatives,

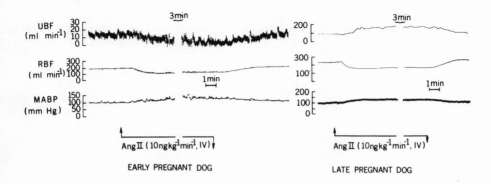

Fig. 2. Effect of intravenous administration of angiotensin II
         (Ang II) in early (left and late (right) pregnancy on
         uterine blood flow (UBF), renal blood flow (RBF), and
         mean aortic blood pressure (MABP) in chloralose-
         anesthetized dogs.

prostacyclin and thromboxane A_2, having powerful and opposite biological activities, are formed by blood vessels and platelets, considerably enlarged the sphere of action on arachidonic acid metabolites arising from enzymic transformation by cyclo-oxygenase. Prostacyclin prevents platelet aggregation and relaxes blood vessels

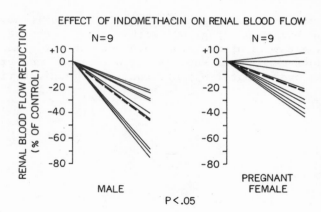

Fig. 3.   Differential effect of indomethacin: 2 mg/kg, i.v. in
         the male dogs decreased renal blood flow by 42%, whereas
         a dose of 20 mg/kg, i.v. in the pregnant female reduced
         the renal blood flow by only 18%.

         n = number of experiments.

whereas thromboxane A_2 constricts blood vessels (21-23) and
aggregates blood platelets (24). As some of the fetal and maternal
circulatory adjustments to pregnancy may be related to a prostaglandin mechanism, we have studied in vitro the capacity of bovine
vascular tissues obtained from mother and the corresponding fetus
to convert $(1-^{14}C)$ arachidonic acid to radiolabeled prostaglandins.
We were particularly interested in the ability of these vascular
tissues to synthesize prostacyclin as this prostaglandin may have
a special role in blood vessels because of its antithrombotic
vasodilator action (19,22-24).

     All blood vessels thus far studied have been shown to be
capable of converting $(1-^{14}C)$ arachidonic acid to radiolabeled
prostaglandins. Blood vessels, cut in fine rings, were incubated
without co-factors in Kreb's solution for 3 h with $(1-^{14}C)$
arachidonic acid (25). The capacity of vascular rings obtained
from pregnant cows and their fetuses and non-pregnant cows to
metabolize arachidonic acid via the cyclo-oxygenase pathway is
shown in Table 1. Fetal vascular tissues generated tenfold more
prostacyclin, as indicated by recovery of 6 keto-$PGF_{1\alpha}$, than PGE_2;
almost half of the total radioactivity recovered from the incubate
was 6 keto-$PGF_{1\alpha}$. In contrast, blood vessels of adult animals
released less 6 keto-$PGF_{1\alpha}$, and more unreacted arachidonic acid
was found in the incubating medium. A finding of possible
importance is the large capacity of major resistance blood vessels,
the mesenteric and renal obtained from both pregnant and non-pregnant

TABLE I

BIOSYNTHESIS OF PROSTAGLADINS FROM (1-^{14}C) ARACHIDONIC ACID*
BY SLICES OF BOVINE VASCULAR TISSUES

	TISSUES	PGF$_{2\alpha}$	6 KETO-PGF$_{1\alpha}$	PGE$_2$	ARACHIDONIC ACID
FETAL	Aorta	5.5 ± 1.0	23.8 ± 0.7	2.6 ± 0.3	52.8 ± 2.8
	Pulmonary Artery	6.0 ± 1.0	29.8 ± 1.9	3.2 ± 0.5	45.4 ± 2.4
	Ductus Arteriosus	6.3 ± 1.6	20.0 ± 2.3	2.0 ± 0.0	56.6 ± 1.3
MATERNAL	Aorta	1.7 ± 0.3	6.8 ± 0.7	1.4 ± 0.1	81.6 ± 0.2
	Pulmonary Artery	2.8 ± 0.2	10.2 ± 0.7	0.6 ± 0.3	75.5 ± 1.5
	Mesenteric Artery	5.8 ± 1.0	20.9 ± 2.1	4.2 ± 0.5	54.5 ± 6.6
NON-PREGNANT	Aorta	2.9 ± 0.1	6.1 ± 0.7	1.3 ± 0.1	80.0 ± 1.2
	Pulmonary Artery	2.5 ± 0.2	5.2 ± 0.4	1.3 ± 0.1	82.6 ± 0.3
	Mesenteric Artery	8.6 ± 0.5	19.5 ± 4.1	3.7 ± 1.0	51.9 ± 6.5

*Percent of total radioactivity recovered from incubation fluid

cows, to form prostacyclin, a potent vasodilator compound (26).
On the basis of this study, we conclude that the high prostacyclin
biosythetic capacity of fetal blood vessels is not restricted to
the ductus arteriosus and suggest that prostacyclin fulfills a
general function for the fetal vasculature as an antithrombotic
and vasodilator agent (27) and may contribute to the resistance of
fetal blood to clotting (28) and to the high cardiac output and
low total vascular resistance which characterize the fetal
circulation (3).

ACKNOWLEDGEMENTS

        This work was supported by USPHS, NHLBI (HL 25406), American
Heart Association (77-894) and Tennessee Heart Association Grants.
We thank Ms. Nancy Gentile and Ms. Lillian Delgado for secretarial
help.

REFERENCES

1.   J. Metcalfe, S. L. Romney, J. R. Swartwout, D. M. Pitcairn,
     A. N. Lethin Jr. and D. H. Barron, Uterine blood flow and
     oxygen consumption in pregnant sheep and goats. Am. J. Physiol.,
     197: 929-934 (1959).
2.   P. V. Dilts, C. R. Brinkmann III, T. H. Kirschbaum and N. S.
     Assali, Uterine and systemic hemodynamic interrelationships
     and their response to hypoxia. Am. J. Obstet. Gynecol.,
     103: 138-157 (1969).
3.   A. M. Rudolph, The course and distribution of the foetal
     circulation. In: "Foetal Automony",Ciba Foundation Symposium,
     G. E. W. Wolstenholme and M. O'Connor, eds., J. A. Churchill
     Ltd.,London, pp.147-161 (1969).
4.   F. S. Greiss, Pressure-flow relationship in the gravid uterine
     vascular bed. Am. J. Obstet., Gynecol., 93: 41-47 (1966).
5.   C. Ladner, C. R. Brinkmann III, P. Weston and N. S. Assali,
     Dynamics of uterine circulation in pregnant and nonpregnant sheep.
     Am. J. Physiol., 218: 257-263 (1970).
6.   T. F. Ferris, J. H. Stein and J. Kauffman, Uterine blood flow
     and uterine renin secretion. J. Clin. Invest., 51: 2827-
     2833 (1972).
7.   N. S. Assali and A. Westersten, Regional flow-pressure
     relationship in response to angiotensin in the intact dog and
     sheep. Circ. Res., 9: 189-193 (1961).
8.   R. Abdul-Karim and N. S. Assali, Pressor response to angiotonin
     in pregnant and nonpregnant women. Am. J. Obstet. Gynecol.,
     82: 246-251 (1961).
9.   A. J. Lonigro, H. D. Itskovitz, K. Crowshaw and J. C. McGiff,
     Dependency of renal blood flow on prostaglandin synthesis in
     the dog. Circ. Res., 32:712-717 (1973).

10. N. G. Bowery, G. P. Lewis and J. Matthews, The relationship between functional vasocilatation in adipose tissue and prostaglandin. Brit. J. Pharmacol., 40: 437-445 (1970).

11. M. A. Williamson, J. B. Lee and K. K. F. Ng, Prostaglandin-like substances appearing in canine renal venous blood during renal ischemia: their partial characterization by pharmacologic and chromatographic procedures. Circ. Res., 27: 765-782 (1970).

12. J. C. McGiff, K. Crowshaw, N. A. Terragno and A. J. Lonigro, Renal prostaglandins: possible regulators of the renal actions of pressor hormones. Nature, 227: 1255-1257 (1970).

13. F. R. Blatchley, B. T. Donovan, N. L. Poyser, E. W. Horton, C. J. Thompson and M. Los, Identification of prostaglandin F_2 in the utero-ovarian blood of guinea-pig after treatment with osetrogen. Nature, 230: 243-244 (1971).

14. N. L. Poyser, E. W. Horton, C. J. Thompson and M. Los, Identification of prostaglandin F_2 released by distension of guinea-pig uterus in vitro. Nature, 230: 526-528 (1971).

15. D. A. Terragno, K. Crowshaw, N. A. Terragno and J. C. McGiff, Prostaglandin synthesis by bovine mesenteric arteries and veins. Circ. Res., 36, 37: (Suppl. I), I-76 - I-80 (1975a).

16. N. A. Terragno, D. A. Terragno, D. Pacholczyk and J. C. McGiff, Prostaglandins and the regulation of uterine blood flow in pregnancy. Nature, 249: 57-58 (1974).

17. N. A. Terragno, D. A. Terragno and J. C. McGiff, The role of prostaglandins in the control of uterine blood flow. In: Hypertension in Pregnancy.M.D. Lindheimer, A. A. Katz and F. P. Zuspan, eds., John Wiley and Sons, New York, pp.391-398 (1976).

18. R. A. Johnson, D. R. Morton, J. H. Kinner, R. R. Gorman, J. C. McGuire, F. F. Sun, N. Whittaker, S. Bunting, J. Salmon, S.Moncada and J.R. Vane, The chemical structure of prosta-glandin X (prostacyclin). Prostaglandins, 12: 915-928 (1976).

19. N. A. Terragno, A. Terragno, J. C. McGiff and D. J. Rodriquez, Synthesis of prostaglandin, by the ductus arteriosus of the bovine fetus. Prostaglandins, 14: 721-727 (1977).

20. N. A. Terragno, A. Terragno, D. S. Jennings and J. C. McGiff, Bradykinin stimulates prostaglandin synthesis in human umbilical blood vessels. Society for Gynecologic Investigation, 6:18 (Abstract) (1975b).

21. R. J. Gryglewski, S. Bunting, S. Moncada, R. J. Flower and J. R. Vane, Arterial walls are protected against deposition of platelet thrombi by a substance (prostaglandin X) which they make from prostaglandin endoperoxides. Prostaglandins, 12: 683-713 (1976).

22. S. Bunting, R. Gryglewski, S. Moncada and J. R. Vane, Arterial walls generate from prostaglandin endoperoxides a substance (prostaglandin X) which relaxes strips of mesenteric and coeliac arteries and inhibits platelet aggregation. Prostaglandins, 12: 897-913 (1976a).

23. S. Bunting, S. Moncada and J. R. Vane, The effects of prosta-
     glandin endoperoxides and thromboxane A_2 on strips of rabbit
     coelic artery and certain other smooth muscle preparations.
     Brit. J. Pharmacol., 57: 462P–463P (1976b).
24. M. Hamberg, J. Svennson and B. Samuelsson, Thromboxanes:
     A new group of biologically active compounds derived from
     prostaglandin endoperoxides. Proc. Natn. Acad. Sci. U.S.A.,
     72: 2994–2998 (1975).
25. N. A. Terragno, J. C. McGiff, M. Smigel and A. Terragno,
     Patterns of prostaglandin production in the bovine fetal and
     maternal vasculature. Submitted to J. Clin. Invest. (1978).
26. S. Moncada, In: 1977 Winter Prostaglandin Conference Report.
     Prostaglandins, 14: 204–205 (1977).
27. S. Moncada, E. A. Higgs and J. R. Vane, Human arterial and
     venous tissues generate prostacyclin (prostaglandin X),
     a potent inhibitor of platelet aggregation. Lancet i, 18–20
     (1977).
28. A. J. Aballi and S. De Lamerens, Coagulation changes in the
     neonatal period and in early infancy. Pediat. Clin. N. Amer.,
     9: 785–817 (1962).

GONADAL FUNCTION

N.L. Poyser and Christine A. Phillips

Department of Pharmacology
Unversity of Edinburgh, 1 George Square
Edinburgh, Scotland, U.K.

The original discovery of "prostaglandin" (PG) in human semen has meant that the role of prostaglandins in reproduction has always received much attention. The actions of PGE and PGF of both the 1- and 2- series on reproductive tissues have been extensively studied. With the development of radioimmunoassays (RIA) for prostaglandins, measurements into the amounts of PGE and PGF synthesised by and released from reproductive tissues in relation to physiological events has been possible, and many significant changes have been observed. The physiological roles of PGE_2 and $PGF_{2\alpha}$ in reproduction were summarised at the first NATO Advanced Study Institute on Prostaglandins (1). With the discovery of the PG endoperoxides, thromboxanes (TX) and prostacyclin (PGI_2), it has become unsatisfactory to study only PGE_2 and $PGF_{2\alpha}$ when investigating prostaglandin action on and release from reproductive tissues. However, information regarding the action of PG endo-peroxides and TXA_2 on reproductive tissues is very limited due, no doubt, to the unstable nature of these compounds with their inherent difficulty in handling especially when one is looking for chronic effects. TXA_2 can be measured as its stable metabolite TXB_2, by RIA or gas chromatography – mass spectrometry (GC-MS). Thromboxane production by reproductive tissues may, therefore, be measured. Prostacyclin is somewhat more stable so its actions on tissues can be examined. However, the effects of chronic treatment in vivo may be more difficult to investigate, though stable analogues will undoubtedly make this easier. Prostacyclin synthesis by and release from reproductive tissues can be estimated by measuring its metabolite, $6\text{-oxo-PGF}_{1\alpha}$ by RIA or GC-MS. Consequently, the actions of prostacyclin on reproductive tissues is being examined, and the production of thromboxanes and prostacyclin by these tissues is being investigated. This article will attempt to

301

summarise some of the data which is known. There is little
information regarding the male, so the female of the species will
be discussed exclusively.

OVARY

Prostacyclin (measured as 6-oxo-PGF$_{1\alpha}$ by RIA) is the major
prostaglandin produced by homogenates of rat ovaries (Fiona Scott
and N. L. Poyser, unpublished results). PGF$_{2\alpha}$, PGD$_2$ and PGE$_2$ are
produced in that order in somewhat smaller quantities, while
thromboxane production is minimal. In the human ovary, 6-oxo-PGF$_{1\alpha}$
is the major product formed by homogenates of the follicles and
stromal cells, together with smaller quantities of PGF$_{2\alpha}$ and PGE$_2$
(2). Homogenates of the corpus luteum, on the other hand, synthesise
PGE$_2$ as the major product, followed by 6-oxo-PGF$_{1\alpha}$ and PGF$_{2\alpha}$.
Thromboxane production was not measured. These results would
indicate that different tissues within the ovary synthesise
prostaglandins in different ratios. However, the cow and horse
corpus luteum are reported to synthesise 6-oxo-PGF$_{1\alpha}$ as the major
product from PGH$_2$ (3), so there may be a species difference.
Nevertheless, it is clear that smashed cell preparations of ovaries
have a high capacity to synthesise prostacyclin, but an extremely
low capacity to synthesise thromboxanes. Whether the ovaries produce
and secret prostacyclin in vivo needs studying.

One of the earliest actions of PGE$_2$ on the ovary to be
discovered was its ability to stimulate steroidogenesis and
progesterone production (4). This action is independent of
luteinizing hormone (LH) or LH receptors, but is achieved in a
similar manner to LH by stimulating adenyl cyclase and increasing
c.AMP levels (5). Prostacyclin has been reported by several
research groups to increase c.AMP levels in several tissues,
especially platelets. Not surprising, therefore, prostacyclin
increase c.AMP levels in granulosa cells obtained from rat ovarian
follicles, in vitro (6). Prostacyclin is apparently less potent
than PGE$_2$, though its stability in the incubation system in not
known. Although it has not been specifically reported, prostacyclin,
by increasing ovarian c.AMP levels, will presumably stimulate
steroidogenesis and progesterone production. However, it is
unlikely that prostacyclin, not PGE$_2$, have a physiological role in
stimulating steroidogenesis, since LH-induced progesterone secretion
by the ovary is not blocked by indomethacin treatment.

Another process induced by LH in the ovary is ovulation, and
this is blocked indomethacin treatment. PGE and PGF levels in
follicular fluid increase just prior to ovulation in the rat, rabbit
and pig (7,8,9). It would be relevant to know whether prostacyclin
levels also increase prior to ovulation in follicular fluid.
Furthermore, it is not really known which of the prostaglandins
produced by the follicle is the "active one" in ovulation, and

what its precise role is in the ovulatory process. Prostacyclin
may have a role in ovulation, but further study is needed.

Other changes occurring in the ovarian follicle, such as
follicular growth and ovum maturation are independent of prostaglandin involvement. Notwithstanding PGE_2 will induce final
ovum maturation, again showing that it is a LH mimic (10).
It would be interesting to know whether prostacyclin has a similar
pharmacological action.

In several non-primate species (e.g. sheep, guinea-pig, rat)
the cessation of progesterone secretion and regression of the
corpus luteum (luteolysis) is brought about by $PGF_{2\alpha}$ secreted from
the uterus. The uterus has therefore an important role in ovarian
function.

Uterus

During studies into the mechanism by which ovarian steroidal
hormones affect prostaglandin production by the uterus, it was
discovered that the major prostaglandin produced by homogenates
of the pseudopregnant rat uterus was $6\text{-oxo-PGF}_{1\alpha}$ (11). The uterus
of other species, namely sheep, guinea-pig, rabbit, monkey and
human, have also been shown to synthesise $6\text{-oxo-PGF}_{1\alpha}$ as a major
product (3,12). Consequently, in the uterus as in the ovary, the
prostacyclin biosynthetic pathway is potentially a major route
for PGH_2 metabilism.

The uterus consists of two layers, the secretory tissue
(endometrium) and muscular tissue (myometrium). There is a
difference in the prostaglandin synthesising capacity and in the
major prostaglandin formed between the two layers. Homogenates
of sheep endometrium, synthesise predominantly $PGF_{2\alpha}$, whith lesser
quantities of prostacyclin and PGE_2, while homogenates of sheep
myometrium synthesis much smaller quantities of $PGF_{2\alpha}$ and PGE_2 (S.N.
Alwachi, K.P. Bland and N.L. Poyser, unpublished results). The
myometrium from the pregnant rat uterus has a higher capacity to
synthesise prostacyclin than the endometrium (13).

In the study in the pseudopregnant rat uterus (11), prostaglandin production was highest on day 5. Subsequent studies on the
pregnant rat uterus have revealed that prostaglandin production is
also highest on day 5, with prostacyclin being the major product
formed (Christine A. Phillips and N. L. Poyser, unpublished results).
The possible significance of these findings is that day 5 is the
day of implantation in the rat. Complimentary studies have shown
that prostaglandin levels are highest at the implantation site
compared with other areas in the pregnant rat uterus, and that
these levels are higher on day 5 than day 6. Prostacyclin is the
most abundant in these implantation sites (14,15). These findings

suggest that prostaglandins, possibly prostacyclin, are important
in implantation, especially as indomethacin prevents or seriously
interferes with implantation in the rat (14, Christine A. Phillips
and N. L. Poyser, unpublished results). The role of prostaglandins
in implantation may be to cause the local increase in capillary
permeability at the implantation site, either directly or by
potentiating the effect of histamine. The role of prostaglandins,
especially prostacyclin, in implantation merits further study.

Another process in which uterine prostaglandins have
been implicated is parturition. In vitro, prostacyclin contracts
the term pregnant rat uterus (free of conceptuses), though it is
less potent than PGE_2 and $PGF_{2\alpha}$ (16, Christine A. Phillips and
N. L. Poyser, unpublished results). In addition, prostacyclin
sensitises the uterus to the spasmogenic action of oxytocin, and
is more potent than $PGF_{2\alpha}$ (16). It may be thought that since
prostacyclin is produced by the myometrium, it may have a role in
increasing uterine contractility at term both by its direct and
indirect actions on the myometrium. However, indomethacin treatment
of rats does not inhibit spontaneous or oxytocin-induced contractions
of the pregnant rat uterus at term (17). These findings cast doubt
on the postulate that myometrial prostacyclin production is essential
for contractions of the uterus during parturition. Nevertheless,
it has been observed in sheep that the level of $6\text{-oxo-PGF}_{1\alpha}$ increases
in utero-ovarian venous plasma, foetal venous plasma and amniotic
fluid during dexamethasone-induced parturition (18). A small
increase in the level of $6\text{-oxo-PGF}_{1\alpha}$ in amniotic fluid also occurs
prior to parturition in the monkey (19). From these limited number
of observations, it is apparent that prostacyclin production by
the pregnant uterus does increase prior to parturition. The role
of the prostacyclin may be to dilate the cervix rather than contract
the uterus. However, PGE_2 is also thought to have a role in dilating
the cervix, so obviously further study is required on this area.

Regarding thromboxane production by the pregnant uterus, there
is not increase in TXB_2 levels in utero-ovarian venous plasma
or amniotic fluid during adrenocorticotrophin (ATCH)-induced
parturition in sheep (20). Variable levels of TXB_2 have been found
in amniotic fluid during human labour, though there is no correlation between the level of TXB_2 and the degree of cervical dilatation
(21). A small increase in the level of TXB_2 has been observed
before delivery in pregnant monkeys (19), though the significance
of this finding is not clear.

Endometrial tissue obtained from pregnant rats on the day of
parturition has the ability to synthesise low amounts of thromboxane,
in vitro (22). A uterine horn removed from a pregnant rat uterus
at term and freed of conceptuses exhibits spontaneous activity when
suspended in an organ bath, in vitro. Significant quantities of
thromboxane are released into the bathing fluid surrounding the

uterine horn (Christine A. Phillips and N. L. Poyser, unpublished results). The pregnant rat uterus is therefore able to synthesise and release thromboxanes, in vitro. Whether, this occurs in vivo needs further study. A possible role of TXA$_2$ produced by the endometrium is to constrict the uterine blood vessels after birth, thereby preventing excessive uterine bleeding though this, at present, is pure speculation.

Returning to ovarian function, it is doubtful whether prosta-cyclin on thromboxanes produced by the uterus have any affect on processes occurring within the ovary. Only PGF$_{2\alpha}$ is important in this respect in so far as causing luteolysis in several non-primate species (23).

CONCLUSION

The ovaries ane uterus have a high capacity for synthesising prostacyclin, though differences exist between different tissues within these organs. In the ovary, prostacyclin stimulates c.AMP synthesis, but it is doubtful whether this is of any physiological significance. Uterine prostacyclin production may have a role in implantation and parturition. Thromboxane production by both the ovary and uterus is low, though the action of thromboxanes or thromboxane analogues on reproductive processes merits examination.

REFERENCES

1. N. L. Poyser, Physiological Roles of Prostaglandins in Reproduction. In: "Prostaglandins and Thromboxanes", F. Berti, B. Samuelsson and G. P. Velo, eds., p.205, Plenum Press, New York (1977).
2. M. P. Liedtke and B. Seifert, Biosynthesis of Prostaglandins in Human Ovarian Tissue, Prostaglandins, 16:825 (1978).
3. F. F. Sun, J. P. Chapman and J. C. McGuire, Metabolism of Prostaglandin Endoperoxides in Animal Tissues, Prostaglandins, 14:1055 (1977).
4. L. Speroff and P. W. Ramwell, Prostaglandin Stimulation of in vitro Progesterone Synthesis, J. Clin. Endocr. Metab., 30: 345 (1970).
5. J. M. Marsh, The Stimulatory Effect of Prostaglandin E$_2$ on Adenyl Cyclase in the Bovine Corpus Luteum, FEBS Letters, 7:283 (1970).
6. A. K. Goff, J. Zamecnik, M. Ali and D. T. Armstrong, Prostaglandin I$_2$ Stimulation of Granulosa Cell Cyclic AMP Production, Prostaglandins, 15:875 (1978).
7. W. J. LeMaire, R. Leidner and J. M. Marsh, Pre and Post Ovulatory Changes in the Concentration of Prostaglandins in Rat Graafian Follicles, Prostaglandins, 9:221 (1975).

8. N. S. T. Yang, J. M. Marsh and W. J. LeMaire, Prostaglandin
    Changes Induced by Ovulatory Stimuli in Rabbit Graafian
    Follicles. The Effect of Indomethacin, Prostaglandins, 4:
    395 (1973).
9. B. K. Tsang, L. Ainsworth, B. R. Downey and D. T. Armstrong,
    Pre-Ovulatory Changes in Cyclin AMP and Prostaglandin
    Concentration in Follicular Fluid of Gilts, Prostaglandins,
    17:141 (1979).
10. A Tsafriri, H. R. Lindner, U. Zor and S. A. Lamprecht,
    In vitro Induction of Meiotic Division in Follicle-Enclosed
    Oocytes by LH, cyclin AMP and Prostaglandin E_2, J. Reprod.
    Fert., 31:29 (1972).
11. L. Fenwick, R. L. Jones, B. Naylor, N. L. Poyser and N. H.
    Wilson, Production of Prostaglandins by the Pseudo-pregnant
    Rat Uterus, in vitro and the Effect of Tamoxifen with the
    Identification of 6-keto-Prostaglandin $F_{1\alpha}$ as a Major Product,
    Br. J. Pharmac., 59:191 (1977).
12. R. L. Jones, N. L. Poyser and N. H. Wilson, Production of 6-
    oxo-Prostaglandin $F_{1\alpha}$ by Rat, Guinea-pig and Sheep Uteri,
    in vitro, Br. J. Pharmac., 59:436P (1977).
13. K. I. Williams, A. Dembinskakiec, A. Zmuda and R. J.
    Gryglewski, Prostacyclin Formation by Myometrial and Decidual
    Fractions of Pregnant Rat Uterus, Prostaglandins, 15:343
    (1978).
14. T. G. Kennedy, Evidence for a Role of Prostaglandins in the
    Initiation of Blastocyst Implantation in the Rat, Biol.
    Reprod., 16:286 (1977).
15. T. G. Kennedy and J. Zamecnik, Concentration of 6-Keto-
    Prostaglandin F_1 alpha is Markedly Elevated at Site of
    Blastocyst Implantation in Rat, Prostaglandins, 16:599 (1978).
16. K. I. Williams, K. E. H. El-Jahir and E. Marcinkiewicz, Dual
    Actions of Prostacyclin (PGI_2) on the Rat Pregnant Uterus,
    Prostaglandins, 17:667 (1979).
17. A-R. Fuchs, Hormonal Control of Myometrial Function During
    Pregnancy and Parturition, Acta Endocr., 89: Suppl. 221, 9
    (1978).
18. M. D. Mitchell, D. A. Ellwood, A. B. M. Anderson and A. C.
    Turnbull, Elevated Concentrations of 6-Keto-Prostaglandin
    $F_{1\alpha}$ in Fetal and Maternal Plasma and in Amniotic Fluid during
    Ovine Parturition, Prostaglandins and Medicine, 1:265 (1978).
19. J. S. Robinson, R. Natale, L. Clover and M. D. Mitchell,
    Prostaglandin E, Thromboxane B_2 and 6-Oxo-Prostaglandin
    $F_{1\alpha}$ in Amniotic Fluid and Maternal Plasma of Rhesus Monkeys
    (Macaca Mulatta) during the Latter Third of Gestation, J.
    Endocr., 81:345 (1979).
20. M. D. Mitchell, B. R. Hicks and J. S. Robinson, Thromboxane
    B-2 in the Plasma and Amniotic Fluid of Late Pregnant and
    Peripartuient sheep, J. Reprod. Fert., 55:147 (1979).

21. M. D. Mitchell, M. J. N. C. Keirse, A. B. M. Anderson and A. C. Turnbull, Thromboxane B_2 in Amniotic Fluid Before and During Labour, Br. J. Obstet. Gynaec., 85:442 (1978).

22. K. I. Williams and I. Downing, Prostaglandin and Thromboxane Production by Rat Decidual Microsomes, Prostaglandins, 14: 813 (1977).

23. N. L. Poyser and E. W. Horton, Uterine Luteolytic Hormone: A Physiological Role for Prostaglandin $F_{2\alpha}$, Physiol. Rev., 56:595 (1976).

REGULATION OF PROSTAGLANIDN $F_{2\alpha}$ RELEASE FROM THE UTERUS DURING THE ESTROUS CYCLE

Hans Kindahl
Department of Obstetrics and Gynaecology
College of Veterinary Medicine
Swedish University of Agricultural Sciences
750 07 Uppsala, Sweden

INTRODUCTION

Already in 1923, Loeb (1) demonstrated that an utero-ovarian relationship existed by performing hysterectomy in guinea pigs and showing that these animals got persistent corpora lutea. Phariss and Wyngarden (2) postulated that the luteolytic substance from the uterus might be prostaglandin $F_{2\alpha}$, and McCracken et al. (3) identified release of $PGF_{2\alpha}$ into the utero-ovarian vein concomitant with regression of corpus luteum in the sheep. Several different types of prostaglandins and thromboxanes can be produced in the uterus (4), however, $PGF_{2\alpha}$ seems to be the far dominating substance which is released into the venous drainage of the uterus and regulating the life-span of the corpus luteum.

The purpose of the following article is to give a brief account of the hormonal mechanisms involved in the regulation of $PGF_{2\alpha}$ release from the uterus during the estrous cycle and early pregnancy.

RELEASE OF $PGF_{2\alpha}$ DURING NORMAL ESTROUS CYCLES AND EARLY PREGNANCY

Primary $PGF_{2\alpha}$ can be measured in the venous drainage of the uterus before entering the peripheral circulation and further metabolism. However, this experimental design requires fairly major surgical intervention, and it is known that this can result in long anestral periods after the insertion of the catheter (cf. 5). Instead the easiest and most reliable method is to quantitate $PGF_{2\alpha}$'s major blood plasma metabolite, 15-keto-13,14-dihydro-$PGF_{2\alpha}$, in peripheral blood plasma samples. This metabolite has a half-life in the circulation of about 8 min, and is not formed during the blood collection.

    The sequential changes in the levels of 15-keto-13,14-dihydro-PGF$_{2\alpha}$ and progesterone were studied in heifers during estrous cycles and early pregnancy. In the first study (6), samples were collected every three hours during the greater part of the estrous cycle. The levels of this PGF$_{2\alpha}$ metabolite varied in a pulsatile manner during luteolysis concomitantly with the decreases in progesterone levels (Fig. 1). However, the peaks often consisted of only one elevated value. In a more detailed study (7), samples

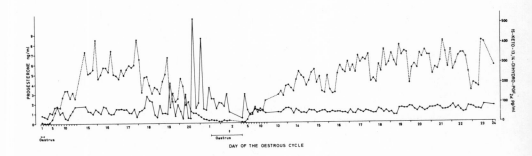

Fig. 1.   Peripheral plasma levels of progesterone (●---●) and
          15-keto-13,14-dihydro-PGF$_{2\alpha}$ (o——o) during one estrous
          cycle and early pregnancy in an heifer. Arrow denotes
          time of mating.

were collected every hour starting on day 16 of the estrous cycle. It was found that the prostaglandin release occurs during 2-3 days as rapid pulses with a duration of 1-5 hours prior to and during luteolysis (Fig.2, upper panel). From an experiment with an early pregnant heifer (6) it was shown that the rescue of the corpus luteum during pregnancy is at least partly due to inhibition of prostaglandin secretion from the pregnant uterus (Fig. 1). Similar results have been found in the early pregnant sheep (8).

From the study where one hour sampling has been performed it
can easily be shown that very varying pictures of the prostaglandin
release can be obtained if samples are not collected very frequently.
The lower panels of Fig. 2 illustrate the four different possibilities
that would have been obtained if samples had been collected only
every fourth hour during this particular luteolytic period. None
of the panels show a true picture of the luteolytic prostaglandin
release, and panel b) shows indeed a very insufficient and misleading
picture not reflecting $PGF_{2\alpha}$ production. However, to spare the
animals and not cause unnecessary stress we have chosen a three
hour sampling interval, which gives a good idea about increased
release of $PGF_{2\alpha}$ into the blood stream.

Measurements of 15-keto-13,14-dihydro-$PGF_{2\alpha}$ have also been
performed in cycling sheep (9) and mares (10), and rather similar
patterns compared to the cow have been obtained. Measurements of
primary $PGF_{2\alpha}$ in swine from the venous drainage (5,11) or
measurements of 15-keto-13,14-dihydro-$PGF_{2\alpha}$ in peripheral plasma
(12) have indicated increased release of $PGF_{2\alpha}$ after days 11-12 and
for about six days (Fig. 3, upper panel). Thus the endogenous
release correlate well in time when the corpus luteum in the swine
becomes sensitive and regresses after exogenously administered $PGF_{2\alpha}$
(13). During early pregnancy the prostaglandin release is
depressed with only transient elevations for about 36 hours (Fig. 3,
lower panel). This is consistent with an antiluteolytic mechanism
initiated by a signal from the conceptus at about day 11 of
pregnancy.

For ethical and practical reasons it can sometimes be a
problem to collect sufficiently frequent blood sampling for
example on humans or small laboratory animals. In these cases
urine samples are more suitable for studies of prostaglandin release.
The major drawback of measuring prostaglandin metabolites in
urine is that no rapid pulses of prostaglandin release can be seen,
however, it can be sufficient to know whether the daily production
of $PGF_{2\alpha}$ is increased or decreased during a physiological event.

The excretion of the main urinary $PGF_{2\alpha}$ metabolite ($5\alpha,7\alpha$-
dihydroxy-11-ketotetranorprostanoic acid) was followed in female
guinea pigs during estrous cycles (14). An elevation in the
metabolite levels was seen, beginning at days 11-13 with very high
levels during the two last days of the cycle and the first day of
the following cycle (Fig. 4, upper panel). This is in agreement
with earlier obtained results when $PGF_{2\alpha}$ was measured in utero-
ovarian venous blood (15). In this latter study it was only
possible to obtain one blood sample from each animal and not study
the release during several days. During early pregnancy this
increase in the prostaglandin productin is totally abolished
indicating an antiluteolytic action of the blastocysts (Fig. 4,
lower panel).

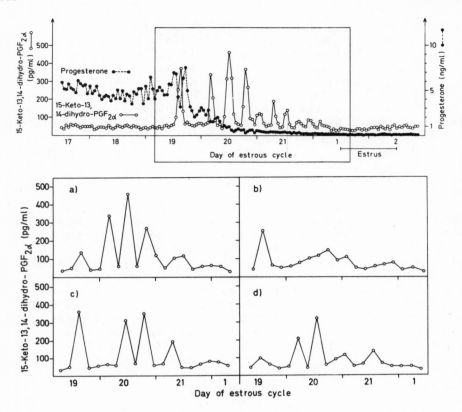

Fig. 2.　Peripheral plasma levels of 15-keto-13,14-dihydro-PGF$_{2\alpha}$
(o———o) and progesterone (•---•) during regression of
the corpus luteum in an heifer. The upper panel shows
the results obtained by analysing hourly samples while
the lower panels show four different profiles of
prostaglandin metabolite levels when only 6 samples a
day were obtained for analysis.

　　　　The release of prostaglandins during the estrous cycle is
very precise and control the length of the estrous cycle in a
manner typical for the species. The uterus can produce several
prostaglandins (4), but contains very strong prostaglandin endoperoxide F$_{2\alpha}$ reductase activity (16). The reducing factor seems
to be unique for the uterus and provides PGF$_{2\alpha}$ whenever prostaglandin endoperoxides are available. Inthe same uterine preparation an inhibiting factor of the fatty acid cyclooxygenase is
present, and its role is probably important for the regulation
of the prostaglandin release. Several more factors (e.g. for
control of phospholipase activity) might be present in the uterus
and together contributing to the very typical pulsatile pattern
of PGF$_{2\alpha}$ release.

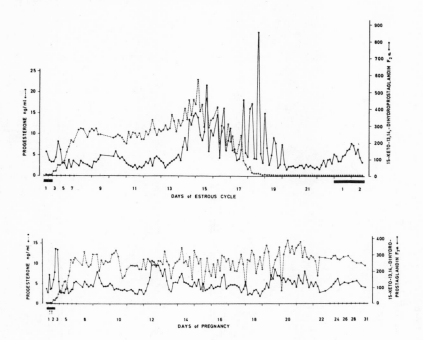

Fig. 3.   Concentrations of progesterone and 15-keto-13,14-dihydro-
          $PGF_{2\alpha}$ in peripheral plasma during the estrous cycle (upper
          panel) and early pregnancy (lower panel) in a gilt.
          Estrous is indicated by the horizontal black bar.   Arrows
          denote time of insemination.

RELEASE OF $PGF_{2\alpha}$ DURING EXPERIMENTAL ESTROUS CYCLES

Intrauterine iodine infusions, a common treatment of sub-
clinical endometritis in e.g. cows, cause a necrotizing endometritis
and alter the estrous cycle length dependent on when the infusions
are done (17).   In general, uterine infusions performed early in
the estrous cycle shortened the cycle length and infusions late
in the cycle lengthened it, while infusions during mid-cycle
appeared to have no effect.   Measurements of the $PGF_{2\alpha}$ metabolite
have shown that 1) prostaglandins are not released immediately
following the iodine infusions 2) release of prostaglandins starts
3-5 days after the iodine infusions concomitant with the repair
of the endometrium 3) progesterone priming is necessary before
$PGF_{2\alpha}$ can be released (18) (see Table 1 and Fig. 5, upper and
lower panels).   It is possible that, during repair, a time-lag
exists between the re-establishment of the above mentioned
prostaglandin inhibitory system (16) as compared to the prostaglandin
synthesizing system.

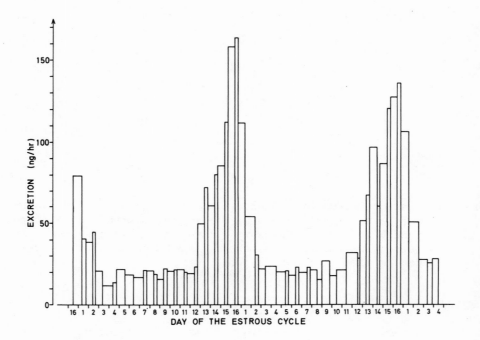

Fig. 4.   Excretion of 5α,7α-dihydroxy-11-ketotetranorprostanoic
          acid in the urine of a guinea pig during the estrous
          cycle (upper panel) and during pregnancy (lower panel).

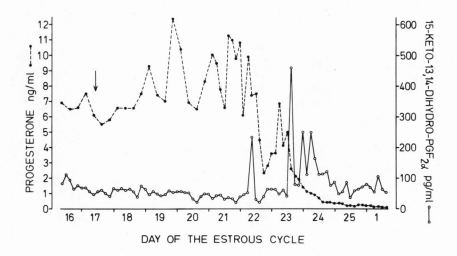

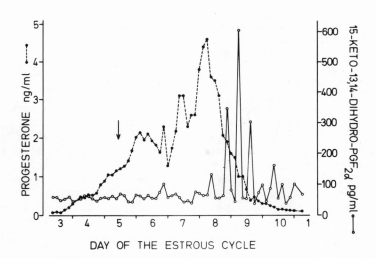

Fig. 5. Peripheral plasma levels of 15-keto-13,14-dihydro-PGF$_{2\alpha}$ (o——o) and progesterone (•---•) in cows subjected to intrauterine iodine infusions on day 5 (upper panel) and day 17 (lower panel), respectively, of the estrous cycle. Arrows denote time of the infusion.

Table 1.

Day of infusion	Cow no.	Pretreatment cycle (days)	Treatment cycle (days)	Posttreatment cycle (days)	Interval from infusion to PG release (hours)	Interval from infusion to estrus (days)
Early						
5	1	22	10	22	N.D.	5
5	2	23	10	22	N.D.	5
5	1	23	9	23	54	4
5	2	23	10	22	69	5
5	3	22	23	21	33	18
Middle						
11	1	23	19	22	147	8
12	2	22	19	23	120	7
Late						
16	1	22	23	23	117	7
17	2	22	25	23	117	8
20	4	21	26	22	93	6
20	3	23	21	N.D.	—	—

N.D. = Not determined.

In the mare $PGF_{2\alpha}$ release can be provoked by intrauterine infusion of physiological saline (19). The release is immediate and cause premature regression of the corpus luteum. Such a treatment is ineffective in e.g. cows and does not alter the estrous cycle length.

Several studies have investigated the role of exogenous progesterone and estradiol in provoking $PGF_{2\alpha}$ release in oophorectomized animals (8,20,21). The progesterone withdrawal in itself has also been suggested as a stimulus for prostaglandin release in cycling ewes (22). However, this release was insignificant (maximum 1/10 of that during normal luteolysis in sheep (cf. 3)). In a study performed in cycling cows, the progesterone withdrawal was performed by enucleation of corpus luteum or injections of cloprostenol (cloprostenol is not in the dose given interfering with the $PGF_{2\alpha}$ metabolite assay). Animals treated before around days 12-13 showed no release of $PGF_{2\alpha}$ (Fig. 6). Animals in which luteolysis was induced later in the estrous cycle showed a small and shortlasting elevation in the prostaglandin metabolite levels (Fig. 7). Both the early and late treated animals showed heat within 2-4 days (with the exception of one aminal), had a contracted uterus and ovulated at the expected time after estrus (23). The prostaglandin release in the animals treated late during the cycle is much smaller than that seen during normal luteolysis (Figs. 1 and 2) both concerning the magnitude and the frequency of the prostaglandin peaks. Thus the findings here do not support the idea that the progesterone withdrawal alone

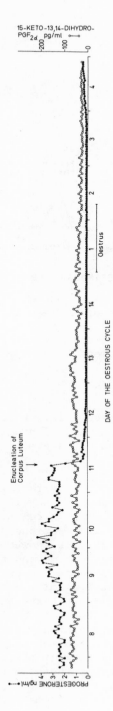

Fig. 6. Peripheral plasma levels of 15-keto-13,14-dihydro-PGF$_{2\alpha}$ (o——o) and progesterone (●--●) in a heifer subjected to manual enucleation of the corpus luteum on day 11 of the estrous cycle.

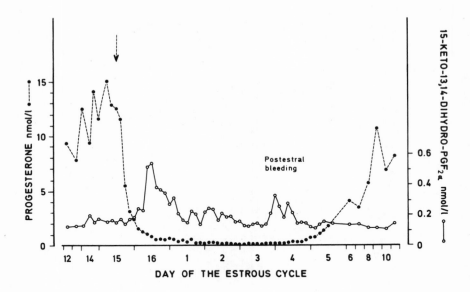

Fig. 7.   Peripheral plasma levels of 15-keto-13,14-dihydro-PGF$_{2\alpha}$
(o——o) and progesterone (•---•) in a cow treated with
cloprostenol on day 15 of the estrous cycle.   Arrow
denote time of the treatment.

plays an important role during luteolysis. Probably the induced
luteolysis is too rapid and effective, and progesterone levels
decrease very rapidly, and no need for a prostaglandin release can
be seen.

    Our last experiment was performed by inserting progesterone
implants subcutaneously in three cows on day 12 of the estrous
cycle. The implants were known to give a relatively constant
release of progesterone resulting in a peripheral blood plasma level
of about 1 ng/ml. All the three animals showed a normal luteolytic
release of prostaglandins at expected time and the progesterone
levels declined, but due to the presence of the implants progesterone
was maintained at a level of about 1 ng/ml. However, the release
of prostaglandins continued and did not cease until the implants
were removed. The animals showed heat two days after removal of
the implants (Fig. 8) (24). Thus, maintenance of the release of
prostaglandin seems to be an all-or-none phenomenon, meaning that
the progesterone level by itself maintains the release once it has
been initiated, but does not regulate the height, duration and
frequency of prostaglandin peaks. It is not known if progesterone
alone or in combination with estrogens from the ovary possess this

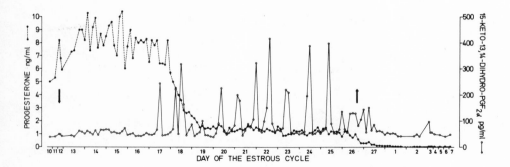

Fig. 8.   Peripheral plasma levels of 15-keto-13,14-dihydro-PGF$_{2\alpha}$
          (o———o) and progesterone (•---•) in a heifer subjected
          to progesterone implants. Arrow denote time of
          insertion (↓) and removel (↑) of progesterone implants,
          respectively.

triggering effect on the prostaglandin synthesis and release.
Furthermore, the low progesterone level seems to be crucial for
inhbition of the prostaglandin release.

        A higher level of circulating progesterone from implants
should probably give a similar result, since the progesterone
level was chosen to about 1 ng/ml because it is a normal (but
very low) level found in the cow (6). A similar experiment has
been done by Smith et al. (25) in the cow. Instead of progesterone
implants Provera-impregnated intravaginal sponges were used. They
observed that during decrease in progesterone levels after removal
of the sponges a prostaglandin release was seen, however they
never studied an eventual prostaglandin release during the
regression of the corpus luteum and the whole period of artificial
progesterone support. It is obviously very likely that PGF$_{2\alpha}$
also in this experiment has been released over the whole period
of progesterone support, and that they only observed the last
prostaglandin metabolite peaks. Thus the progesterone withdrawal
in itself is of no importance for initiating prostaglandin release.

ACKNOWLEDGEMENTS

        These studies have been supported by grants from the World
Health Organization and from the Swedish Council for Forestry
and Agricultural Research.

REFERENCES

1. L. Loeb, The effect of extirpation of the uterus on the life
   and function of the corpus luteum in the guinea pig, Proc.
   Soc. Exptl. Biol. Med., 20:441 (1923).
2. B. B. Phariss and L. J. Wyngarden, The effect of prostaglandin
   $F_{2\alpha}$ on the progestogen content of ovaries from pseudopregnant
   rats, Proc. Soc. Exptl. Biol. Med., 130:92 (1969).
3. J. A. McCracken, J. C. Carlson, M. E. Glew, J. R. Goding, D. T.
   Baird, K. Green and B. Samuelsson, Prostaglandin $F_{2\alpha}$ identified
   as a luteolytic hormone in sheep, Nature New Biol., 238:
   129 (1972).
4. N. L. Poyser, this publication 1980.
5. A. R. Gleeson, G. D. Thorburn and R. I. Cox, Prostaglandin
   F concentrations in the uteroovarian venous plasma of the sow
   during the late luteal phase of the oestrous cycle,
   Prostaglandins, 5:521 (1974).
6. H. Kindahl, L.-E. Edqvist, A. Bane and E. Granstrom, Blood
   levels of progesterone and 15-keto-13,14-dihydroprostaglandin
   $F_{2\alpha}$ during the normal oestrous cycle and early pregnancy in
   heifers, Acta Endocrinol., 82:134 (1976).
7. H. Kindahl, L.-E. Edqvist, E. Granstrom and A. Bane, The
   release of prostaglandin $F_{2\alpha}$ as reflected by 15-keto-13,14-
   dihydroprostaglandin $F_{2\alpha}$ in the peripheral circulation during
   normal luteolysis in heifers, Prostaglandins, 11:871 (1976).
8. J. S. Roberts, B. Barcikowski, L. Wilson, R. C. Skarnes and
   J. A. McCracken, Hormonal and related factors affecting the
   release of prostaglandin $F_{2\alpha}$ from the uterus, J. Steroid
   Biochem., 6:1091 (1975).
9. H. Kindahl, E. Granström, L. E. Edqvist and P. Eneroth,
   Prostaglandin levels in peripheral plasma during the reproductive
   cycle. In" "Advances in Prostaglandin and Thromboxane Research",
   vol. 2, B. Samuelsson and R. Paoletti, eds., Raven Press (1976),
   667.
10. G. H. Stabenfeldt, L.-E. Edqvist, H. Kindahl, B. Gustafsson
    and A. Bane, Physiological concepts in female reproduction and
    their practical implications. J. Amer. Vet. Med. Ass., 172:
    667 (1978).
11. M. P. E. Moeljono, W. W. Thatcher, F. W. Bazer, M. Frank, L.
    J. Owens and C. J. Wilcox, A study of prostaglandin $F_{2\alpha}$ as
    the luteolysin in swine : II. Characterization and comparison
    of prostaglandin F, estrogens and progestin concentrations in
    utero-ovarian vein plasma of non-pregnant and pregnant
    gilts, Prostaglandins, 14:543 (1977).
12. V. M. Shille, I. Karlbom, S. Einarsson, K. Larsson, H. Kindahl
    and L.-E. Edqvist, Concentrations of progesterone and 15-keto-
    13,14-dihydroprostaglandin $F_{2\alpha}$ in peripheral plasma during the
    estrous cycle and early pregnancy in gilts, Zbl. Vet. Med. A.,
    26:169 (1979).

13. D. M. Hallford, R. P. Wetteman, E. J. Turman and I. T. Omtvedt, Luteal function in gilts after prostaglandin $F_{2\alpha}$, J. Anim. Sci., 41:1706 (1975).

14. E. Granstrom and H. Kindahl, Radioimmunoassay for urinary metabolites of prostaglandin $F_{2\alpha}$, Prostaglandins, 12:759 (1976).

15. F. R. Blatchley, B. T. Donovan, E. W. Horton and N. L. Poyser, The release of prostaglandins and progestin into the utero-ovarian venous blood of guinea-pigs during the estrous cycle and following estrogen treatment, J. Physiol., 223:69 (1972).

16. P. Wlodawer, H. Kindahl and M. Hamberg, Biosynthesis of prostaglandin $F_{2\alpha}$ from arachidonic acid and prostaglandin endoperoxides in the uterus, Biochim. Biophys. Acta, 431:603 (1976).

17. B. E. Seguin, D. A. Morrow and T. M. Louis, Luteolysis, luteostasis, and the effect of prostaglandin $F_{2\alpha}$ in cows after endometrial irritation, Amer. J. Vet. Res., 35:57 (1974).

18. H. Kindahl, E. Granstrom, L.-E. Edqvist, B. Gustafsson, G. Astrom and G. Stabenfeldt, Progesterone and 15-keto-13,14-dihydroprostaglandin $F_{2\alpha}$ levels in peripheral circulation after intrauterine iodine infusions in cows, Acta Vet. Scand., 18:274 (1977).

19. D. P. Neely, G. H. Stabenfeldt, H. Kindahl, J. P. Hughes and J. W. Kendrick, Effect of intrauterine saline infusion during the late luteal phase on the estrous cycle and luteal function of the mare, Am. J. Vet. Res., 40:665 (1979)

20. B. V. Caldwell, S. A. Tilson, W. A. Brock and L. Speroff, The effects of exogenous progesterone and estradiol on prostaglandin F levels in ovariectomized ewes, Prostaglandins, 1:217 (1972).

21. T. M. Louis, D. M. Parry, J. S. Robinson, G. D. Thorburn and J. R. G. Challis, Effects of exogenous progesterone and oestradiol on prostaglandin F and 13,14-dihydro-15-oxo prostaglandin $F_{2\alpha}$ concentrations in uteri and plasma of ovariectomized ewes, J. Endocr., 73:427 (1977).

22. J. R. G. Challis, C. S. Forster, B. J. A. Furr, J. S. Robinson and G. D. Thorburn, Production of prostaglandin F_α in ewes following luteal regression induced with a prostaglandin analogue, Estrumate (cloprostenol ; I.C.I. 80996), Prostaglandins, 11:537 (1976).

23. H. Kindahl, L.-E. Edqvist and J.-O. Lindell, On the control of prostaglandin release during the bovine estrous cycle, Abstr. International Prostaglandin Conference, Washington, (1979), 61.

24. H. Kindahl, J.-O. Lindell and L.-E. Edqvist, On the control of prostaglandin release during the bovine estrous cycle. Effects of progesterone implants, Prostaglandins, (1979) in press.

25.   J. F. Smith, R. J. Fairclough and A. J. Peterson, Plasma
      levels of progesterone, Provera, oestradiol-17β, and
      13,14-dihydro-15-keto-prostaglandin F in cows treated with
      Provera-impregnated intravaginal sponges, J. Reprod. Fert.
      55:359 (1979).

ACTION OF PROSTAGLANDINS AND OTHER ARACHIDONIC ACID METABOLITES ON AIRWAY FUNCTION

*M. F. Cuthbert and **P. J. Gardiner,

*Department of Pharmacology and Therapeutics
London Hospital Medical College, London and
Chest Unit, Department of Medicine
Kings College Hospital, London, England

The prostaglandins were first isolated from the lungs by Bergstrom and his co-workers in 1962 (1). More recently other metabolites of arachidonic acid have also been isolated from the lungs, namely, thromboxanes (2,3) and prostacyclin (4). It is now established that the prostaglandins, thromboxanes and prostacyclin (prostanoids) have powerful effects on both respiratory and vascular smooth muscle and that the lungs have an important function in their metabolic degradation. The most important enzyme in this respect is 15-prostaglandin dehydrogenase and some 90% of most infused prostaglandins except the PGA's and PGI_2 are removed in a single passage through the pulmonary circulation in both animals and man (5,6). It is understandable that these findings have led to considerable speculation on the possible physiological and pathological role of the prostanoids on respiratory function and has raised the possibility that prostaglandins of the E series or their metabolites, or substances that interfere with the synthesis of action of the prostanoids, might be of therapeutic value in the treatment of certain respiratory disorders, notably in bronchial asthma.

In this article it is intended to review the actions of the prostanoids on airways function. An experimental section is also included which describes recent studies on the paradoxical effect of some prostanoids on isolated smooth muscle preparations from the guinea-pig and man.

**Research Department, Miles Laboratories Limited, Stoke Poges, Slough, Berks., England.

EFFECTS OF PROSTAGLANDINS ON RESPIRATORY SMOOTH MUSCLE FUNCTION

Animal Studies

Prostaglandins of both E and F series have marked activity
on isolated smooth muscle preparations. Prostaglandin $F_{2\alpha}$ ($PGF_{2\alpha}$)
usually causes contraction of preparations from a number of
species (7) while prostaglandin E_1 (PGE_1) causes relaxation (8).
These effects appear to be directly on smooth muscle, the relaxant
effects of the E prostaglandins being mediated through the cyclic
AMP system. More recently (9) paradoxical effects, particularly
of prostaglandin E_2 (PGE_2) have been described and these will be
referred to later.

Studies in anaesthetised animals have in general confirmed
the findings in isolated tissues, $PGF_{2\alpha}$ increasing bronchial
resistance whereas PGE_1 antagonises the increase in bronchial
resistance due to histamine or vagal stimulation and sometimes
reduces resting tone (8,10). Rosenthale and his co-workers (11,12)
showed that both PGE_1 and PGE_2 by aerosol can prevent the
bronchoconstriction produced by histamine or anaphylaxis although
their relative potency compared with isoprenaline depended on the
species used.

In a comparative study in the guinea-pig (13) it has been
shown that although PGE_1 and isoprenaline have similar activity by
the intravenous route, when given by aerosol PGE_1 had 10-100 times
the activity of isoprenaline. The difference in the activity of
PGE_1 by the intravenous and aerosol route may be because infused
prostaglandins are rapidly inactivated by the lungs (5,6).

Human Studies

In 1968, Sweatman & Collier (14) showed that human bronchial
muscle has intrinsic tone and that $PGF_{2\alpha}$ causes contraction
whereas both PGE_1 and PGE_2 cause relaxation. Initial studies in
asthmatics with a freon-activated preparation of PGE_1 using simple
spirometry (15) showed bronchodilatation with an inhaled dosage
of 55 µg which was comparable in degree and duration to that of
500µg isoprenaline. The free acid of PGE_1 was found consistently
to cause coughing and retrosternal soreness in normal subjects and
so the neutral triethenolamine salt was used in all studies in
asthmatics. More recent studies using total body pletysmography
(16) have shown both PGE_1 and PGE_2 to be effective bronchodilators
causing a fall in airways resistance and a rise in specific airways
conductance.

When inhaled by healthy subjects $PGF_{2\alpha}$ is known to be a potent
bronchoconstrictor of short duration (17) which can be effectively
reversed by isoprenaline or PGE_2 inhalation (16,18). Pretreatment

of the subjects with several possible prostaglandin antagonists, flufenamic acid, disodium cromoglycate and atropine, failed to modify $PGF_{2\alpha}$-induced bronchoconstriction (16) although Patel (19) has shown atropine pretreatment to reduce $PGF_{2\alpha}$-induced bronchoconstriction in asthmatics, probably indicating a cholinergic component in these patients.

In 1973, Mathe and his co-workers (20) drew attention to the possible role of $PGF_{2\alpha}$ in bronchial asthma. Using total body plethysmography, asthmatics were found to be about 10 times more sensitive to histamine inhalation than healthy subjects but approximately 8000 times more sensitive to $PGF_{2\alpha}$ inhalation than healthy subjects. This led the authors to suggest that hypersensitivity to endogenous $PGF_{2\alpha}$ may contribute to increased airways resistance and that local release of $PGF_{2\alpha}$ might explain the precipitation of an asthmatic attack by a variety of stimuli. The hypersensitivity of asthmatics to inhaled $PGF_{2\alpha}$ has been confirmed (16) but shows marked individual variation, some asthmatics being no more sensitive than healthy subjects. Variation in sensitivity was not correlated with any particular feature of asthma or its treatment.

Both PGE_2 and $PGF_{2\alpha}$ have been shown to affect airways function when given intravenously (16,21). As expected, $PGF_{2\alpha}$ increases airways resistance in healthy subjects, whereas PGE_2 reduces airways resistance in healthy subjects but has variable effects in asthmatics. The role of $PGF_{2\alpha}$ and other prostanoids in bronchial asthma is discussed in a later section.

RECENT DEVELOPMENTS

Following the discovery of further metabolites of the arachidonic acid cycloxygenase cascade and of the prostaglandins, these new substances were examined for bronchomotor activity in animals and in some cases man.

Animal Studies

In vitro. Most of this work has been performed using the superfused guinea-pig trachea. It can be seen in Table 1 that all of the naturally occurring metabolites of arachidonic acid except PGE_2 and $PGF_{2\beta}$, the synthetic isomer of $PGF_{2\alpha}$, contract the trachea.

The relative contractant potencies of these substances to $PGF_{2\alpha}$ differ greatly, with thromboxane A_2 (TXA_2) being the most potent and thromboxane B_2 (TXB_2) the weakest. The two prostaglandin isomers, prostaglandin D_2 (PGD_2), the naturally occurring isomer of PGE_2, and $PGF_{2\beta}$ had opposite effects to their counterparts.

TABLE 1

Relative Bronchomotor Activity of Some Metabolites of Arachidonic Acid
in the Guinea-Pig in vitro and in vivo

Metabolite	Relative bronchomotor activity in vitro ($PGF_{2\alpha} = 1$)	Reference	Relative bronchomotor activity in vivo ($PGF_{2\alpha} = 1$)	Reference
TXA_2	45	3, 22	30 – 500	3, 22
TXB_2	1/14	23	1/10 – 1/100*	23*
PGI_2	weak contractant	4, 24	relaxant	25
PGG_2) PGH_2) PGD_2)	5 – 10	31	5 – 10	31
PGE_2	relaxant	8	relaxant	8
$PGF_{2\beta}$	relaxant	26	relaxant	26

*in dogs

Some of the metabolites of prostaglandin E_2 and $F_{2\alpha}$ have also been tested for relative bronchomotor activities to their parent compounds (Table 2).

All of these metabolites had similar qualitative activities to their parents but their relative potencies differed, with the 15-oxo derivatives being equipotent and the others generally being markedly less potent.

Prostacyclin (PGI$_2$) unlike the other metabolites of arachidonate and prostaglandins, appears less distinct in its type of bronchomotor activity on the guinea-pig trachea. PGI$_2$ has been found to act as a weak contractant of the trachea at basal inherent or acetylcholine-induced tone levels (4,24). In contrast, PGI$_2$ has been shown to inhibit carbachol-induced contractions of the guinea-pig trachea (25). 6 oxo-PGF$_{1\alpha}$, the main degradation product of PGI$_2$, was inactive in all of these studies.

<u>In vivo</u>. It can be seen in Table 1 that the rank order of contractant potency of the prostanoids in the guinea-pig <u>in vivo</u> correlates with that <u>in vitro</u>.

Endoperoxides administered by aerosol to guinea-pig produced both a transient increase followed by antagonism of induced tracheal insufflation pressure. It was suggested that this mixed action of the endoperoxides was a result of their conversion to prostaglandins mainly of the E-type. As TXA$_2$ is very unstable (t$\frac{1}{2}$-about 30S in aqueous medium at 37°C) it has not been tested by aerosol administration.

Prostaglandin $F_{2\beta}$ (PGF$_{2\beta}$) was shown to be an effective bronchodilator protecting anaesthetised guinea-pigs and cats against acetylcholine and PGF$_{2\alpha}$-induced bronchoconstriction (26). In contrast to PGE$_1$ and PGE$_2$, however, PGF$_{2\beta}$ was a relatively weak bronchodilator by aerosol although it was as active as isoprenaline or salbutamol. Similarly PGD$_2$ had the opposite bronchomotor activity to its isomer PGE$_2$ in anaesthetised dogs and guinea-pigs (30,31).

The primary and tertiary metabolites of PGF$_{2\alpha}$ and PGE$_2$ were shown to be markedly less active than their parent compounds in inducing or inhibiting bronchoconstriction in anaesthetised guinea-pigs (27). The 13,14 dihydro derivatives of PGE$_{2\alpha}$ and E_2, however, were approximately equipotent with their parent compounds.

The bronchomotor activities of the prostanoids <u>in vivo</u> have as yet correlated with their effects on the isolated tracheo-bronchial tissues. In contrast prostacyclin which appeared to have little or no bronchomotor activity <u>in vitro</u> has been shown to inhibit PGF$_{2\alpha}$-induced bronchoconstriction in the dog and histamine-

TABLE 2

Relative Bronchomotor Potency of Some Metabolites
of PGE_2 and $PGF_{2\alpha}$ on the Isolated Guinea-Pig Trachea

PG Metabolite	Relative bronchomotor potency ($PGF_{2\alpha}$ and PGE_2 = 1)	Reference
15-oxo $PGF_{2\alpha}$	1.1, 2-3	27, 28
13,14,dihydro $PGF_{2\alpha}$	1.2	27
13,14,dihydro,15-oxo $PGF_{2\alpha}$	0.08	27
15-oxo PGE_2	0.16, 1.3	27, 29
13,14,dihydro PGE_2	0.12, 0.1-0.2	27, 29
13,14,dihydro,15-oxo PGE_2	0.06, 0.01	27, 29

or antigen-induced bronchoconstriction in guinea-pigs (25).
Surprisingly PGI_2 was active by both the intravenous and aerosol
routes of administration. The latter result was unexpected as
PGI_2 quickly degrades to its stable degradation product, 6-oxo-
$PGF_{1\alpha}$, which is inactive or markedly less active in this test
model.

Human Studies

In vitro. It was generally believed from earlier studies
that E and F prostaglandins relaxed and contracted human isolated
bronchial muscle respectively. However, a more detailed study
of the parent prostaglandins actions revealed that PGE_2 was capable
of inducing both contraction and relaxation of human bronchial
muscle probably by stimulation of the PGF contractant or the PGE
relaxant receptor (32,33). These results were confirmed by
Strandberg and Hedqvist (34). Of the remaining studies on
human isolated bronchial muscle only the endoperoxides, PGD_2
and the primary metabolite of $PGF_{2\alpha}$ have been tested (28,35). All
of these substances contracted human bronchial muscle with
similar potencies to that of $PGF_{2\alpha}$.

In vivo. The poor stability and the high potential risk
involved in testing inhaled TXA_2, endoperoxides and PGD_2 have
restricted recent clinical research to the use of PGE_1, E_2, $F_{2\alpha}$,

I_2 and $F_{2\beta}$. Generally the aims of these studies were to clarify the direct tracheobronchial smooth muscle activity of the prostanoids and to investigate their full range of therapeutic uses in the respiratory tract.

$PGF_{2\alpha}$. Patel found that inhalation of $PGF_{2\alpha}$ by healthy volunteers resulted in two distinct responding groups (36), those who only showe ‹signs of large airway constriction (as seen by changes in airways conductance SG_{AW} only) and those in which peripheral airways constriction only occurred (as seen by changes in closing volume). All asthmatics showed both large and small airways constriction to varying degrees. Initially it appeared that aspirin-sensitive asthmatics seemed to tolerate much higher doses of inhaled $PGF_{2\alpha}$ than aspirin-insensitive patients (37). A similar study by Orehek et al (38), however, found that large numbers of aspirin-sensitive asthmatics were highly sensitive to inhaled $PGF_{2\alpha}$. This cast confusion on the previous workers hypothesis which stated that airway regulation in aspirin-sensitive asthmatics is more dependent upon endogenous prostaglandins than aspirin-insensitive patients.

Orehek et al also showed that SCH 1000, an anticholinergic drug, inhibited the immediate bronchoconstrictor effect of $PGF_{2\alpha}$ but it failed to prevent either coughing or the more severe late (30 min) bronchoconstriction (38). These results confirmed those of Patel and of Mathé & Hedqvist (19,39) and taken together suggest that the immediate bronchoconstriction induced by $PGF_{2\alpha}$ is probably the result of stimulation of the lung irritant receptors whereas the late severe response is probably produced by a different process, which might be stimulation of a specific prostanoid receptor(s).

PGE_1 and E_2. Recent studies have shown that the prostaglandins in addition to their direct activity on the smooth muscle of the airways may have significant physiological or pathophysiological roles on some important cells lining the airways. The mast cells lining the airways are thought to play a major role in airway constriction in asthma. A number of stimuli are thought to degranulate mast cells resulting in the release of their contents amongst which are found two potent bronchoconstrictor agents, histamine and SRS-A or leukotriene C. Following a study of the bronchomotor activity if inhaled PGE_1 and E_2 in asthmatics Pasargiklian et al (40) showed that premedication of asthmatics with these two prostaglandins resulted in significant protection against non-specific water mist, esercise and allergen-induced bronchoconstriction. These results, although limited, seem to strengthen earlier observations (41) that E prostaglandins inhibit human lung mast cell degranulation in vitro and consequently have the potential to protect the patient against the offending stimulus.

There are indications that PGE_1 may also directly affect
the surface epithelial secretory cells (goblet, epithelial serous
and Clara cells) of the tracheobronchial tract. These cells are
responsible for tracheobronchial mucus secretion which in asthma
generally seems as yet to be an area of underestimated pathophysiological importance. Most of the early work concerning
prostaglandin involvement in mucus secretion (42,43) was performed
using rats, hamsters, cats and monkeys. More recently a study
has been carried out on mucociliary clearance in asthmatics after
inhaling PGE_1 (44). Although the majority of the patients showed
definite signs of imporvement in mucociliary action 30 min after
drug treatment, this was not thought to be significant. Further
larger studies of these new potential therapeutic roles of
prostaglandins in asthma are needed before conclusions can be
reached.

PGI_2. It has recently been shown in healthy volunteers and
asthmatic subjects (45,46) that, although inhaled PGI_2 or its
stable 20-methyl isomer (250µg-500µg) were inactive with respect
to bronchomotor activity, the former induces slight pharyngeotracheal
irritation with some coughing. Both compounds administered 6-7
min prior to non-specific H_2O mist or exercise-induced asthma
completely prevented the expected bronchoconstrictor response
as did disodium cromoglycate. These results seemed at the time to
suggest that PGI_2 may be inhibiting mast cell degranulation.
This suggestion has recently been rejected (47) since similar doses
of PGI_2 provided no protection against antigen-induced bronchoconstriction.

$PGF_{2\beta}$. A recent study in healthy and asthmatic volunteers
(48) showed slight bronchoconstriction, tightness of the chest
and initial coughing following the inhalation of $PGF_{2\beta}$, the most
severe symptoms occurring in asthmatics. These results were
disappointing in view of the bronchodilator activity seen in
experimental animals but seem to emphasise the poor predictive
value of such observations in animals for the qualitative activity
of some of the prostanoids in the tracheobronchial tract of man.

PARADOXICAL ACTIVITY OF PROSTANOIDS IN VITRO

A series of experiments has recently been performed using
two isolated tracheobronchial preparations to clarify the
bronchomotor activities of some of the previously mentioned
prostanoids. The two tissues used were the isolated guinea-pig
trachea zig zag strip as described by Piper (49) and the human
isolated bronchial muscle strip as described by Collier & Sweatman
(50). A cumulative dosing procedure was used for all of the
drugs with a 5 min contact time except in the case of PGI_2 which
was 10 min. Tissue movement was recorded by an isotonic transducer
with a load of 250mg. The tissues were allowed to equilibrate at

which point they possessed inherent tone. Drug responses were
measured as either a reduction or an increase in this natural
inherent level of tone. A wide range of drug concentrations
were used on both tissues. Isoprenaline and histamine acted as
reference relaxant and contractant agents respectively. It can
be seen from Fig. 1 that the rank order of relaxant potency for
the drugs using the guinea-pig trachea was isoprenaline>PGE_1>$PGF_{2\beta}$
>PGI_2>PGE_1>$PGF_{2\alpha}$ although $PGF_{2\alpha}$ generally acted as a weak
contractant. Further scrutiny of these results (Table 3), however,
reveals that unlike isoprenaline or histamine, which produced
consistent relaxant or contractant responses respectively, the
prostanoids produced a high incidence of unexpected effects on
some preparations. The incidence of these paradoxial effects
varied greatly, although PGE_1 and $PGF_{2\beta}$ predominantly produced
relaxant responses. In contrast to their effects on the guinea-pig

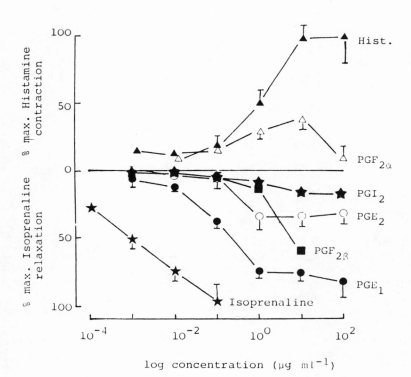

Fig. 1.   Mean effects of reference prostaglandins on the isolated
          guinea-pig trachea. Each point represents the mean of
          at least 4 observations and the vertical lines represent
          the standard error of the means.

TABLE 3

Paradoxical Effects of Reference Prostaglandins
on the Isolated Guinea-Pig Trachea

PG	Conc'n $\mu g\ ml^{-1}$	Total no. of observations made	Percent incidence contraction (C) or relaxation (R)
E_1	0.01	212	1.4 (C)
E_2	0.001	6	66.6 (C)
	0.01	25	36.0 (C)
	0.1	49	24.4 (C)
	1.0	47	6.3 (C)
	10.0	41	9.7 (C)
$F_{2\alpha}$	0.01	61	16.4 (R)
	0.1	104	13.5 (R)
	1.0	120	8.4 (R)
	10.0	89	15.7 (R)
I_2	0.001	9	22 (C)
	0.01	9	33 (C)
	0.1	9	11 (C)
	1.0	9	0 (C)
	10.0	8	0 (C)
	100.0	3	0 (C)

trachea, only two of the prostanoids, PGE_1 and PGI_2, acted
consistently as relaxants of human isolated bronchial muscle
(Fig. 2). The remainder contracted the tissue with the following
rank order of potency $PGF_{2\alpha} > PGE_2 > PGF_{2\beta}$: Again, further scrutiny
of these results also reveals that isoprenaline and histamine
produced responses of one type only, this was not so far the
prostanoids (Table 4). Although PGE_1 virtually always relaxed
the preparations, the other prostanoids produced a significant
number of contractant responses at most dose levels.

As expected human isolated bronchial muscle is a very useful
tissue in predicting the qualitative activity of prostanoids in
man. It seems of little value, however, in predicting the
quantative activity of the prostanoids in man in that PGE_1 appears
markedly less active than isoprenaline in vitro but on inhalation

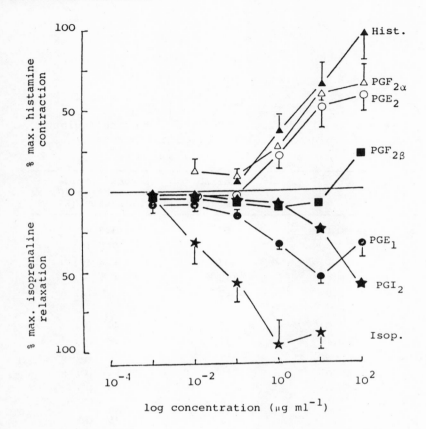

Fig. 2.   Mean effects of reference prostaglandins on human
          isolated bronchial muscle. Each point is the mean of at
          least 4 observations and the vertical lines represent
          the standard error of the mean.

by man the order of relative potencies are reversed with PGE_1 being
far superior to isoprenaline. Unexpectedly, however, the guinea-
pig trachea which in the past was highly predictive of the bronchodilator activities of sympathomimetics and methylxanthines
proved of no value in predicting bronchodilator activity of
prostanoids in man. This latter point is especially emphasised
by the findings for $PGF_{2\beta}$ which contracts both human airways
in vitro and in vivo. Many suggestions can be proposed to explain
the discrepancy between the guinea-pig and human airway
responsiveness to prostanoids eg, species differences, location of
tissue within the tracheobronchial tract etc. One explanation
which appealed to us and which we have investigated was a possible
difference in the endogenous substances responsible for the
regulation of inherent tone of each tissue.

TABLE 4

Paradoxical Effects of Reference Prostaglandins
on Human Isolated Bronchial Muscle

PG	Conc'n $\mu g\ ml^{-1}$	Total no. of observations made	Percent incidence contraction (C) or relaxation (R)
E_1	0.01	67	3.3 (C)
	0.1	179	0.5 (C)
	1.0	187	1.6 (C)
	10.0	176	1.5 (C)
	100.0	17	11.7 (C)
E_2	0.01	5	20 (C)
	0.1	31	58 (C)
	1.0	39	80 (C)
	10.0	33	91 (C)
	100.0	4	100 (C)
$F_{2\alpha}$	0.01	4	25 (R)
	0.1	29	17.2 (R)
I_2	0.001	8	25.0 (C)
	0.01	11	36.4 (C)
	0.1	11	27.3 (C)
	1.0	8	25.0 (C)
$F_{2\beta}$	0.01	8	62.5 (C)
	0.1	9	44.4 (C)
	1.0	9	44.4 (C)
	10.0	10	30.0 (C)
	100.0	4	50.0 (C)

It has already been shown by Orehek et al (51) that endogenous prostaglandins are responsible for the regulation of the inherent tone of the guinea-pig trachea in vitro. This work has been extrapolated by many workers to human tracheobronchial smooth muscle but as yet no experiments have been performed to confirm this suggestion. Consequently we have used the two tracheobronchial muscle preparations previously described (guinea-pig trachea and human bronchial muscle) to investigate this area of uncertainty. Three non-steroidal anti-inflammatory agents were separately added to the guinea-pig trachea using a cumulative dosing procedure with a 30 min contact time. These agents reduced the inherent tone of the tracheal preparation (Fig. 3) with a similar rank order of potency to that of inhibition of prostaglandin synthetase (52) which seemed to confirm the results of Orehek et al. We then repeated this work using human isolated bronchial muscle and unlike the trachea this tissue failed to relax to either mefenamic acid or indomethacin except at very high concentrations which probably bear no relation to their effectiveness in the inhibition of prostaglandin synthesis (Fig. 4). Similar findings have been reported by Brink et al (53) using indomethacin. Consequently it appears that unlike their role in the guinea-pig trachea endogenous prostaglandins play little or no role in the regulation of inherent tone of human isolated bronchial muscle and this may help to explain the poor predictiveness of the guinea-pig trachea with respect to the PG bronchodilator activity in man.

These two groups of experiments formed the foundation for a wider study of prostanoid activity in the tracheobronchial tract (9) which resulted in the differentiation of three prostanoid receptors in the airways. These receptors were the χ - PG receptor for contraction, the ψ - PG receptor for relaxation and ω - PG receptor for irritancy or cough. The first two receptors were mainly studied using the guinea-pig trachea and human bronchial muscle preparations. In contrast the ω - PG receptor was studied by monitoring the responsiveness of restrained conscious cats to inhaled prostaglandins (54). It must be recognised, however, that many prostanoids remain untested and that they may also interact with these receptors or they may have their own specific receptors.

SUMMARY AND CONCLUSIONS

1. In vitro studies using guinea-pig and human respiratory smooth muscle show that prostaglandins $F_{2\alpha}$, G_2, H_2, D_2 and thromboxanes A_2 and B_2 usually cause a contraction whereas prostaglandins E_1, E_2, $F_{2\beta}$ and I_2 (prostacyclin) usually cause a relaxation although a large number of paradoxical effects for PGE_2, PGI_2 and $PGF_{2\beta}$ have been shown on human isolated bronchial muscle.

2.   In anaesthetised guinea-pigs, PGE_1 and PGE_2 are approximately
     equipotent as bronchodilators relative to isoprenaline while
     $PGF_{2\alpha}$ is a weak bronchoconstrictor.   In contrast to their
     quantitative activities <u>in vitro</u> and by intravenous

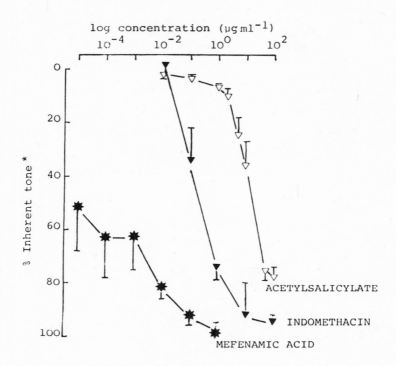

Fig. 3.   Reduction in the inherent tone of the guinea-pig
          trachea by 3 non-steroidal anti-inflammatory drugs.
          Each point is the mean of at least 5 observations and
          the vertical lines represent the standard error of the
          mean.   *, 100% inherent tone is the maximum relaxation
          obtained with isoprenaline.

administration to guinea-pigs, both PGE_1, E_2 and $F_{2\alpha}$ were
significantly more potent than isoprenaline or histamine when
given by aerosol.   These findings may be related to rapid
enzymatic degradation by the lung and the level of smooth
muscle affected.   Although PGG_2, H_2 and D_2 are potent broncho-
constrictors when given iv in the guinea-pig limited data
suggests that TXA_2 is by far the most potent bronchoconstrictor studied in the prostanoid series.

3.   In healthy and asthmatic volunteers, effective doses of PGE_1
      and E_2 by aerosol usually cause bronchodilation as seen by a
      fall in airway resistance and an increase in specific airways
      conductance comparable in duration and degree to that of
      isoprenaline but superior in potency although a valid dose
      comparison has not been performed. Some workers have found
      PGE_2 to cause bronchoconstriction in asthmatic subjects.

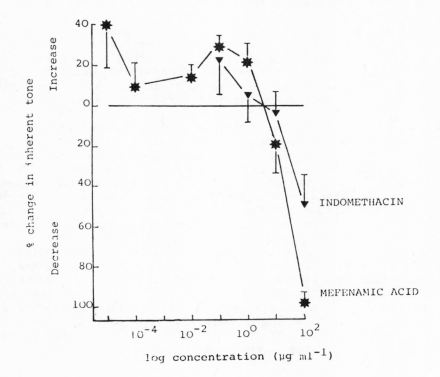

Fig. 4.   Reduction in the inherent tone of human isolated
           bronchial muscle by 2 non-steroidal anti-inflammatory
           agents. Each point represents the mean of at least
           five observations and the vertical lines represent the
           standard error of the mean. % decrease in inherent
           tone is the maximum relaxation obtained with isoprenaline.
           Increase in inherent tone is the maximum contraction
           obtained with histamine.

4. $PGF_{2\alpha}$ cause bronchoconstriction in healthy subjects which is
      readily reversible. Some workers have shown atropine to
      inhibit $PGF_{2\alpha}$-induced bronchoconstriction but most have
      reported no modifying action of flufenamic acid, atropine or

disodium cromoglycate. Some asthmatics are extremely sensitive to $PGF_{2\alpha}$, possibly indicative of an involvement in the aetiology of bronchial asthma.

5. Naturally-occurring prostaglandins now seem unlikely to prove to be bronchodilators of therapeutic value since all those tested to date are irritant to the upper respiratory tract and the E compounds are chemically unstable. A better understanding of in vitro and in vivo techniques predictive of both the qualitative and quantitative activity of PGs in man taken together with the conscious restrained cat method for investigating irritancy or other alternative irritancy test models, however, should prove useful in the search for therapeutically useful potent, stable, long-acting and non-irritant prostaglandin E bronchodilator analogues.

6. The actions on the respiratory system of endoperoxides, thromboxanes and prostacyclin (PGI_2) have not as yet been explored fully in man. The present results show that PGI_2 usually relaxes guinea-pig and human isolated respiratory muscle although in general there is poor correlation between the quantitative action of PGI_2 on these preparations and in healthy or asthmatic human subjects. Some interesting results with prostacyclin and some other prostaglandins indicate that they may have prophylactic protective effects in some asthmatics and may also aid mucus clearance. An equally promising approach to the therapy of respiratory diseases such as asthma lies in the development of synthetic compounds which can specifically inhibit the synthesis of endogenous prostanoids or antagonise their action at the smooth muscle receptor(s). This line of work must inevitably also help to elucidate the physiological and/or the pathophysiological role of prostanoids in the human respiratory tract.

REFERENCES

1. S. Bergstrom, F. Dressler, L. Krabisch, R. Ryhage and J. Sjövall, The isolation and structure of a smooth muscle stimulating factor in normal pig and sheep lungs. Arkiv fur Kemi., 20:63 (1962).
2. P. J. Piper and J. R. Vane, Release of additional factors in anaphylaxis and its antagonism by anti-inflammatory drugs. Nature, 223:29 (1969).
3. M. Hamberg, J. Svensson and B. Samuelsson, Thromboxanes. A new group of biologically active compounds derived from prostaglandin endoperoxides. Proc. Nat. Acad. Sci. USA., 72:2994 (1975).

4. S. Moncada, R. Gryglewski, S. Bunting and J. R. Vane, An enzyme
    isolated from arteries transforms prostaglandin endoperoxides
    to an unstable substance that inhibits platelet aggregation.
    Nature, 263:663 (1976).
5. P. J. Piper, J. R. Vane and J. H. Wyllie, Inactivation of
    prostaglandins by the lung. Nature, 225:600 (1970).
6. P. Jose, U. Niederhauser, P. J. Piper, C. Robinson and A. P.
    Smith, Inactivation of prostaglandin $F_{2\alpha}$ in the human pulmonary
    circulation. Brit. J. Clin. Pharmacol., 3:342 (1976).
7. E. Anggard and S. Bergström, Biological effects of an unsaturated
    tri-hydroxy-acid ($PGF_{2\alpha}$) from normal swine lung. Acta. Physiol.
    Scand., 58:1 (1963).
8. I. H. M. Main, The inhibitory actions of prostaglandins on
    respiratory smooth muscle. Brit. J. Pharmacol., 22:511 (1964).
9. P. J. Gardiner and H. O. J. Collier, Specific receptors for
    prostaglandins in the airways. Prostaglandins (in preparation)
    (1979/80).
10. P. A. Berry and H. O. J. Collier, Bronchoconstrictor action
    for antagonism of a slow reacting substance from anaphylaxis
    of guinea-pig isolated lung. Brit. J. Pharmacol., 23:201
    (1964).
11. M. E. Rosenthale, A. Dervinis, A. J. Begany, M. Lapidus
    and M. I. Gluckman, Bronchodilator activity of prostaglandin
    E_2 when administered by aerosol to three species. Experientia.,
    26:1119 (1970).
12. M. E. Rosenthale, A. Dervinis and J. Kassarich, Bronchodilator
    activity of the prostaglandins E_1 & E_2. J. Pharmacol. Exp.
    Ther., 178:541 (1971).
13. B. J. Large, P. F. Leswell and D. R. Maxwell, Bronchodilator
    activity of prostaglandin E_1 in experimental animals.
    Nature, 224:78 (1969).
14. W. J. F. Sweatman and H. O. J. Collier, Effects of prosta-
    glandins on human bronchial muscle. Nature, 217:69 (1968).
15. M. F. Cuthbert, Effect on airways resistance of prostaglandin
    E_1 given by aerosol to healthy and asthmatic volunteers.
    Brit. Med. J., 4:723 (1969).
16. A. P. Smith, M. F. Cuthbert and L. S. Dunlop, Effects of inhaled
    prostaglandins E_1, E_2 and $F_{2\alpha}$ on airways resistance in
    healthy and asthmatic man. Clinical Science, 48:421 (1975).
17. P. Hedqvist, A. Holmgren and A. A. Mathé, Effect of prosta-
    glandin $F_{2\alpha}$ on airways resistance in man. Acta. Physiol.
    Scand., 82:29a (1971).
18. A. P. Smith and M. F. Cuthbert, The antagonistic action of
    prostaglandins $F_{2\alpha}$ and E_2 aerosols on bronchial muscle tone
    in man. Brit. Med. J., 3:212 (1972).
19. K. R. Patel, Atropine, sodium cromoglycate and thymoxamine
    in $PGF_{2\alpha}$ induced bronchoconstriction in extrinsic asthma.
    Brit. Med. J., 2:360 (1975).
20. A. A. Mathé, P. Hedqvist, A. Holmgren and N. Svanborg, Bronchial
    hyperreactivity to prostaglandin $F_{2\alpha}$ and histamine in patients
    with asthma. Brit. Med. J., 1:193 (1973).

21. A. P. Smith, A comparison of the effects of prostaglandin E_2 and salbutamol by intravenous infusion on the airways obstruction of patients with asthma. Brit. J. Clin. Pharmacol., 1:399 (1974).

22. J. Svensson, K. Strandberg, T. Tuvemo and M. Hamberg, Thromboxane A : Effects on airway and vascular smooth muscle. Prostaglandins, 14:425 (1977).

23. M. A. Wasserman and R. L. Griffin, Thromboxane B_2 : comparative bronchoactivity in experimental systems. Eur. J. Pharmacol., 46:303 (1977).

24. C. Omini, S. Moncada and J. R. Vane, The effects of prostacyclin (PGI_2) on tissues which detect prostaglandins. Prostaglandins, 14:625 (1977).

25. M. A. Wasserman, D. W. Du Charme, R. L. Griffin, M. G. Wendling and G. L. De Graaf, Bronchial and cardiovascular actions of prostacyclin (PGI_2). Pharmacologist, 19:145 (1977).

26. M. E. Rosenthale, A. Dervinis, J. Kassarich, S. Singer and M. I. Gluckmann, Comparative studies on the bronchodilating properties of prostaglandin $F_{2\beta}$. Adv. Biosc., 9:229 (1973).

27. P. Y. Lo, Effects of pulmonary metabolites of prostaglandins E_2 and $F_{2\alpha}$ on guinea-pigs respiratory tract. J. Pharm. Pharmacol., 29:752 (1977).

28. W. Dawson, R. L. Lewis, R. E. McMahon and W. J. F. Sweatman, Potent bronchoconstrictor activity of 15-keto-prostaglandin $F_{2\alpha}$. Nature, 250:331 (1974).

29. D. J. Crutchley and P. J. Piper, Comparative bioassay of prostaglandin E_2 and its three pulmonary metabolites. Brit. J. Pharmacol., 54:397 (1975).

30. M. A. Wasserman, D. W. Du Charme, R. L. Griffin, G. L. De Graaf and F. G. Robinson, Bronchopulmonary and cardiovascular effects of prostaglandin D_2 in the dog. Prostaglandins, 13:255 (1977).

31. M. Hamberg, P. Hedqvist, K. Strandberg, J. Svensson and B. Samuelsson, Prostaglandin endoperoxides IV Effects on smooth muscle. Life Sci., 16:451 (1975).

32. H. O. J. Collier and P. J. Gardiner, Pharmacology of airways smooth muscle. In: "Evaluation of Bronchodilator Drugs", D. M. Burley, S. W. Clarke, M. F. Cuthbert, J. W. Paterson and J. H. Shelley, eds., Trust Education and Research in Therapeutics. London (1974).

33. P. J. Gardiner, The effects of some natural prostaglandins on isolated human circular bronchial muscle. Prostaglandins, 10:607 (1975).

34. K. Strandberg and P. Hedqvist, Bronchial effects of some prostaglandin E & F analogues. Acta. Physiol. Scand., 100:172 (1977).

35. P. Hedqvist, K. Strandberg and M. Hamberg, Bronchial and cardiovascular actions of prostaglandin endoperoxides and an endoperoxide analogue. Acta. Physiol. Scand., 103:299 (1978).

36. K. R. Patel, Effect of prostaglandin $F_{2\alpha}$ on lung mechanics
     in intrinsic asthma. Postgrad. Med. J., 52:275 (1976).
37. A. Szczeklik, R. J. Gryglewski and G. Grerniawska-Mysik,
     Participation of prostaglandins in pathogenesis of aspirin-
     sensitive asthma. Naunyn-Schmiedebergs' Arch. Pharmacol.,
     297:599 (1977).
38. J. Orehek, P. Gayrard, C. Grimaud and J. Charpin, Bronchial
     reactivity to inhaled prostaglandin $F_{2\alpha}$ in patients with
     common or aspirin-sensitive asthma. J. Allergy Clin. Immunol.,
     59:414 (1977).
39. A. A. Mathe and P. Hedqvist, Effect of prostaglandin $F_{2\alpha}$ and
     E_2 on airways conductance in healthy subjects and asthmatic
     patients. Am. Rev. Resp. Dis., 111:313 (1975).
40. M. Pasargiklian, S. Bianco and L. Allegra, Clinical, functional
     and pathogenetic aspects of bronchial reactivity to prosta-
     glandins $F_{2\alpha}$, E_1 & E_2.In:"Adv. Prostaglandin & Thromboxane Res.
     B. Samuelsson & R. Paoletti, eds., 1:461, Raven Press (1976).
41. J. L. Walker, The regulatory role of prostaglandins in the
     release of histamine and SRS-A from passively sensitised human
     lung tissue. In: "Advances in the Biosciences",   S. Bergstrom,
     and S. Bernhard, eds.,
42. J. Iravani and G. N. Melville, Mucociliary activity in the
     respiratory tract as influenced by prostaglandin E_1.
     Respiration, 32:305 (1975).
43. J. Irvani, G. N. Melville and H. G. Richter, Mucus production
     influenced by drugs: An electron microscope study.
     Pneumonologic Suppl.,267 (1976).
44. H. J. Biersak, J. R. Hedde, R. Felix and C. Winkler,
     Mukoziliare Clearance under Prostaglandin E_1 Inhalation.
     Prax. Pneumol., 32:105 (1978).
45. S. Bianco, M. Robuschi, R. Cesarani and C. Gandolfi, Prevention
     of aspecifically induced bronchoconstriction by prostacyclin
     (PGI_2) in asthmatic subjects. IRCS Med. Science. Clin. Med;
     Clin. Pharmacol. & Ther.; Resp. Sys.,6:256 (1978).
46. A. Szczeklik, R. J. Gryglewski, E. Nizankowska, R.
     Nizankowski and J. Musial, Pulmonary and anti-platelet
     effects of intravenous and inhaled prostacyclin in man.
     Prostaglandins, 16:651 (1978).
47. M. Pasargiklian and S. Bianco, Ventilatory and cardio-
     vascular effects of Pl and 6-keto-$PGF_{1\alpha}$ by inhalation. Fourth
     International Prostaglandin Conference (in press) (1979).
48. P. Hamosh and T. Da Silva, The effect of prostaglandin $F_{2\beta}$
     on expiratory flow rates. Prostaglandins, 10:599 (1975).
49. P. J. Piper, Release of catecholamine and other substances
     by antigen and mediators of the anaphylactic reaction.
     PhD thesis. University of London (1969).
50. H. O. J. Collier and W. J. F. Sweatman, Antagonism by
     fenamates of prostaglandin $F_{2\alpha}$ and of slow reacting substance
     on human bronchial muscle. Nature, 219:864 (1968).

51. J. Orehek, J. S. Douglas, A. J. Lewis and A. Bouhuys,
     Prostaglandin regulation of airway smooth muscle tone.
     Nature, 245:84 (1973).
52. E. L. Tolman and R. Partridge, Multiple sites of interaction
     with prostaglandins and non-steroidal anti-inflammatory
     agents. Prostaglandins, 9:349 (1975).
53. C. Brink, C. Grimaud, C. Guillot and J. Orehek, The interaction
     between indomethacin and contractile agents on isolated human
     airway smooth muscle. Brit. J. Pharmacol. (in press)
     (1979/80).
54. P. J. Gardiner, J. L. Copas, R. D. Elliot and H. O. J.
     Collier, Tracheobronchial irritancy of inhaled prostaglandins
     in the conscious cat. Prostaglandins, 15:303 (1978).

ARACHIDONIC ACID METABOLISM IN THE LUNGS: EFFECT OF HISTAMINE

AND SLOW-REACTING-SUBSTANCE OF ANAPHYLAXIS

G. C. Folco, C. Omini, L. Sautebin and F. Berti

Institute of Pharmacology, School of Pharmacy
University of Milan
20129 Milan, Italy

INTRODUCTION

Since the discovery of prostaglandins from pig and sheep lungs by Bergström (1), the description of their pharmacological activity upon bronchial smooth muscle (2) and pulmonary vessels (3) has stimulated investigation on the role of these lipidic compounds in the physiopathology of the respiratory system. Interest in the prostaglandin field increased remarkably when, in 1975, Thromboxane-A_2 (TXA$_2$) was identified, and its potent vasoconstrictor and thrombogenic activity was established (4). The potential clinical importance of TXA$_2$ began to be more considered when it was demonstrated that this "ephemeral substance", which is made by platelets, could be also generated in the lungs as a main metabolite of arachidonic acid (AA) (5). In fact release of prostaglandins and mainly rabbit-aorta contracting substance (RCS), now identified as a mixture of TXA$_2$ and a small amount of endoperoxides was shown by Piper and Vane, when studying chemical mediators in anaphylactic guinea-pig lungs (6). TXA$_2$ is a dangerous agent which displays a powerful contracting capacity on the bronchial smooth muscle. Intravenous injection of TXA$_2$ in anaesthetized guinea-pigs brings about a sustained increase in the airways resistence, an effect which is 40 folds higher than that of prostaglandin endoperoxide PGH$_2$ and 500 times that of PGF$_{2\alpha}$ (7). In spite of the high sensitivity to the spasmogenic action of TXA$_2$, the smooth muscle of the main airways does not seem to generate TXA$_2$. In this respect, Orehek et al. (8) reported that the effluent of contracting trachea does contain RCS-activity. Furthermore it has been proved that thracheal spirals in resting tonus condition can produce both PGE$_2$ and PGF$_{2\alpha}$ whereas, in increased tonus condition, they mainly form prostaglandins

of the E type which are responsible for relaxation (9). This
phenomenon is explained by Gryglewski as "the self-defence of
smooth muscle against the overdone bronchoconstriction".
Regarding TXA$_2$ generation in the guinea-pig lungs, Gryglewski et
al. (10), working with subpleural strip, free from bronchial
smooth muscle, suggested that the contractile protein in alveolar
interstitial cells may be an excellent source of TXA$_2$, which
is formed and released in massive amount upon challenge. As a
matter of fact it has already been demonstrated by several
authors that histamine, SRS-A and other mediators of anaphylaxis
are capable to induce TXA$_2$ formation when perfused through
guinea-pig lung, being the phenomenon more pronounced in sensitized
tissue (10,11). These observations reinforce the concept that
TXA$_2$ may have a role in guinea-pog anaphylaxis and speak in favour
of the hypothesis of Gryglewski emphasizing anatomical
localization for AA metabolism in lungs.

    SRS-A, an acidic lipidic-like mediator, which is generated
by a number of tissues during immunologic reactions (12) is a
selective peripheral airways-constrictor. This is supported by
the differential effect of partially purified preparations of
SRS-A on guinea-pig tracheal spirals and parenchimal strips (13).
SRS-A has been recently identified from mouse mastocytoma cells
as a product of AA via lipoxygenase pathway, and its chemical
structure proposed by Samuelsson and coworkers (14). The
pharmacological action of SRS-A has been so far explored with
partially purified preparations and since structurally defined
material has now become available, a reinterpretation of the
data will be necessary. Another interesting point is that products
of the lipoxygenase pathway (fatty acid hydroperoxides) promote
a marked increase of the anaphylactic release of SRS-A (15). This
in connection with the capability of SRS-A to increase the
generation of TXA$_2$ in the lungs, might be of some importance
on the understanding of the mechanism underlying a sundrome known
as aspirin-sensitive asthma (16).

    These and other observations prompted us to investigate the
possibility to control with autonomic drugs the generation and
release of TXA$_2$ from isolated lungs of the guinea-pig. Our
effort has been centred particularly on two spasmogens, histamine
and SRS-A, which are involved in allergic phenomena in connection
with the metabolism of AA via the thromboxane-A$_2$ synthetase
pathway. In addition to this, the ability of the two primary
mediators of anaphylaxis to stimulate the lipoxygenase pathway
in normal and sensitized lungs of the guinea-pig has been also
considered.

METHODS

In these experiments normal and ovalbumin sensitized (17) guinea-pigs (male, 350-450 g) were utilized. The lungs were removed and perfused through the pulmonary artery with Krebs-bicarbonate solution, as previously described by Piper and Vane (6). The pulmonary effluent superfused a bank of isolated tissues in cascade, including spirally cut strips of rabbit aorta (RbA), rabbit mesenteric artery (RbMA), circular fibers of rabbit stomach (RbSS) and rat stomach (RSS) in order to detect arachidonate-metabolite-like activity. These tissues were treated with a mixture of receptor antagonists and indomethacin in order to increase their sensitivity (18). The isolated lungs were challenged with histamine, specific H_1 and H_2-histamine receptor agonists, SRS-A and carbachol. Their capacity to increase generation of TXA_2 has been studied in presence of various autonomic compounds. The importance of activation or blockade of adrenergic, histaminergic and muscarinic receptors in the formation of TXA_2 has been considered. In some experiments the amount of TXA_2 present in the pumonary outflow was evaluated following the radioimmunoassay method described by Granström (19).

Particularly the lung perfusates were collected for 30 sec. after injection or perfusion of the lungs with the different compounds: during this time, biological activity was already shown by the bioassay tissues. After the collection of the perfusate for TXA_2 determination, additional 4 min. collections were carried out and 12-L-hydroxy-5,8,10,14 eicosatetraenoic acid (HETE) was determined according to Sautebin et al. (20). The perfusates, after addition of known amount of octadeuterated HETE as internal standard, were acidified and extracted with peroxide free ethyl ether. The extracts were evaporated to dryness under nitrogen and analyzed by mass-fragmentography as methyl ester-TMS derivatives.

SRS-A was prepared in our laboratory according to the method described by Orange (21).

Experimental data were analyzed following the method of factorial analysis of variance for completely reandomized design with two factors at two levels; multiple comparison according to Duncan (22) was also performed.

RESULTS

Histamine H_1 and H_2-Receptors in the Generation of TXA_2

Two types of histamine receptors, termed H_1 and H_2, are responsible for various physiological and pathological actions of histamine (23). Their function in the lung airway smooth muscle is still a debated question, however the availability of H_2-receptor agonists and antagonists allowed the elucidation of some actions of the two distinct histamine receptors. Yen et al. (24) showed that the activation of H_1-receptors in sensitized guinea-pig lungs is mainly characterized by formation of $PGF_{2\alpha}$, whereas H_2-receptor stimulation causes generation of PGE_2.

These findings seem to suggest a protective function of H_2-histamine receptors which induce formation of bronchodilating prostaglandins (PGE_2). This type of prostaglanidns may in turn control histamine release from sensitized mast cells by activation of an adenylate cyclase (25).

Although the pathophysiological production of TXA_2 by the lungs is not clear, it is known that the compound may be generated in this tissue by histamine, but the specificity of histamine receptors involved in this process has not been studied. With the aim to verify the physiological importance of the two histamine receptors on TXA_2 release, experiments were carried out on guinea-pig isolated lungs using specific agonists and antagonists of histamine receptors.

The injection of histamine (1 µg) or 2 methyl-histamine (10 µg) through the pulmonary artery of the isolated lungs of normal guinea-pigs, increased the appearance of TXA_2-like activity in the effluent, as revealed by the contraction of RbA strip in the bioassay cascade (Fig. 1).

The small contraction of RSS indicated that prostaglandin-like activity was released (Fig. 1). During perfusion of the lungs with pyrilamine, a specific antagonist of H_1-receptor, histamine and 2-methyl-histamine almost completely lost their capacity to generate TXA_2-like activity from the lungs. On the contrary during perfusion of the tissues with cimetidine, a specific H_2-receptor antagonist, 2-methyl-histamine fully retained its capacity to stimulate the generation of TXA_2-like substance.

When 4-methyl-histamine or dimaprit, specific agonists for histamine H_2-receptors, were administered as a bolus injection (100 µg), neither prostaglandin-like material nor TXA_2 were present in the pulmonary outflow (Fig. 1). In similar experiments using ovalbumin sensitized guinea-pig lungs, the activation of H_1-receptor was associated with a marked generation of TXA_2-like activity as shown by the contraction of RbA.

In the same tissue dimaprit and 4-methyl-histamine (100 µg) caused a modest release of TXA_2-like material, an effect which was antagonized by pyrilamine. In order to confirm the results obtained using the cascade system, the amount of TXA_2 present in the pulmonary effluent was quantitatively evaluated by a specific

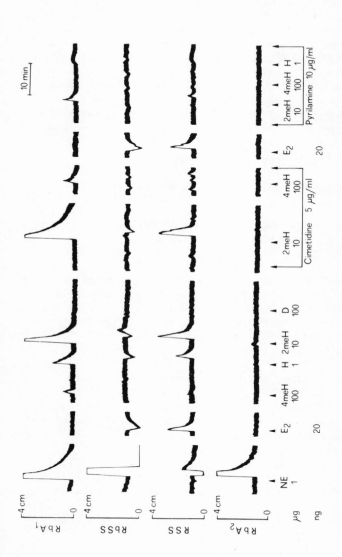

Fig. 1. Prostaglandin-like material and thromboxane A_2 (TXA_2) generation by specific activation of H_1 and H_2-receptors on isolated lungs of normal guinea-pigs. The assay tissues were rabbit aortic strips (RbA_1 and RbA_2), rabbit stomach strip (RbSS) and rat stomach strips (RSS). Sensitivity of the bioassay tissues was checked with noradrenaline (NA) before superfusion with the antagonist mixture. Between the first rabbit aortic strip and the other bioassay tissues a delay coil (120 s) was inserted in order to cause inactivation of TXA_2 (half life of TXA_2 in aqueous medium at 37°C = 32.5 s). The agonists, histamine (H), 2-methylhistamine (2meH), 4-methylhistamine (4meH) and dimaprit (D) were injected as a bolus through the lungs. The antagonists cimetidine and Pyrilamine were continuously infused through the lungs as indicated in the figure. Contractions of the tissues in cascade were matched by prostaglandin E_2 (E_2).

radioimmunoassay technique after identification by thin-layer
chromatography. The results obtained with these experiments
(Fig. 2) indicate that stimulation of H_2-receptors by dimaprit and
4-methyl-histamine did not increase the rate of formation of
TXA_2 from normal guinea-pig lungs. On the contrary, histamine
or 2-methyl-histamine were effective in augmeting the formation
of TXA_2. Using sensitized lungs a greater increase of TXA_2
formation was observed with histamine and 2-methyl-histamine.
The H_2-antagonists again were ineffective.

From these experiments it is concluded that there is no
direct relationship between H_2-receptor activation and formation
of TXA_2 in the perfused guinea-pig lungs, although a modulatory
role of H_2-receptor on thromboxane formation cannot be ruled out

Activation and Blockade of Adrenergic Receptors

The perfusion of isolated lungs from normal guinea-pigs
with isoproterenol (10 ng/ml min^{-1}) reduces significantly the
increased production of TXA_2-like activity and prostaglandin-like
material promoted by histamine (1 µg) and SRS-A (0.1 U): the
inhibitory activity of isoproterenol is antagonized by
β-adrenoceptor blocking drugs.

The results obtained using the cascade system were confirmed
identifying the TXA_2 present in the pulmonary effluent following
a specific radioimmunoassay technique. The data (Fig. 3) clearly
show that isoproterenol diminishes the capacity of both histamine
an d SRS-A to increase the generation of TXA_2. The effect of
isoproterenol is reversed by sotalol.

In order to obtain information on the role of β_1 and β_2-
adrenoceptors in modulating the generation of TXA_2 induced by
histamine and SRS-A, the activity of practolol and ICI-118-551
was studied. This last compound is known to act selectively on
the β_2-adrenoceptor at ng levels (26), whereas practolol is less
potent (µg levels) and more specific for β_1-adrenoceptors (27).
The experimental data show that both practolol and ICI-118-551
partially restore the ability of histamine to generate TXA_2 in
normal guinea-pig lungs. In fact while practolol, perfused through
the lungs at the rate of 1 µg/ml min^{-1}, restores the effect of
histamine in the order of 50%, ICI-118-551 at the concentration
rate of 50 ng/ml min^{-1} was more effective, being the difference
between the two blockers highly significant. This, however, does
not imply that the uβl-receptor is less involved than the β_2- in
modulating the effect of histamine (Table 1).

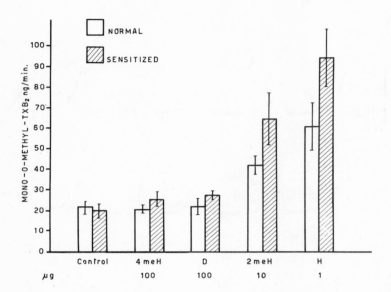

Fig. 2.   Thromboxane A_2 (TXA$_2$) measured as mono-O-methyl-TXB$_2$,
          generation by normal (open columns) and sensitized
          (hatched columns) guinea-pig lungs induced by bolus
          injection of histamine (H), 2-methylhistamine (2meH),
          4-methylhistamine (4 meH) and dimaprit (D).   TXA$_2$
          expressed as ng/min, refers to the total amount present
          in the effluent from individual lungs collected for
          2 min after drug injection.   Each column represents the
          mean of 4 experiments.   Vertical bars show s.e. mean.

          Duncan's test carried out on the experimental data
          gives the following results of the comparison between
          each two means: control vs 4-methylhistamine = NS
          ($P > 0.05$); control vs dimaprit = NS ($P > 0.05$); control
          vs 2-methylhistamine = highly significant ($P < 0.01$);
          control vs histamine = highly significant ($P < 0.01$);
          normal 2-methylhistamine vs sensitized 2-methylhistamine
          = NS ($P > 0.05$); normal histamine vs sensitized-
          histamine = significant ($0.01 < P < 0.05$).

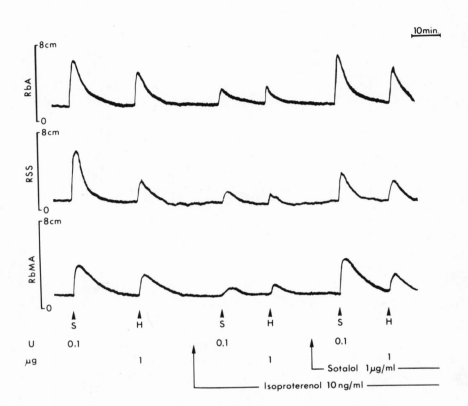

Fig. 3.   Effect of isoproterenol on the generation of TXA_2-like
          activity and prostaglandins induced by histamine (H)
          and SRS-A (S) in normal perfused lungs of the guinea-pig.
          Lung outflow superfused a bank of assay tissues as
          described in Fig. 1.

          Histamine (1 µg) and SRS-A (0.1 U) were injected as a
          bolus through the lungs. Isoproterenol and sotalol
          were perfused through the lungs at the concentration
          rate of 10 ng/ml min^{-1} respectively.

TABLE 1

Effect of Beta-adrenergic blockers in restoring the
capacity of histamine to generate TXA_2 in normal
isolated guinea-pig lungs inhibited by isoproterenol

COMPOUNDS	TXA_2 (ng/min ± S.E.)
Control	5.07 ± 0.23 (30)
Histamine (H)	63.02 ± 4.19 (15)
Isoproterenol (I)	5.60 ± 0.40 (25)
I + H	14.00 ± 2.70 (12)
Practolol (PRCT)	4.92 ± 0.97 (10)
ICI-118-551 (ICI)	5.12 ± 0.43 (10)
PRCT + H	65.00 ± 5.20 (10)
ICI + H	60.90 ± 3.80 (9)
PRCT + I + H	33.03 ± 4.40 (10)
ICI + I + H	46.60 ± 3.40 (9)

Histamine: bolus injection, 5 µg;
Isoproterenol: perfusion, 10 ng/ml min^{-1};
Practolol: perfusion, 1 µg/ml min^{-1};
ICI-118-551: perfusion, 50 ng/ml min^{-1};
In brackets the number of experiments.

When TXA_2 biosynthesis was caused by bolus injections of SRS-A
through normal guinea-pig lungs, the amount of TXA_2 in the pulmonary
effluent raised from control values of 5 ng/min to 152 ng/min:
again isoproterenol was significantly effective in reducing this
increase. Pretreatment of the lungs with both practolol or
ICI-118-551 partially restored the capacity SRS-A to increase
TXA_2 generation (Table 2).

Although the difference between the two blockers in reversing
the effect of isoprenaline was found to be statistically significant,
no definite conclusion can be drawn concerning a prevailing effect
of β_1 or β_2-adrenoceptor in the pulmonary tissue.

TABLE 2

Effect of Beta-adrenergic blockers in restoring the capacity
of SRS-A to generate TXA$_2$ in normal isolated guinea-pig
lungs inhibited by isoproterenol.

COMPOUND	TXA$_2$ (ng/min ± S.E.)
Control	5.07 ± 0.23 (30)
SRS-A	152.90 ± 15.90 (15)
Isoproterenol (I)	5.60 ± 0.40 (25)
I + SRS-A	12.90 ± 2.10 (13)
Practolol (PRCT) + SRS-A	154.00 ± 14.20 (8)
ICI-118-551 + SRS-A	151.00 ± 13.30 (9)
PRCT + I + SRS-A	61.01 ± 9.90 (8)
ICI-118-551 + I + SRS-A	29.40 ± 3.27 (9)

SRS-A: bolus injection, 0.1 U;
Isoproterenol: perfusion, 10 ng/ml min^{-1};
Practolol: perfusion, 1 µg/ml^{-1};
ICI-118-551: perfusion, 50 ng/ml min^{-1}.
In brackets the number of experiments.

In order to activate specifically the α-adrenoceptor, the
isolated lungs of normal guinea-pigs were also perfused with
phenylephrine (5 ng/ml min^{-1}); in these experiments the effect of
histamine and SRS-A in producing TXA$_2$ was not impaired.

Activation and Blockade of Cholinergic Receptor

The injection of histamine and SRS-A into the isolated lungs
of guinea-pigs is followed by formation and release of arachidonate metabolites particularly of TXA$_2$. However, when a
sustained activation of the muscarinic receptors is induced with
carbachol (1-10 µg) in normal and ovalbumin sensitized lungs,
the release of arachidonate metabolites in the pulmonary effluent
does not occur (Fig. 4). Furthermore perfusion of the sensitized
lungs with carbachol (1 µg/ml min^{-1}) does not interfere with the
capacity of histamine and SRS-A to generate TXA$_2$-like material.
The accumulation of acetylcholine at the cholinergic sites of
the isolated lungs caused by neostigmine (1 µg/ml min^{-1}) was
without effect as well.

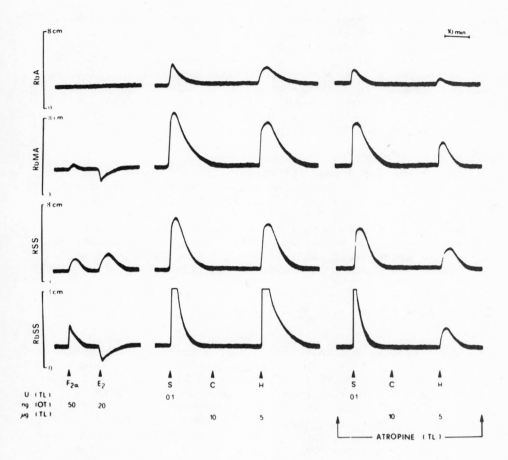

Fig. 4. Effect of atropine on the generation of prostaglandin-like
         substances and thromboxane A_2 in normal perfused lungs
         of the guinea-pig. Lungs outflow superfused a bank of
         assay tissues consisting of: rabbit aorta (RbA),
         rabbit mesenteric artery (RbMA), rat stomach strip (RSS),
         and rabbit stomach trip (RbSS). The following agonist
         were injected as a bolus through the lungs (TL): SRS-A
         (S) 0.1 U, carbachol (C) 10 µg; histamine (H) 5 µg.
         Atropine was perfused TL at the concentration of 1 µg/ml
         min^{-1}. Prostaglandin F2 ($F_{2\alpha}$, 50 ng) and prostaglandin E_2
         (E_2, 20 ng) were injected directly over the tissues (OT)
         in cascade.

The perfusion of the lungs with atropine (1 µg/ml min^{-1}) clearly impairs the capacity of histamine and SRS-A to increase the formation of TXA$_2$-like substance and other prostaglandins. Similar results were obtained with ipratropium bromide, a synthetic anticholinergic compound, which possesses a certain degree of bronchoselectivity (28). The conversion of arachidonic acid in the lungs into prostaglandin-like material and TXA$_2$ was completely normal in presence of atropine. The results obtained with the cascade system were proved by the radioimmunological determination of TXA$_2$ in the pulmonary effluent of normal and ovalbumin sensitized lungs (Fig. 5).

From these experiments it appears that atropine (1 µg/ml min^{-1}) and carbachol (10 µg bolus injection) do not modify signficantly the basal rate of formation of TXA$_2$ from the isolated lungs.

Atropine, in both normal and ovalbumin sensitized lungs, markedly reduces the formation of TXA$_2$ induced by histamine and SRS-A: the antagonistic activity of atropine is significantly more pronounced against histamine in sensitized lungs.

Effect of Histamine and SRS-A on the Generation of Lipoxygenase Products

Lipoxygenase has been isolated from human platelets (29) and guinea-pig lungs (30). This enzyme, involved in arachidonic acid metabolism, is not inhibited by aspirin-like drugs and it generates 12-L-hydroxy-5,8,10,14-eicosatetraenoic acid (HETE) through the intermediate formation of the corresponding hydroperoxide (HPETE). The biological importance of HPETE and 12-HETE is far from being elucidated, however it is known that HETE stimulates chemotaxis for polimorphonuclear leukocytes, and that fatty acid hydroperoxides play a role in the anaphylactic mediator release (15). In this respect several investigators have shown that non steroidal anti-inflammatory compounds increase the release of histamine and SRS-A from sensitized lung tissues (31): this phenomenon seems to be explained by the augmented generation of HPETE and HETE and not by preferential formation of natural prostaglandins and, to a lesser extent, thromboxanes biosynthesis (32). With these observations in mind, the ability of histamine and SRS-A to stimulate cyclo-oxygenase and lipoxygenase pathways in normal and ovalbumin sensitized lungs was studied.

When isolated unsensitized lungs are challenged with SRS-A (0.1 U), the amount of HETE in the pulmonary outflow is almost doubled. In contrast both histamine (5 µg) and carbachol (10 µg) do not alter the basal rate of production of the fatty acid hydroperoxide (data not shown).

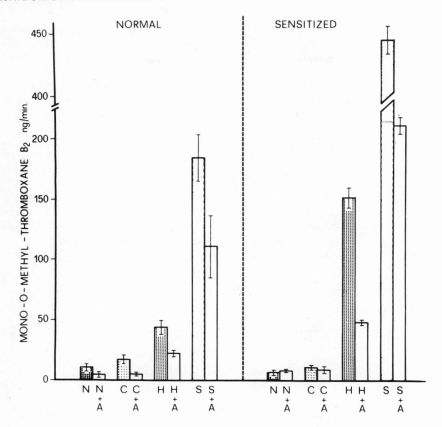

Fig. 5.   Effect of atropine (A) on TXA$_2$ generation (measured as
          mono-0-methyl TXB$_2$) induced by carbachol (C), histamine
          (H) and SRS-A (S) in perfused lungs of normal and ovalbumin
          sensitized guinea-pigs. Columns represent the amount
          (ng min^{-1}) of TXA$_2$ in 10 ml of perfusate after (60 sec.)
          the bolus injection of the various challengers. Carbachol
          (10 µg), histamine (1 µg) and SRS-A (0.1 U) were injected
          separately and after 15 min. perfusion of the lungs with
          atropine (1 µg/ml min^{-1}). N denotes control lungs and
          each bar represents the mean value ± S.E.M. of six
          experiments.

          Duncan test gives the following results for the comparison
          between each two means:
          Normal and sensitized
          N. vs C. = not significant (P>0.5)
          N. vs H = highly signficant (P<0.01)
          N. vs S. = highly significant (P<0.01)
          H. vs H + A = highly significant (P<0.01)
          S. vs S + A = highly significant (P<0.01)

In the experiments with isolated lungs from sensitized guinea-pigs, the effect of SRS-A is largely amplified (almost 4 times above the control levels), while histamine and carbachol again do not interfere with the lipoxygenase pathway. When the antigen, (ovalbumin, 1 mg), was injected through the sensitized lungs, a significant increase of HETE in the pulmonary effluent was observed.

TABLE 3

Determination of HETE and TXA_2 in the perfusate of isolated lungs from ovalbumin sensitized guinea-pigs under different challengers.

CHALLENGER	HETE ng/min ± S.E.	TXA ng/min ± S.E.
Control	4.3 ± 0.5	13 ± 1.6
Histamine 5 µg	3.6 ± 0.6	123 ± 15.0
Carbachol 10 µg	3.7 ± 0.6	14 ± 1.8
SRSA 0.1 U	15.9 ± 3.2	445 ± 16.5
Ovalbumin 1 mg	8.0 ± 1.3	667 ± 41.5

The data represent the mean values of at least ten experiments. TXA_2 was measured as mono-0-methyl-thromboxane B_2.

Measuring at the same time both HETE and TXA_2 formation from the sensitized lungs under different challengers it has been observed that ovalbumin and SRS-A are capable to stimulate the formation of the two unstable arachidonate metabolites, whereas histamine enhances only the content of TXA_2 in the pulmonary effluent. Carbachol is uneffective on both arachidonate metabolic pathways (Table 3).

DISCUSSION

The outstanding capacity of the pulmonary tissue to metabolize arachidonic acid (AA), suggested thepossibility that the variety of arachidonate metabolites may have a role in the lung tissue under physiological conditions. The discovery that AA metabolites, such as endoperoxides, TXA_2, TXB_2, HHT and HETE, are recovered from lung perfusates of sensitized guinea-pigs during antigen challenge, indicated that these compounds may participate also in pathological processes in the lung. Furthermore the original observation of Mathé (33) that the peak outflow of histamine preceded that of prostanoic metabolites during the anaphylactic-shock is consistent with the hypothesis that these compounds are "secondary mediators" of anaphlyaxis. This is further supported by the capacity of both histamine and SRS-A to release mainly TXA_2 a phenomenon which is particularly amplified in sensitized lungs. However, considering the potent contractile action of TXA_2 on the smooth muscle of the respiratory tract, it is very difficult to understand the object for a positive feed-back mechanism through which histamine and SRS-A liberate from the lungs an even more dangerous substance. Regarding the spasmogenic activity of TXA_2, we provide direct evidence on the capacity of this unstable compound to contract helical strips of human pulmonary lobar artery and human bronchus. As shown in Fig. 6, 100 and 280 ng/ml of TXA_2, measured by radioimmunoassay in the pulmonary outflow, formed during AA infusion into the isolated perfused guinea pig lungs, bring about a dose dependent contraction of the isolated artery along with brisk contraction of a strip of human bronchus. It is interesting to note that $PGF_{2\alpha}$, which has been shown to increase pulmonary arterial pressure and airway resistence in several animal species is ineffective in doses as high as 200 ng/ml. Considering that TXA_2 is generated by blood platelets and in view of its vasoconstrictor activity, it is reasonable to suggest that this endoperoxide metabolite could play a role in the pathogenesis of pulmonary hypertension associated with thromboembolic phenomena.

We have also observed that PGI_2 (100-200 ng) reduces the tonus of the isolated human bronchus, an effect which is the opposite of that obtained in the guinea-pig tracheal chain preparation (Fig. 6). The bronchodilator activity of PGI_2 provides an explanation for the results of Pasargiklian and Bianco (34), who observed that inhaled PGI_2, prevents bronchoconstriction in humans induced by exercise.

Regarding the capacity of histamine to generate TXA_2, the presence of H_1 and H_2-receptors, particularly in the pulmonary vascular bed of the dog (35) and guinea-pig lungs (36), raised the question of the type of histamine receptors involved in this process. The results from our experiments, indicating that only

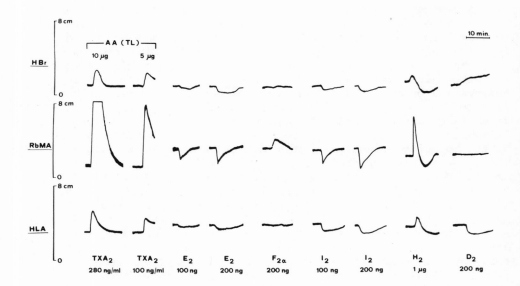

Fig. 6.   Effect of TXA$_2$, PGI$_2$ and other arachidonic acid metabolites (PGF$_2$, PGH$_2$ and PGD$_2$) on superfused helical strips
of human pulmonary lobar artery (HLA) and human
bronchus (HBr).

Isolated lungs of guinea-pig were perfused with Krebs-
bicarbonate solution (10 ml/min) according to Piper
and Vane. The pulmonary outflow superfused a cascade of
isolated tissue including HBr, rabbit mesenteric artery
(RbMA) and HLA. The superfused tissues were treated
with Indomethacin and with a mixture of antagonists as
suggested by Gilmore et al.

Arachidonic acid (AA) was injected as a bolus (5,10 μg)
through the lungs (TL) and the amount of TXA$_2$ present
in the pulmonary effluent (responsible for the biological
activity) was determined as mono-O-methyl-TXB$_2$ by
radioimmunoassay. Prostacyclin and other prostaglandins
were injected as a bolus directly over the tissues in
cascade.

H_1-receptor activation is responsible for substantial production
of natural prostaglandins along which TXA_2, cast some doubt on the
functional significance of H_2-receptors in guinea-pig lungs.

Furthermore the analysis of the pulmonary perfusates during
H_2-receptor activation did not show any PGE_2 and $PGF_{2\alpha}$ formation,
in clear contrast with the finding of Yen et al. (24). In fact,
these investigators suggested a correlation between H_2-receptor
stimulation and PGE_2 production, in spite of their inability to
demonstrate a significant increase of PGE_2 generation from
lungs during challenge with histamine in presence of pyrilamine.
In agreement with Gryglewski (10), it is conceivable that histamine,
in connection with H_1-receptor activation, may generate from
lung parenchyman (alveolar cells?) TXA_2 and from respiratory smooth
muscle the relaxing PGE_2: in this way a "self-defense" mechanism
may be accomplished.

Activation of the β-adrenoceptor represents another pharmacological approach which controls the worsening of the effect of
"primary mediator" of anaphylaxis. In fact isoproterenol and
salbutamol strongly counteract this amplifier mechanism, preventing
the generation of TXA_2 induced by histamine and SRS-A in the
guinea-pig lungs. This is further reinforced by the ability of
β-adrenoceptor blockers, devoid of quinidine-like properties,
such as sotalol and practolol to restore the TXA_2 generating capacity
of the lungs depressed by isoproterenol.

The protective role for β-adrenoceptor activation may be
explained by an accumulation of intracellular cyclic-AMP (37),
however other mechanisms than activation of adenyl-cyclase may
come into play (38). Concerning the type of β-adrenoceptor
involved in the reduction of TXA_2 generation from the lungs,
our results do not permit any conclusion; a prominent role of
either receptor is therefore pure speculation. On this respect
we are investigating the formation of TXA_2 using normal or
sensitized guinea-pig lungs desensitized to $β_2$-adrenoceptor
activation. This area is undoubtedly an important one, in which
further development will prove exciting.

In our experimental model we have explored the possible
influence of α-adrenoceptor activation on the formation of TXA_2.
The results obtained seem to indicate that α-adrenoceptors do not
play a role in this phenomenon at least in non sensitized
guinea-pig lungs. It is worth-testing the activation and
blockade of α-adrenoceptors in lungs from ovalbumin sensitized
guinea-pigs, since enhanced α-adrenergic responses have been
shown in asthmatic patients (39).

Although previous studies (40) suggest that target cells in human lungs,involved in the immunologic release of mediators, possess cholinergic sites, we failed to demonstrate a relationship between activation of cholinergic receptors and secondary formation of TXA_2 in normal or in sensitized guinea-pig lungs. In fact carbachol and cholinoesterase inhibitors, which are very potent in contracting smooth muscles of this respiratory system, do not induce generation of arachidonate metabolites from isolated lungs. On the other hand the finding that atropine and ipratropium-bromide (SCH-1000) prevent the generation of TXA_2 and other prostaglandin-like substances induced by histamine and SRS-A represents a new interesting aspect particularly from the therapeutical point of view. Despite mild side effects, atropinic compounds, either alone or in combination with an adrenergic drug, may have a place in the treatment of severe reversible airway obstruction not adequately controlled by conventional treatment.

The mechanism of action of atropine and SCH-1000 in reducing TXA_2 generation from the lungs is at the moment very difficult to explain. The two drugs may act at the phospholipase A_2 site preventing arachidonic acid cleavage from membrane phospholipids, since normal conversion of AA in lung takes place during blockade of the cholinergic receptor. Whatever the mechanism, our results provide evidence for a new site of action of atropine along with their well known ability to control the reflex efferent cholinergic discharge which adversely affects the asthmatic subject. Another point of interest arising from our experiments is represented by the difference between the two primary mediators of anaphylaxis, histamine and SRS-A in promoting AA transformation in the lungs. Our data clearly indicate in normal and particularly in sensitized lungs that SRS-A increases the arachidonate metabolites from both lipoxygenase (HETE) and cyclo-oxygenase (TXA_2) pathways, whereas histamine enhances only the production of metabolites from the cyclo-oxygenase system. Furthermore the effect of SRS-A in generating HETE from isolated lungs is rather specific, since activation of cholinergic receptors does not stimulate AA metabolism. The ability of SRS-A to activate the lipoxygenase pathway deserves particular attention since it is known that fatty acid hydroperoxides seem to enhance the immunological release from tissues treated with aspirin-like drugs. As a consequence, SRS-A, but not histamine, will lead to a deleterious vicious cycle stimulating via HETE its own release from the sensitized cells. An extention of these observations would be that fatty acid hydroperoxides, which are increased when cyclo-oxygenase is no longer competing for available substrate, may represent a crucial moment in the pathogenesis of aspirin-sensitive asthma. This is in agreement with Parker (41) who has already pointed out that SRS-A should be considered a "prime candidate" as a mediator of bronchospasm in this syndrome.

REFERENCES

1. S. Bergström, F. Dressler, L. Krabisch, R. Ryahge and J.
    Sjövall, The isolation and structure of a smooth muscle
    stimulating factor in normal sheep and pig lungs. Ark. Kemi.,
    20: 63-72 (1962).
2. M. Hamberg, J. Svensson, P. Hedqvist, K. Strandberg and
    B. Samuelsson, Involvement of endoperoxides and thromboxanes
    in anaphylactic reaction. In: "Advances in Prostaglandin and
    Thromboxane Research". B. Samuelsson and R. Paoletti, eds.,
    Vol. 1, Raven Press, New York, pg. 495-501 (1976).
3. P. J. Kadowitz, W. J. George, P. D. Jainer and A. L. Hyman,
    Effect of Prostaglandins E_1 and $F_{2\alpha}$ on adrenergic responses
    in the pulmonary circulation. Adv. Biosci., 9: 501-506 (1973).
4. M. Hamberg, J. Svensson and B. Samuelsson, Thromboxanes: a
    new biologically active compounds derived from prostaglandin
    endoperoxides. Proc. Natl. Acad. Sci. USA., 72: 2994-2998
    (1975).
5. J. R. Vane, Inhibitors of prostaglandin, prostacyclin and
    thromboxane synthesis. In: "Advances in Prostaglandin and
    Thromboxane Research". B. Samuelsson and R. Paoletti, eds.,
    Vol. 4, Raven Press, New York, pg. 27-44 (1978).
6. P. J. Piper and J. R. Vane, Release of additional factors
    of anaphylaxis and its antagonism by anti-inflammatory drugs.
    Nature, 223: 29-35 (1969).
7. B. Samuelsson, G. C. Folco, E. Granström, H. Kindahl, C.
    Malmsten, Prostaglandins and hromboxanes: iochemical and
    hysiological considerations. In: "Advances in Prostaglandin
    and Thromboxane Reserach". B. Samuelsson and R. Paoletti,
    eds., ol. 4, Raven Press, New York, pg. 1-25 (1978).
8. J. Orehek, J. S. Douglas and A. Bouhuys, Contractile responses
    of the guinea-pig trachea in vitro: modification by
    prostaglandin synthesis inhibiting drugs. J. Pharmacol., 194:
    554-564 (1975).
9. L. Grodzinska, B. Panczenko and R. J. Gryglewski,Generation
    of Prostaglandin E-like material by the guinea-pig trachea
    contracted by histamine. J. Pharm. Pharmacol., 27:88-91
    (1975).
10. R. J. Gryglewski, Kiec-Dembinska and L. Grodzinska, Generation
    of prostaglandin and thromboxane-like substances by large
    airways and lung parenchyma. In: "Prostaglandins and
    Thromboxanes". F. Berti, B. Samuelsson and G. P. Velo, eds.,
    Plenum Press, New York, pg. 165-178 (1977).
11. D. M. Engineer, P. J. Piper and P. Sirois, Release of
    prostaglandins and rabbit aorta contracting substance (RCS)
    from guinea-pig lung by slow-reacting substance of anaphylaxis.
    Brit. J. Pharmacol., 59:444P (1977).
12. W. E. Brockelhurst, The release of histamine and formation
    of slow-reacting substance of anaphylaxis (SRS-A) during
    anaphylactic shock. J. Physiol., 151: 416-435 (1960).

13.   J. M. Drazen, R. A. Lewis,S. I. Wasserman, and P. Orange,
      Differential effects of partially purified preparation of
      slow-reacting substance of anaphylaxis on guinea-pig trachea
      spirals and parenchymal strips. J. Clin. Invest., 63:
      1-5 (1979).
14.   B. Samuelsson, P. Borgeat, S. Hammarström and R. C. Murphy,
      Introduction of a nomenclature: Leukotrienes. Prostaglandins,
      17: 785-786 (1979).
15.   J. J. Adcock, L. G Garland, S. Moncada, and J. A. Salmon
      The mechanism of enhancement by fatty acid hydroperoxides
      of anaphylactic mediator release. Prostaglandins, 16:
      179-187 (1978).
16.   R. J. Gryglewski, A. Szczeklic and E. Nizankowska, Aspirin-
      sensitive asthma: its relationship to inhibition of
      prostaglandin biosynthesis. In: "Prostaglandins and
      Thromboxanes". F. Berti, B. Samuelsson and G. P. Velo,
      eds., Plenum Press, New York, pg. 191-203 (1977).
17.   D. M. Engineer, P. J. Piper and P. Sirois, Interaction
      between the release of SRS-A and of Prostaglandins. Brit. J.
      Pharmac., 57: 460-461P (1976).
18.   N. Gilmore, J. R. Vane and J. H. Willie, Prostaglandins
      released by the spleen. Nature, 218: 1135-1140 (1968).
19.   E. Granström, H. Kindhal and B. Samuelsson, A method for
      measuring the unstable thromboxane A_2: radioimmunoassay of
      the derived mono-0-methyl thromboxane B_2. Prostaglandins, 12:
      929-941 (1976).
20.   L. Sautebin, G. Spagnuolo, C. Galli and G. Galli, A mass
      fragmentographic procedure for the simultaneous determination
      of HETE and $PGF_{2\alpha}$ in the central nervous system. Prostaglandins,
      16: 985-988 (1979).
21.   R. P. Orange, R. C. Murphy, M. L. Karnovsky, F. K. Austen,
      The physico-chemical characteristics and purification of
      slow-reacting substance of anaphylaxis. J. Immun., 110:
      760-770 (1973).
22.   D. B. Duncan, Multiple range and multiple F. tests.
      Biometrics II: 1-42 (1955).
23.   J. W. Black, W. A. M. Duncan, C. J. Durant, C. R. Ganellin
      and E. M. Parsons, Definition and antagonism of histamine
      H_2-receptors. Nature, Lond.,236: 385-390 (1972).
24.   S. S. Yen, A. A. Mathé and J. J. Dugan. Release of
      prostaglandins from healthy and sensitized guinea-pig lung
      and trachea by histamine. Prostaglandins II: 227-239
      (1976).
25.   M. E. Rosenthale, A. Dervinis and D. Strike, Actions of
      prostaglandins on the respiratory tract of animals. In:
      "Advances in Prostaglandin and Thromboxane Reasearch". B.
      Samuelsson and R. Paoletti, eds., Raven Press, New York,
      pg. 477-494 (1976).
26.   A. J. Coleman, A. R. Somerville, The selective action of β-
      adrenoceptor blocking drugs and the nature of β_1 and β_2
      adrenoceptors. Br. J. Pharmacol., 59: 83-93 (1977).

27. C. Omini, A. R. Somerville, G. C. Folco, G. Rossoni and L. Puglisi, Interaction between β_1 and β_2 adrenoceptors in the isolated guinea-pig trachea. Pharmacol. Res. Comm., 11: 529-535 (1979).

28. A. Engelhardt and H. Klupp, The pharmacology and toxicology of a new tropane alkaloid derivative. Postgraduate Med. J., 51:(suppl. 7) 82-84 (1975).

29. M. Hamberg and B. Samuelsson, Prostaglandin endoperoxides. Novel transformation of arachidonic acid in human platelets. Proc. Natl. Acad. Sci. USA., 71: 3400-3404 (1974).

30. M. Hamberg and B. Samuelsson, Prostaglandin endoperoxides. VII. Novel transformation of arachidonic acid in guinea-pig lung. Biochem. Biophys. Res. Comm., 61: 942-949 (1974).

31. D. M. Engineer, U. Niederhauser, P. J. Piper and P. Sirois, Release of mediators of anaphylaxis: inhibition of prostaglandin synthesis and the modification of release of slow-reacting substance of anaphylaxis and histamine. Brit. J. Pharmac., 62: 61-66 (1978).

32. J. R. Boot, A. D. J. Brockwell, W. Dawson and W. J. F. Sweatman, The relationship between prostaglandin like substances and SRS-A released from immunologically challenged lungs. Brit. J. Pharmac., 59:444P (1977).

33. A. Mathé, Prostaglandins and the lung. In: "Prostaglandins" Vol. 3, P. W. Ramwell, ed., Plenum Press, New York, pg.169-224 (1977).

34. M. Pasargiklian and S. Bianco, Ventilatory and cardiovascular effects of PI and 6-keto-$PGF_{1\alpha}$ by inhalation. Fourth International Prostaglandin Conference Abstracts. Washington D.C., May 27-31 (1979) g.91.

35. A. Tucker, E. K. Weir, J. T. Reeves and R. F. Grover, Histamine H_1-and H_2-receptors in pulmonary and systemic vasculature of the dog. Am. J. Physiol., 229: 1008-1013 (1975).

36. R. K. Turker, Presence of H_2-receptors in the guinea-pig pulmonary vascular bed. Pharmacology, 9: 306-311 (1973).

37. R. P. Orange, G. W. Austen and K. F. Austen, Immunological release of histamine and slow-reacting substance of anaphylaxis. I. Modulation by agents influencing cellular levels of cyclic AMP. J. Exp. Med., 134: (Suppl.) 136s (1971).

38. M. J. Berridge, The interaction of cyclic nucleotides and calcium in the control of cellular activity. In: "Advances in Cyclic Nucleotide Research". P. Greengard and G. A. Robison, eds., Raven Press, New York, Vol. 6, pg. 1-98 (1975).

39. W. R. Henderson, J. Shelhamer, D. B. Reingold, L. J. Smith, R. Evans III and M. Kaliner Alpha-adrenergic hyper-responsiveness in asthma. Analysis of vascular and pupillary responses. New Engl. J. Med., 300: 642-647 (1979).

40. M. Kaliner, R. P. Orange and F. K. Austen, Immunological
     release of histamine and slow-reacting substance of anaphylaxis
     from human lung. J. Exp. Med., 136: 556-567 (1972).
41. C. W. Parker, Aspirin-sensitive asthma. In: "Asthma".
     L. M. Lichtenstein and F. K. Austen, eds., Academic Press Inc.,
     pg. 301-313 (1977).

IDENTIFICATION AND DISTRIBUTION OF ARACHIDONIC ACID METABOLITES IN THE HUMAN GASTROINTESTINAL TRACT, AND THE WAYS IN WHICH SOME OF THESE AFFECT THE LONGITUDINAL MUSCLE

Alan Bennet, Christopher N. Hensby*, Gareth J. Sanger and Ian F. Stamford

Department of Surgery, King's College Hospital
Medical School, London, England and
Department of Clinical Pharmacology
Royal Postgraduate Medical School
London, England

Prostaglandins (PGs) may have various roles in gastrointestinal function. They have also been implicated as contributors to various gastrointestinal diseases, including gastritis, gastric ulcer formation, ulcerative colitis, irritable bowel syndrome, idiopathic intestinal pseudo-obstruction, food intolerance, and radiation-induced and other forms of diarrhoea (1-8). In contrast, PGs administered as drugs may be useful in the treatment of peptic ulceration, prevention of aspirin- or indomethacin-induced gastric mucosal damage (9) and reversal of post-operative ileus (10). Knowledge of the types of compounds formed from the C20-unsaturated fatty acids eicosatrienoic, eicosatetraenoic (arachidonic) and eicosapentaenoic acids, and their actions on the human gut, is therefore important. Most studies to date have concerned PGE and PGF_α compounds, but we have now extended this to include other metabolites of arachidonic acid.

CHARACTERISATION OF PROSTANOIDS EXTRACTED FROM HUMAN GUT

The first characterisation of PG-like material (PG-1m) in human gastrointestinal tissues was in extracts of human stomach (11). Subsequent work showed PG-1m in extracts of homogenized tissue from all regions of the human gastrointestinal tract (12). PGE and PGF_α compounds were thought to be the major PGs formed by tissues of all species. More recently however, other prostanoids such as 6-keto-$PGF_{1\alpha}$ and thromboxane (Tx) B_2, formed from prostacyclin (PGI_2) and thromboxane A_2 respectively, have been found in the gut of various laboratory animals (13-16). Human gastric mucosa can form 6-keto-$PGF_{1\alpha}$, PGD_2, PGE_2, $PGF_{2\alpha}$ and TxB_2 (12), and 6-keto-$PGF_{1\alpha}$ occurs in extracts of human rectal

365

mucosa (17).

In previous work (12) the PG-1m extracted from homogenates
of human gut was formally identified in only 2 instances.
Characterisation in the other cases was by biological assay
before and/or after chromatography against PGE_2 on the rat stomach
strip (see Refs. 18 & 19 for detailed methods of extraction,
homogenisation and bioassay). The sensitivity of our assay was
high to PGE_1 and PGE_2, moderate to $PGF_{2\alpha}$ but low to many of the
relatively stable prostanoids that may occur in extracts. Amounts
of any substances of low potency were therefore underestimated.
As found previously (19), mucosa from the stomach tended to form
more PG-1m than did the muscle; the same trend was seen for the
terminal ileum, whereas the reverse occurred in the colon. This
distribtuion of PG-1m in the colon was confirmed by freezing
specimens of colon wall, cutting 100µm sections parallel to the
mucosal surface and extracting groups of 5 x 100µm sections
(Fig. 1).

PGE and PGF_α compounds were tentatively characterised using
chromatography and sensitivity of the PG-1m to inactivation by
alkali (See Refs. 20 & 21 for detailed methodology). PGE_2-like
material together with small amounts of material running with
PGE_1 were found in the extracts of stomach mucosa, whereas
material running with PGE_1, PGE_2, PGE_3 and $PGF_{1\alpha}$ were extracted
from colonic muscle or mucosa; materials running with $PGF_{2\alpha}$
and $PGF_{3\alpha}$ were found only in extracts of colonic mucosa.

A major problem is that PGI_2, TxA_2 and other unstable
metabolites of arachidonic acid are rapidly degraded and would
not survive our extraction process. In addition, 6-keto-$PGF_{1\alpha}$ and
PGE_2 have similar Rf values in the chromatography systems used.
Thus 6-keto-$PGF_{1\alpha}$, which stimulates the rat fundus strip with
potency about 200 times less than PGE_2, would be characterised
and assayed as PGE_2. These problems can be overcome by gas
chromatography - mass spectrometry (GC-MS). The addendum to the
earlier paper (12) reported two studies using GC-MS which
identified mainly 6-keto-$PGF_{1\alpha}$, together with smaller amounts of
PGD_2, PGE_2, $PGF_{2\alpha}$ and TxB_2, in extracts from two specimens of
human gastric mucosa. We now report preliminary data obtained by
GC-MS on the products extracted from homogenates of human stomach,
terminal ileum and sigmoid colon. obtained from surgery at least
6cm from any macroscopic lesion. Mesentery and fat were removed
and the tissue was divided along the submucosal plexus into
one part containing the muscle and serosa, and another part
containing the mucosal layers. After cutting into small pieces
and washing in Krebs solution, weighed amounts were homogenised
at room temperature in Krebs solutions to obtain new synthesis
of PGs from released endogenous precursors (19).

Following chloroform extraction (18) and evaporation, some samples were dissolved in dichloromethane and purified using LH20 column chromatography. Elution was carried out first with dichloromethane to remove non-polar inpurities, and then with methanol to elute the PGs which were then evaporated to dryness. These dried extracts, and others not purified by LH20 column chromatography, were dissolved in 10ml double-distilled water acidified to pH3.0 with hydrochloric acid, percolated through Amberlite XAD-2 columns, and successively eluted with 15ml distilled water, 5ml n-heptane and 10ml methanol.

The methanolic fraction was evaporated at 40°C under nitrogen and then desiccated under vacuum. The residue was redissolved in 200μl of methanol : chloroform (1:1v/v) and applied as a narrow band on a silica gel G thin layer chromatography plate (200 x 100 x 0.2mm Merck; FIV solvent system (22)). Authentic prostanoid standards (Upjohn Co. Ltd.) were applied next to each biological sample. The plates were developed to 15cm from the origin and 1cm zones were eluted twice with 5ml methanol which was then evaporated. Zones corresponding to authentic arachidonic acid (AA) and 12-hydroxy-eicosatetraenoic acid (12-HETE) were pooled and the residues re-chromatographed as described above using diethyl ether:petroleum spirit:acetic acid (50:50:1 by volume). This gave better separation of the zones corresponding to AA and 12-HETE which were eluted as described above.

Chemical derivatisation was as follows:

a)   O-Methyloxime. Residues from prostanoid zones were redissolved in 100μl pyridine containing methyloxime hydrochloride 5mg/ml, and heated to 60-80°C for 1 hour. The pyridine was removed under vacuum desiccation for 30 minutes.

b)   Methylesters. Organic residues of AA, 12-HETE and PGs following O-methyloxime formation (see above) were redissolved in 100μl methanol and treated with 200μl freshly re-distilled diazomethane. After vortexing, the samples were evapoured under nitrogen at room temperature and the procedure repeated.

c)   Trimethylsilyl ether. Vacuum-desiccated residues of 12-HETE, methyl esters and prostanoid O-methyloxime methyl esters were redissolved in 25μl N, N-bis (trimethylsilyl)-tri-fluoro-acetamide (BSTFA:Sigma) and heated at 60°C for 15 minutes.

Gas chromatography-mass spectrometry was performed by injection 10μl samples of standards and samples into a Finnigan 9600 gas chromatograph equipped with a glass column (1.5 x 2mm) packed with 1% SE-30 on Supelcoport (Phase Separation). The chromotograph was interfaced via a glass jet separator with a Finnigan 3200 quadrupole mass spectrometer, and the system was operated using

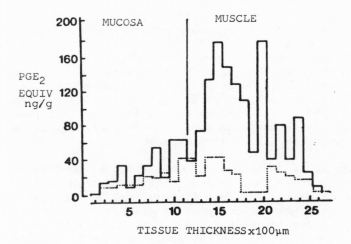

Fig. 1. Prostaglandin-like material extracted from homogenates
         of sections cut through the wall of sigmoid colon (female
         aged 76 years):—homogenates in Krebs solution to allow
         new PG synthesis; ..... homogenates in acid ethanol
         to indicate 'basal' amounts of PG. (After Bennett et
         al., 1977).

a Finnigan 6000 data system. The gas chromatograph was operated
between 175° and 220°C using helium (30ml/min) as the carrier
gas. Settings for the mass spectrometer were 25eV electron
energy, 10^{-7} amps/V pre-amplifier, and 1700 V electron multiplier.

     Only compounds formed from arachidonic acid were detected.
If derivatives 8,11,14-eicosatrienoic acid or 5,8,11,14,17-
eicosapentaenoic acid were present their amounts were probably
at most 80ng recovered/g wet weight tissue. Impurities in some
extracts hindered identification of all the arachidonic acid
metabolites that may have been present. However, all the extracts
of homogenized muscle or mucosa contained 6-keto-$PGF_{1\alpha}$ and TxB_2,
an 'usually contained HETE. PGD_2, PGE_2 and $PGF_{2\alpha}$ were also identified
in specimens of human stomach, but their presence in either the
mucosa or the muscle was not consistent. In the only specimen
of terminal ileum studied, 6-keto-$PGF_{1\alpha}$, TxB_2 and HETE were
identified in both the mucosa and the muscle; PGE_2 was detected
in the muscle and PGD_2 in the mucosa, but other ileal prostanoids
may have been masked by the substantial impurities. Besides the
ubiquitous 6-keto-$PGF_{1\alpha}$ and TxB_2, the 3 specimens of sigmoid
colon yielded PGE_2 and HETE from all specimens of muscle, but
in only 2 specimens of mucosa; PGD_2 was variably found in extracts
from 2 specimens of muscle or mucosa, and $PGF_{2\alpha}$ was not detected.

The number of specimens studies is small, and only a semi-quantitative assessment has been possible so far. Nevertheless it seems clear that, under the conditions used, gut muscle and mucosa can produce PGI_2, TxA_2 and lipoxygenase products, as indicated by the amost consistent identification of their degradation compounds 6-keto-$PGF_{1\alpha}$, TxB_2 and HETE.

Peskar et al (23) confirmed the presence of PGE_2 in extracts of human gastric juice using radioimmunoassay. Using GC-MS and radio-immunoassay, they found that incubates of the microsomal fraction from human gastric mucosa formed more PGE_2 than 6-keto-$PGF_{1\alpha}$ (24). The difference from our findings of more 6-keto-$PGF_{1\alpha}$ might be due to methodology. At least some of the TxB_2 in our homogenates must have come from TxA_2 formed by platelets present in the tissue, and similarly 6-keto-$PGF_{1\alpha}$ may come from PGI_2 formed by the blood vessels. An additional problem, as we found subsequently, is that in some cases we probably eluted substantial amounts of the less-polar prostanoids from our LH20 columns with dichloromethane.

The relative importance of different pathways for arachidonic acid metabolism in human gut is therefore still far from clear. Apart from the problems associated with methodology, other factors may alter arachidonic acid metabolism. These include the diseases for which the specimens were resected, medication, diet, anaesthesia, muscle activity, and endogenous substances which affect prostanoid synthesis and inactivation.

The Effects and Interactions of Prostanoids on Longitudinal Muscle Strips from the Human Gastrointestinal Tract

PGE_2 or $PGF_{2\alpha}$ usually contract the longitudinal muscle of human isolated gastrointestinal tissue, whereas in the circular muscle $PGF_{2\alpha}$ and PGE_2 usually cause contraction and relaxation respectively (25-29). We now report studies with other prostanoids, using specimens of human stomach, terminal ileum and sigmoid colon obtained as described previously. The mucosa and sub-mucosa were cut away, and muscle strips approximately 4mm wide and 3cm long were cut parallel to the longitudinal muscle fibres (the taeniae were used in the colon). Each strip was suspended in 10ml Krebs solution (37ºC; 5% CO_2 in O_2; 1g load)/and responses were registered using an isotonic transducer.

PGD_2, PGE_2, $PGF_{2\alpha}$ and the (15s)-hydroxy-9α,11α- (epoxymethano) prosta-5Z, 13E-dienoic acid analogue of PGH_2 (U-46619) caused dose-dependent contractions of all tissues. PGI_2 relaxed gastric and colonic specimens, but usually caused weak contractions of strips from the terminal ileum. Responses to 6-keto-$PGF_{1\alpha}$, 6,15-diketo-$PGF_{1\alpha}$ or TxB_2 were generally weak and variable (Table 1). The effect of PGI_2 on the human stomach contrasts with the contraction of the longitudinal

TABLE 1

Effects and approximate threshold concentrations of prostanoids on longitudinal muscle from human stomach, terminal ileum and colon.

PROSTANOID	STOMACH			TERMINAL ILEUM			TAENIA COLI		
	Response	Threshold ng/ml	n	Response	Threshold ng/ml	n	Response	Threshold ng/ml	n
PGD_2	Weak contraction	20–1000	3	Contraction	100–2000	3	Contraction	10–1000	3
PGE_2	Contraction	0.5–10	3	Contraction	1	2	Contraction	10–100	2
$PGF_{2\alpha}$	Contraction	1–10	3	Contraction	10	3	Contraction	100–1000	2
U–46619	Contraction	0.0001–1	3	Contraction	0.001–5	3	Contraction	1–10	3
PGI_2	Relaxation	50–200	3	Weak contraction / Weak relaxation	10–1000 / 10000	2 / 1	Relaxation	1000–10000	4
6–keto–$PGF_{1\alpha}$	Weak contraction	100	3	Weak contraction	10000	1	Weak contraction or relaxation	1000–10000	3
6,15–diketo–$PGF_{1\alpha}$	Weak contraction or relaxation	10000	3	Contraction / No effect	100 / –	1 / 1	Weak contraction	1000	2
TxB_2	Contraction / No effect	1000 / –	1 / 2	Weak contraction	100	2	Weak contraction / No effect	1000 / –	2 / 1

muscle of rat gastric fundus and rabbit stomach (30,31). In rat
colon, PGI_2 causes either weak contraction or relaxation of the
longitudinal muscle (30).

In general, the sensitivity to prostanoids was: stomach>
terminal ileum>taenia coli. U-46619 was the most potent
excitatory prostanoid in these tissues, particularly with gastric
muscle which contracted to concentrations as low as 0.1pg/ml-
1ng/ml (Table 1). Gastric tissue was also the most responsive
to PGI_2, but the greater relaxation of stomach muscle than that
of taenia coli (Fig. 2), could be due at least partly to a
greater stomach muscle tone.

The contraction of human terminal ileum muscle to PGI_2
contrasts with the consistent relaxant effect in the stomach and
colon. In one specimen of jejunum PGI_2 also caused muscle
relaxation, but other regions of small intestine have not been
studied because they are difficult to obtain.

There are many possible explanations of the differences in
the sensitivity of stomach, ileum and colon to prostanoids.
Such differences also occur with PGE_2, $PGF_{2\alpha}$ and PGI_2 in the
rat stomach and colon (32,30), and other gradients exist in the
gut (e.g. innervation, Ref.33). Other factors such as the type
of disease and extent of inflammation may contribute to small
differences in responses of human tissues (34).

Since PGI_2 can be formed throughout the gastrointestinal
tract and, unlike other prostanoids can relax the longitudinal
muscle, we investigated the interaction of PGI_2 with the contraction
of stomach longitudinal muscle to other prostanoids (35).
After obtaining rough dose-response curves, consistent sub-maximal
contractions were produced with acetylcholine (ACh; 0.05-1µg/ml)
and either PGE_2 (3ng/ml-1µg/ml), $PGF_{2\alpha}$ (0.1-1µg/ml)or U-46619
(5-100ng/ml). PGI_2 1µg/ml was then added to the bathing solution
and new consistent responses to the same doses of excitatory
prostanoid obtained.

The results expressed below are medians with semi-quartile
ranges in parentheses.

PGI_2 lowered muscle tone and this probably explains why
contractions to U-46619 or ACh tended to increase (by 14(7 to
29)% and 6(19 to-26)% respectively, n=6 and 19). However, PGI_2
reduced contractions to PGE_2 or $PGF_{2\alpha}$ by 34(15 to 81)% and
51(20 to 79)% respectively (n=7 and 6; P<0.01 compared with the
effect on ACh or U-46619, Mann Whitney U-test).

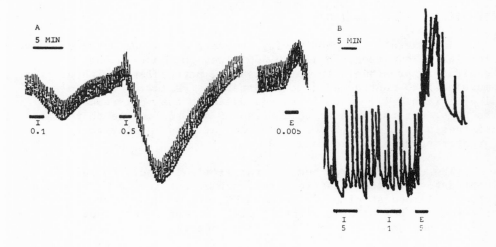

Fig. 2.   PGI$_2$ (I) potently relaxed the longitudinal muscle of
          human stomach (A) but was less effective in human taenia
          coli (B). PGE$_2$ (E) contracted both tissues, whereas
          administration of vehicle had almost no effect (not shown).
          The numbers below I and E represent µg/ml.

      We previously found that in human isolated myometrial strips
PGI$_2$ 1µg/ml reduced contractions to PGF$_{2\alpha}$ and, unlike in the
stomach, it reduced contractions to U-46619 (36). This may
indicate that the types of excitatory prostanoid modulated by
PGI$_2$ vary with the tissue, but the actions of U-46619 are complex
and may involve stimulation of PG synthesis (37), or activation
of TxA$_2$ receptors (38).

      The roles of prostanoids in gastric motility remain to be
fully elucidated, and the type of prostanoid formed will affect
the response. PGI$_2$ may preferentially modulate the effects of
other prostanoids, and this may be of importance both in physiology
and pathology. It seems that the prostanoids which contribute
to the tone in longitudinal muscle strips of human stomach are
mainly excitatory since inhibitors of PG synthesis reduce the
muscle tone (39,40). Similarly, in human isolated intestine,
inhibitors of cyclo-oxygenase lower the longitudinal muscle
tone (29,40,41).

ACKNOWLEDGEMENTS

We thank Miss M. A. Carroll, Miss K. Crowley, Mrs. J. E. Wright and Mr. E. V. Bagshaw for their help, and the MRC and Wellcome Trust for support.

REFERENCES

1. H. O. J. Collier. Prostaglandin synthetase inhibitors and the gut. In: Prostaglandin Synthetase Inhibitors. H. J. Robinson and J. R. Vane, eds., pp.121-133, Raven Press, New York (1974).
2. A. T. Mennie, V. Dalley, L. C. Dinneen and H. O. J. Collier. Treatment of radiation-induced gastrointestinal distress with acetylsalicylate. Lancet, 2: 942-943 (1975).
3. J. R. Luderer, L. M. Demers, E. M. Bonnem, A. Saleem and G. H. Jeffries. Elevated prostaglandin E in idopathic intestinal pseudo obstruction. New England J. Med., 295: 1179 (1976).
4. S. R. Gould, A. R. Brash and M. E. Conolly. Increased prostaglandin production in ulcerative colitis. Lancet, 2: 198 (1977).
5. W. Schlegel, K. Wenk, H. C. Dollinger and S. Raptis. Concentrations of prostaglandin A-, E- and F-like substances in gastric mucosa of normal subjects and of patients with various gastric diseases. Clin. Sci. Mol. Med., 52: 255-258 (1977).
6. P. D. Buisseret, L. J. F. Youlten, D. I. Heinzelmann and M. H. Lessof. Prostaglandin-synthesis inhibitors in prophylaxis of food intolerance. Lancet, 1: 906-908 (1978).
7. D. W. Harris, P. R. Smith and C. H. J. Swan. Determination of prostaglandin synthetase activity in rectal biopsy material and its significance in colonic disease. Gut, 19: 875-877 (1978).
8. J. Rask-Madsen and K. Bukhave. Indomethacin-responsive diarrhoea in irritable bowel syndrome. Gut, 19: A448 (1978).
9. M. M. Cohen and J. M. Pollett. Prostaglandin E_2 prevents aspirin and indomethacin damage to human gastric mucosa. Surg. Forum., 27: 400-401 (1976).
10. M. J. Ruwart, M. S. Klepper and B. D. Rush. The beneficial effects of prostaglandins in post-operative ileus. Gastroenterology, 74: 1088 (1978).
11. A. Bennett, J. G. Murray and J. H. Wyllie. Occurrence of prostaglandin E_2 in the human stomach, and a study of its effects on human isolated gastric muscle. Br. J. Pharmac., 32: 339-349 (1968).
12. A. Bennett, I. F. Stamford and H. L. Stockley. Estimation and characterization of prostaglandins in the human gastrointestinal tract. Br. J. Pharmac., 61: 579-586 (1977).

13. C. Pace-Asciak and L. S. Wolfe. A novel prostaglandin
     derivative formed from arachidonic acid by rat stomach
     homogenates. Biochemistry, N.Y., 10: 3657-3664 (1971).
14. C. Pace-Asciak. Isolation, structure and biosynthesis of
     6-keto prostaglandin $F_{1\alpha}$ in the rat stomach. Am. Chem. Soc.,
     98: 2348-2349 (1976).
15. M. Ali, J. Zamecnik, A. L. Cerskus, A. J. Stoessl, W. H.
     Barnett and J. W. D. McDonald. Synthesis of thromboxane
     B_2 and prostaglandins by bovine gastric mucosal microsomes.
     Prostaglandins, 14: 819-827 (1977).
16. S. Moncada, J. A. Salmon, J. R. Vane and B. J. R. Whittle.
     Formation of prostacyclin and its product 6-oxo-$PGF_{1\alpha}$ by
     the gastric mucosa of several species. J. Physiol., 275:
     4P (1978).
17. H. Sinzinger, K. Silberbauer, M. Winter and H. Seyfried.
     Human rectal mucosa generates prostacyclin. Lancet, 2:
     1253 (1978).
18. W. G. Unger, I. F. Stamford and A. Bennett. Extraction of
     prostaglandins from human blood. Nature, Lond., 233:
     336-337 (1971).
19. A. Bennett, I. F. Stamford and W. G. Unger. Prostaglandin
     E_2 and gastric acid secretion in man. J.Physiol., 229:
     349-360 (1973).
20. I. F. Stamford and W. G. Unger. Improved purification and
     chromatography of extracts containing prostaglandins.
     J. Physiol., 225: 4-5P (1972).
21. K. Green and B. Samuelsson. Thin layer chromatography of
     prostaglandins. J. Lipids Res., 5: 117-120 (1964).
22. N. H. Anderson. Preparative thin layer and column
     chromatography of prostaglandins. J. Lipid Res., 10: 316-319
     (1969).
23. B. M. Peskar, A. Holland and B. A. Peskar. Quantitative
     determination of prostaglandins in human gastric juice by
     radioimmunoassay. Clin. Chem. Acta., 55: 21-27 (1974).
24. B. A. Peskar, U. Schade, E. Rietschel and B. M. Peskar.
     Synthesis and metabolism of endogenous prostaglandins by
     human gastric mucosa. Abstr. Fourth. Int. Prostaglandin
     Conference, Washington, p.93 (1979).
25. A. Bennett, K. G. Eley and G. B. Scholes. Effects of
     prostaglandins E_1 and E_2 on human, guinea-pig and rat small
     intestine. Br. J. Pharmac., 34: 639-647 (1968).
26. A. Bennett and B. Fleshler. Prostaglandins and the
     gastrointestinal tract. Gastroenterology, 59: 790-800 (1970).
27. B. Fleshler and A. Bennett. Responses of human, guinea-pig
     and rat colonic circular muscle to prostaglandins. J. Lab.
     Clin. Med., 74:872 (1969).
28. A. Bennett and J. Posner. Studies on prostaglandins
     antagonists. Br. J. Pharmac., 42: 584-594 (1971).

29. A. Bennett and H. L. Stockley. The contribution of prosta-
     glandins in the muscle of human isolated small intestine
     to neurogenic responses. Br. J. Pharmac., 61: 573-578 (1977).
30. C. Omini, S. Moncada and J. R. Vane. The effects of prosta-
     cyclin (PGI$_2$) on tissues which detect prostaglandins (PGs).
     Prostaglandins, 14: 625-632 (1977).
31. B. J. R. Whittle, K. G. Mugridge and S. Moncada. Use of the
     rabbit transverse stomach strip to identify and assay
     prostacyclin, PGA$_2$, PGD$_2$ and other prostaglandins. Eur. J.
     Pharmac., 53: 167-172 (1979).
32. N. Gilmore, J. R. Vane and J. H. Wyllie. Prostaglandins
     released by the spleen. Nature, 218: 1135-1140 (1968).
33. A. Bennett and H. L. Stockley. The intrinsic innervation of
     the human alimentary tract and its relation to function. Gut,
     16: 443-453 (1975).
34. J. P. Hughes, P. J. Kadowitz, A. L. Hyman, J. E. Ray and
     P. D. Joiner. Pharmacology of human isolated colonic
     circular and longitudinal smooth muscle from cancer and non-
     cancer patients. Dis. Col. & Rect., 19: 120-125 (1976).
35. A. Bennett and G. J. Sanger. Prostacyclin relaxes the
     longitudinal muscle of human isolated stomach and antagonizes
     contractions to some prostanoids. J. Physiol., (in press)
     (1979).
36. A. Bennett and G. J. Sanger. Prostacyclin and prostaglandin
     E$_2$ selectively antagonize responses of human isolated
     myometrium to excitatory prostaglandins. J. Physiol., 292:
     36-37P (1979).
37. C. Malmsten. Some biological effects of prostaglandin
     endoperoxide analogues. Life. Sci., 18: 169-176 (1977).
38. R. A. Coleman, P. P. A. Humphrey, I. Kennedy, G. P. Levy
     and P. Lumley. U-46619, a selective thromboxane A$_2$-like
     agonist? Br. J. Pharmac., (in press) (1979).
39. H. L. Stockley and A. Bennett. Modulation of activity by
     prostaglandins in human gastrointestinal muscle. In: Fifth
     International Symposium on Gastrointestinal Motility.
     G. Vantrappen, ed., Typoff Press, Belgium, pp.31-36 (1976).
40. A. Bennett, D. Pratt and G. J. Sanger. Antagonism by
     fenamates of prostaglandin action in guinea-pig and human
     alimentary muscle. Br. J. Pharmac., (in press) (1979).
41. D. E. Burleigh. The effects of indomethacin on the tone and
     spontaneous activity of the human small intestine in vitro.
     Arch. Int. Pharmacodyn. Ther., 225: 240-245 (1977).

PROSTANOID AGONISTS AND ANTAGONISTS: DIFFERENTIATION OF PROSTANOID

RECEPTORS IN THE GUT

Gareth J. Sanger and Alan Bennett

Department of Surgery,
King's College Hospital Medical School
London, England

Prostaglandin (PG) E and F compounds have been studied extensively on gastrointestinal muscle from several species, and various antagonists of their actions have been examined (see Ref. 1). However, less is known of the effects of the numerous other substances which can also be formed from arachidonic acid and other C_{20}-unsaturated fatty acids.

We combine in this chapter work in our laboratory (2-9) on prostanoid actions in rat, guinea-pig and human isolated gastrointestinal muscle, and their antagonism by various drugs including several which can be safely given to man.

METHODS

Adult Wistar rats of either sex and male albino guinea-pigs were stunned and bled. Strips of rat gastric fundus approximately 3mm wide and 2cm long were cut parallel to the longitudinal muscle fibres, one from each side of the greater curvature. Segments of guinea-pig distal ileum or colon 2-3cm long, and spiral strips approximately 3mm wide and 3cm long were used to determine longitudinal and circular muscle responses respectively.

Human gastrointestinal muscle was obtained at operation for benign or malignant disease, and a sample was obtained at least 6cm away from any macroscopic lesion. After removal of the mucosal layers, strips of muscle approximately 4-5mm wide and 2-3cm long were cut parallel to the longitudinal muscle fibres. Each strip was suspended under a 1g load in a 10ml organ bath containing Krebs solution (NaCl 7.1; $CaCl_2.6H_2O$ 0.55; KH_2PO_4 0.16; KCl 0.35; $MgSO_4.7H_2O$ 0.29; $NaH O_3$ 2.1; dextrose 1.0g/l) maintained at 37°C

and bubbled with 5% CO_2 in O_2. Isotonic muscle contractions were
recorded with transducers and pen recorders.

Results are expressed as medians with ranges or semi-quartile
ranges in parentheses, and analyzed using the Wilcoxon matched-
pairs test or the Mann-Whitney U-test.

Rat Gastric Fundus

Cumulative dose-response curves were obtained to acetylcholine
(ACh) and to one prostanoid. A drug to be tested as an antagonist
was then added, and at least 30 min later the dose-response curves
were repeated. Measurements were made of the maximum contraction
height and the concentration of agonist producing a response 50%
of maximum (EC50). The drugs tested as antagonists were SC-19220
(10), trimethoquinol, sodium meclofenamate and indomethacin.

All the prostanoids contracted the rat gastric fundus. On the
basis of EC50 values, their relative potencies were PGE_2>U-
46619∿U-44069∿$PGF_{2\alpha}$∿PGH_2>PGD_2∿PGI_2>6-keto-$PGF_{1\alpha}$>6,15-diketo-$PGF_{1\alpha}$>
TxB_2. Addition of the drugs tested as prostanoid antagonists
reduced the muscle tone, so that the subsequent dose-response
curves usually showed greater amplitudes of maximum contraction.
Drug antagonism was therefore evaluated from EC50 values.

SC-19220 5μg/ml produced significantly greater antagonism of
contractions to PGE_2, $PGF_{2\alpha}$, PGI_2, 6-keto-$PGF_{1\alpha}$, or 6-15-diketo-$PGF_{1\alpha}$
than to ACh. Contractions to PGD_2, PGH_2, the epoxymethano
analogues of PGH_2, or TxB_2 were not affected significantly more than
ACh (Fig. 1). The results with PGE_2 and $PGF_{2\alpha}$ confirm previous
observations (11). Since similar concentrations of SC-19220 block
contraction of rat gastric fundus to arachidonic acid (12), PGH_2
formed from arachidonic acid may not contribute substantially to
the contraction. However, it may be more difficult to block
endogenous than exogenous PGH_2.

Trimethoquinol, a β-adrenoceptor stimulant used clinically
in some countries as a bronchodilator (13), antagonizes PGH_2-
induced platelet aggregation and rabbit aorta contraction without
greatly reducing responses to TxA_2 (14). We found that trimethoquinol
was by far the most potent antagonist tested on the rat stomach;
50ng/ml reduced contractions to all the agonists, and except for
PGE_2 the effect on the prostanoids was much greater than on ACh
(Fig. 2).

β-adrenoceptor stimulation may be involved in this antagonism,
since propranolol 1μg/ml prevented the preferential reduction of
$PGF_{2\alpha}$ by trimethoquinol (9) (Fig. 3). Contractions of rat gastric
fundus to PGE_1 and PGE_2 appear to differ in the way they are affected
by β-adrenoceptor stimulants, although their binding sites (15) seem

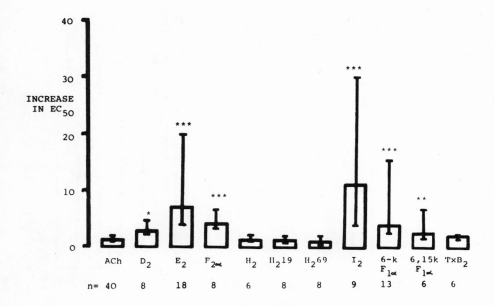

Fig. 1.   SC-19220 5µg/ml preferentially antagonised contractions
          of rat stomach fundus longitudinal muscle to some prostanoids.
          Results are expressed as the increase in concentration
          of agonist required to produce a 50% of maximum response
          (increase in EC50) after addition of SC-19220, and are
          given as medians and semiquartile ranges. The effect of
          SC-19220 on each prostanoid is compared with that on ACh;
          *P<0.1, **P<0.05, ***P<0.01; n=number of experiments.

similar. Whereas trimethoquinol 50ng/ml had little effect on the
contraction to PGE$_2$, it antagonized the contraction to PGE$_1$ by
a propranolol-sensitive mechanism (9) (Fig.3). The β-adrenoceptor
stimulant isoxsuprine also reduce the contraction of rat gastric
fundus to PGE$_1$ with little effect on the response to ACh (16,17).

     Sodium meclofenamate and indomethacin are drugs which may
be given to man, although meclofenamate has not yet been marketed.
Both inhibit fatty acid cyclo-oxygenase (18), but in addition
meclofenamic acid potently antagonises certain prostanoid responses,
at first shown by Collier & Sweatman (19). Sodium meclofenamate
showed a different spectrum of blockade compared with SC-19220 or
trimethoquinol. Meclofenamate 1µg/ml reduced contractions of rat
gastric fundus to all the prostanoids except 6,15-diketo-PGF$_{1\alpha}$ or
TxB$_2$, significantly more than contractions to ACh (Fig. 4). The
effects of meclofenamate 2µg/ml were similar to those with 1µg/ml

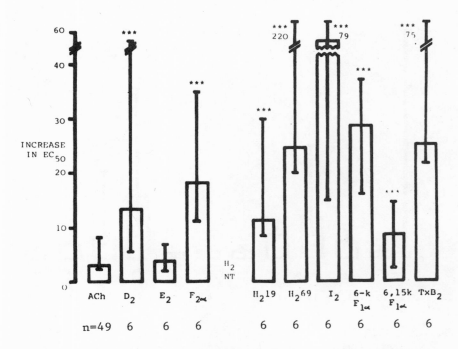

Fig. 2. Trimethoquinol 50mg/ml antagonised contractions of
         longitudinal muscle from rat stomach fundus to various
         prostanoids (PGH₂ was not tested). Results are expressed
         as for Fig. 1.

except that antagonism of PGE₂ and PGI₂ was greater (P<0.007 and
<0.038 respectively), and there was a tendency for a greater block
of PGF₂α and U-46619 (P=0.055 and 0.078 respectively).

Indomethacin 1μg/ml also reduced contractions to PGD₂, the
PGH₂ analogues, or PGI₂ more than contractions to ACh (Fig. 5).
Similar concentrations of indomethacin reduced submaximal
contractions to PGE₁ in gerbil colon (20), although considerably
higher concentrations were needed to cause preferential antagonism
of contractions to PGE or PGFα compounds in guinea-pig ileum
(21-23).

There are various possible explanations of our results with
indomethacin. For example, endogenous prostanoids may potentiate
responses to exogenous agonists (particularly certain prostanoids),
so that the reduction with indomethacin may be due merely to
inhibition of endogenous PG synthesis. Alternatively, indomethacin
may block recpetors for some prostanoids. However, sodium

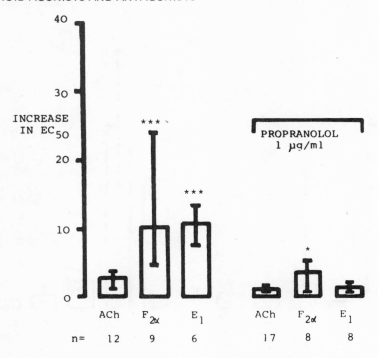

Fig. 3.   Trimethoquinol 50ng/ml preferentially inhibited contrac-
          tions of rat stomach fundus to $PGF_{2\alpha}$ or PGE_1.   The
          inhibition was prevented by propranolol. Results are
          expressed as for Fig. 1.

meclofenamate 1 or 2μg/ml was more effective than indomethacin
1μg/ml in antagonising contractions to the PGH_2 analogues
(p<0.01 with U-44069; Fig. 5), and may therefore block the
receptors on which the analogues act.

        Also in the rat, sodium meclofenamate (and flufenamate and
mefenamate) antagonised the stimulant effect of $PGF_{2\alpha}$ on gastric
secretion, but not the inhibitory effect of PGE_2 (24), and sodium
flufenamate antagonised increases in mesenteric vasoconstriction
obtained with PGE_2 or epoxymethano PGH_2 analogues in the presence
of noradrenaline (25). However, no comparisons were made with
indomethacin.

        We conclude that different spectra of blocking activity with
SC-19220, trimethoquinol and meclofenamate might be explained by
the existence of different types of prostanoid receptor in rat
gastric fundus. None of the drugs antagonized contractions to both
PGE_2 and the PGH_2 analogues, and the results with β-adrenoceptor
stimulants suggest that receptors for PGE_1 and PGE_2 may be different.

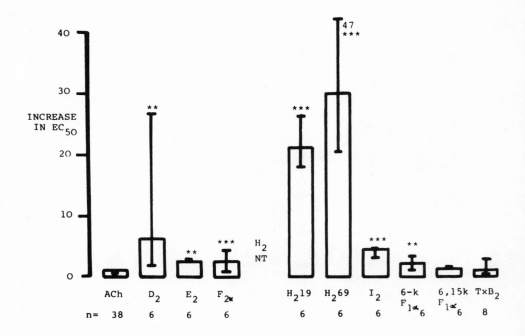

Fig. 4.   Sodium meclofenamate 1µg/ml preferentially antagonised
          contractions of rat stomach fundus to some prostanoids
          (PGH2 was not tested). Results are expressed as for
          Fig. 1.

The drugs which can safely be given to man have other well-defined
actions which may be important in reducing prostanoid responses.
These include inhibition of endogenous prostanoid synthesis with
meclofenamate, and β-adrenoceptor stimulation with trimethoquinol.

Guinea-Pig Intestine

     The longitudinal muscle of guinea-pig isolated ileum contracts
to PGE and PGFα compounds (11,26,27), PGD$_2$ (7,28), 6-keto-PGF$_{1\alpha}$
(29), and the PGH$_2$ epoxymethano analogues (2). We now report
some preliminary studies on prostanoid effects and receptors in
the circular muscle of the guinea-pig ileum and colon.

     No prostanoid tested caused a contraction of ileal circular
muscle except for U-46619 which sometimes caused a very small
contraction. Since this tissue had no intrinsic tone we looked
for an inhibitory effect on consistent submaximal contractions
elicited with KCl. PGE$_2$ 1µg/ml given 1 min prior to KCl always

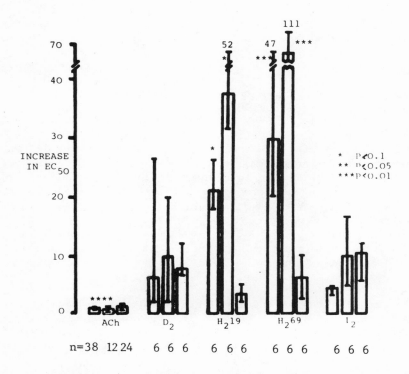

Fig. 5.   Comparison of the effects of sodium meclofenamate and
indomethacin on contractions of rat stomach fundus to
various prostanoids and to ACh. For each agonist, the
columns represent the results for meclofenamate 1 and
2µg/ml and indomethacin 1µg/ml (left to right respectively),
expressed as for Fig. 1. The effect of meclofenamate
on each agonist is compared with that of indomethacin:
*P<0.1, **P<0.05, ***P<0.01.

markedly reduced the contraction, by 92(73 to 100)% (median and
semi-quartile ranges, n=9). PGD_2, U-46619, U-44069 or PGI_2
1µg/ml sometimes had a variable effect, but the median results
showed a slight inhibition of contraction to KCl by respectively
17(5 to 32)%, 11(-28 to 21)%, 19(11-37)% and 7(0 to 45)%
(medians and ranges, n=9, 6, 5 and 5 respectively). $PGF_{2\alpha}$, 6-keto-
$PGF_{1\alpha}$ or TxB_2 had little effect (4(0 to 12)%, 1(-1 to 2)%, or
2(-7 to 3)% reduction, n=7, 4 and 4 respectively). The findings
with PGE_2 and $PGF_{2\alpha}$ confirm previous work (30,31).

In colonic circular muscle PGD_2, $PGF_{2\alpha}$, U-46619, PGI_2 or
6-keto-$PGF_{1\alpha}$ caused contraction whereas PGE_2 caused relaxation.
Approximate threshold concentrations (ng/ml) for the agonists were

respectively 100(10 to 100), 5(4 to 10   10, 55(0.5 to 100) and
100(1 to 100)   (medians and ranges; n=9, 9, 2, 4 and 4 respectively);
TxB_2 1ng/ml-10µg/ml had no effect (n=4). These results for PGE_2
and $PGF_{2\alpha}$ confirm previous observations (32,33).

SC-19220 inhibited contractions of guinea-pig colonic
circular muscle to $PGF_{2\alpha}$ but not the relaxations to PGE_2 (11).
In addition, SC-19220 (80-1000ng/ml) prevented the contraction
to 1µg/ml PGD_2, PGI_2 or 6-keto-$PGF_{1\alpha}$, but it greatly reduced muscle
tone and hampered the detection of relaxation. However, an
inhibitory effect of PGD_2 or PGI_2 1µg/ml was demonstrated by
their reduction of submaximal contractions to ACh (by 32(3-50)% and
8(-4 to 40)% respectively; medians and ranges, n=5 and 4). Thus
in colonic circular muscle PGD_2 or PGI_2 exerted a predominant
excitatory ('$PGF_{2\alpha}$-like') effect which overshadowed an inhibitory
'PGE_2-like response. By contrast, in the presence of SC-19220,
$PGF_{2\alpha}$, 6-keto-$PGF_{1\alpha}$, or TxB_2 1µg/ml did not consistently affect
the ACh-induced contractions (0(18 to 10)%, 0(-10 to 30)% and
0(-14 to 6)% reduction, n=5, 5 and 3). The PGH_2 analogues were
not tested.

Since the circular muscle of guinea-pig ileum was virtually
unresponsive to $PGF_{2\alpha}$, and only an inhibitory response was
detected with PGD_2, PGI_2 and the PGH_2 analogues, we suggest that
there are regional differences in the distribution of prostanoid
receptors in guinea-pig intestine.

In other guinea-pig experiments (7), we examined the effect
of sodium meclofenamate on excitatory responses to PGD_2, PGE_2 or
$PGF_{2\alpha}$ in ileal and colonic longitudinal muscle and colonic
circular muscle. After obtaining rough dose-response curves to
ACh, PGD_2, PGE_2 or $PGF_{2\alpha}$, doses were chosen which gave approximately
equal consistent submaximal contractions. Contact times were
usually 30 seconds with 3-10 minute cycle times. Sodium
meclofenamate was then added to the bath and after a 15-20 minute
contact time, consistent contractions were again obtained.

In the longitudinal muscle of guinea-pig ileum, sodium
meclofenamate 1 or 2.5µg/ml dose-relatedly inhibited contractions
to PGD_2, PGE_2 or $PGF_{2\alpha}$, with little effect on contractions to
ACh (Fig. 6). The antagonists SC-19220 and polyphloretin
phosphate blocked contractions induced by PGE_1, PGE_2 and $PGF_{2\alpha}$ to
about the same extent (10,11,34), and high concentrations of
flufenamic or mefenamic acid (40µg/ml) preferentially reduced
contractions of guinea-pig ileal longitudinal muscle to PGE_2 or
$PGF_{2\alpha}$ (23).

In colonic longitudinal muscle, sodium meclofenamate often
increased the contractions to ACh. This was at least partly due
to the lowering of muscle tone in some preparations,but the
maximal shortening did not seem to be affected. Meclofenamate 2

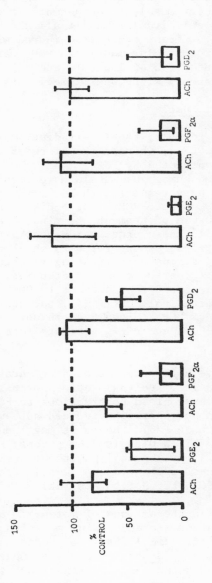
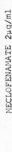

Fig. 6. Antagonism by sodium meclofenamate of PG-induced contractions in guinea-pig ileum longitudinal muscle. Results are expressed as a percentage of control; the columns represent medians, and the bars semiquartile ranges. Compared to ACh, contractions to $PGF_{2\alpha}$, PGE2 or PGD_2 were selectively antagonized by meclofenamate (P<0.01; n=10 for 1μg/ml meclofenamate, n=8 for 2.5μg/ml).

or 10µg/ml reduced contractions to PGE_2 or PGD_2 without blocking
responses to ACh or $PGF_{2\alpha}$, but 1µg/ml meclofenamate had no significant effect (Table 1).

Meclofenamate was studied only against contractions to PGD_2
and $PGF_{2\alpha}$ in the circular muscle of guinea-pig colon; PGE_2 relaxes
this tissue, and in ileal circular muscle all the prostanoids either
inhibit or have no significant effect. Compared with ACh, the
contractions of colonic circular muscle to PGD_2 were not selectively
reduced by meclofenamate 1, 2 or 10µg/ml, and those to $PGF_{2\alpha}$ were
preferentially reduced only with 10µg/ml meclofenamate (Table 1).

Human Gastrointestinal Muscle

As in laboratory animals, the longitudinal muscle is usually
contracted by PGE_2 or $PGF_{2\alpha}$, whereas the circular muscle is usually
relaxed by PGE_2 and contracted by $PGF_{2\alpha}$ (11,30,32,33). The actions
of other prostanoids on human gut muscle have received little study,
except for our preliminary results with PGD_2, an epoxymethano
analogue of PGH_2, PGI_2, 6-keto-$PGF_{1\alpha}$, 6,15-diketo-$PGF_{1\alpha}$ and TxB_2
on the longitudinal muscle of stomach, terminal ileum and colon,
(5,35). In general, all these prostanoids contract the
longitudinal muscle strips, except for PGI_2 which causes relaxation
of gastric and colonic strips by activating receptors which must
therefore differ from those for other prostanoids. In addition, PGI_2
1µg/ml preferentially reduced contractions to PGE_2 or $PGF_{2\alpha}$ in
strips of gastric longitudinal muscle (5), but contractions to an
epoxymethano analogue of PGH_2 (U-46619) were not reduced. These
results may mean that PGE_2 and $PGF_{2\alpha}$ activate receptors different
from those for U-46619.

There are relatively few studies on drug antagonism of PG
responses in the human gut. Polyphloretin phosphate but not
SC-19220 selectively antagonised contractions to PGE_2 or $PGF_{2\alpha}$ (11).
However, polyphloretin phosphate in vivo did not antagonise PGE_2-
or $PGF_{2\alpha}$-induced diarrhoea (36)although it may reduce diarrhoea in
mice caused by PGE_2 (37). N-0164 (sodium p-benzyl-4-(1-oxo-2-(4-
chlorobenzyl)-3-phenylpropyl) phenyl phosphonate) 1-20µg/ml
antagonised contractions of longitudinal muscle from human stomach,
jejunum and ileum to PGE_2 but not to ACh (38).

We have now studied the actions of mefenamic acid, sodium
mefenamate, sodium flufenamate and sodium meclofenamate on
contractions of the longitudinal muscle of human isolated
gastrointestinal tract to PGE_2 or $PGF_{2\alpha}$. The experiments were
similar to those on the guinea-pig intestine, but the PG contract
times and cycle times were longer. Only one fenamate was tested
on each preparation, and where possible the degree of block was
assessed by determining the increase in the dose of agonist
needed to restore the contraction height (dose-ratio).

TABLE 1

Effect of sodium meclofenamate on PG-induced contractions of guinea-pig colonic muscle

Results are expressed as the percentage of control, in median and semiquartile ranges.

*P<0.05, compared with ACh, n = 6 for each.

Concentration of meclofenamate μg/ml	ACh	PGD_2	ACh	PGE_2	ACh	$PGF_{2\alpha}$
LONGITUDINAL MUSCLE						
1	124(128-94)	117(124-109)	124(138-115)	87(110-76)	107(132-103)	98(141-71)
2	112(123-92)	108(110-106)	120(131-115)	73(113-68)*	110(132-101)	74(129-58)
10	110(123-83)	14(33-8)*	121(142-112)	42(62-18)*	115(172-113)	41(106-24)
CIRCULAR MUSCLE						
1	83(121-75)	69(111-61)	NOT TESTED	NOT TESTED	110(123-92)	97(129-82)
2	98(112-88)	119(123-55)	"	"	112(117-105)	97(118-68)
10	97(109-91)	58(95-33)	"	"	103(129-70)	46(103-25)*

Unlike in the guinea-pig, we did not detect regional differences in PG-blocking activity; the results for stomach, ileum and colon are therefore combined. All the drugs reduced muscle tone and this probably explains why some responses were increased. Sodium meclofenamate 1µg/ml reduced contractions to $PGF_{2\alpha}$ (dose-ratio approx. 10, n=3) and higher concentrations (2,5 or 20µg/ml) prevented the response to the original concentration of $PGF_{2\alpha}$. Contractions to ACh or PGE_2 were often increased with 1 or 5µg/ml meclofenamate, presumably because of the fall in muscle tone. Sodium flufenamate 2µg/ml also reduced contractions to $PGF_{2\alpha}$ (dose-ratio 10, n=4), with little effect on those to ACh. Contractions to PGE_2 were not selectively blocked with 5, 10 or 50µg/ml flufenamate (3,2 and 2 experiments respectively).

In contrast, sodium mefenamate 20 or 50µg/ml or mefenamic acid 50 or 100µg/ml often increased contractions to ACh or $PGF_{2\alpha}$, but tended to reduce the contractions to PGE_2 (P=0.05 for the combined results with 50 and 100µg/ml sodium mefenamate and mefenamic acid). Thus, there are differential effects of fenamates on response to PGs, and these may indicate different types of receptor.

CONCLUSIONS

Our results indicate that in various gastrointestinal tissues of man and laboratory animals there are several types of receptor for prostanoids. Differences may occur not only between species, but also between the different regions of the gastrointestinal tract and between longitudinal and circular muscles. Variations in the types and amounts of prostanoid receptors may explain why many tissues respond differently to drugs which act on these receptors.

ACKNOWLEDGEMENT

We thank the MRC for support.

REFERENCES

1. A. Bennett. Prostaglandin antagonists. Adv. Drug Res., 8: 83-118 (1974).
2. A. Bennett, C. Jaroski and D. E. Wilson. A study of receptors activated by analogues of prostaglandin H_2. Br. J. Pharmac., 63: 358P (1978).
3. A. Bennett and G. J. Sanger. The effects of prostaglandin D_2 on the circular muscle of guinea-pig isolated ileum and colon. Br. J. Pharmac., 63: 357P-358P (1978).

4. A. Bennett and G. J. Sanger. Trimethoquinol selectively
    antagonises longitudinal muscle contractions of rat isolated
    gastric fundus to thromboxane B_2 and epoxymethano analogues
    of PHG_2. Br. J. Pharmac., 66:450P (1979).
5. A. Bennett and G. J. Sanger. Prostacyclin relaxes the long-
    itudinal muscle of human isolated stomach and antagonizes
    contractions to some prostanoids. J. Physiol., (in press)
    (1979).
6. A. Bennett and G. J. Sanger, Unpublished.
7. A. Bennett, D. Pratt and G. J. Sanger. Antagonism by fenamates
    of prostaglandin action in guinea-pig and human alimentary
    muscle. Br. J. Pharmac., (in press) (1979).
8. A. Bennett, C. Jarosik, G. J. Sanger and D. E. Wilson,
    Unpublished.
9. S. M. Lacey and G. J. Sanger, Unpublished.
10. J. H. Sanner. Antagonism of prostaglandin E_2 by 1-acetyl-2-
    (8-chloro-10,11-dihydrobenz (b,f) (1,4) oxazepine-10-
    carbonyl) hydrazine (SC-19220). Arch. Int. Pharmacodyn. Ther.,
    180: 45-56 (1968).
11. A. Bennett and J. Posner. Studies on prostaglandin antagonists.
    Br. J. Pharmac., 42: 584-594 (1971).
12. J. A. Splawinski, A. S. Nies, B. Sweetman and J. A. Oates.
    The effects of arachidonic acid, PGE_2 and $PGF_{2\alpha}$ on the
    longitudinal stomach strip of the rat. J. Pharmacol. Exp.
    Ther., 187: 501-510 (1973).
13. Y. Yamamura and S. Kishmoto. Clinical effectiveness of a
    new bronchodilator, Inolin, on bronchial asthma. Annals of
    Allergy, 26: 504-507 (1968).
14. D. E. MacIntyre and A. L. Willis. Trimethoquinol is a potent
    prostaglandin endoperoxide antagonist. Br. J. Pharmac., 63:
    361P (1978).
15. O. V. Miller and W. E. Magee. Specifity of prostaglandin
    binding sites in rat forestomach tissue and their possible use
    as a quantitative assay. In: Advances in Biosciences, 9. S.
    Bergstrom and J. Bernhard, eds., pp.83-89. Pergamon Press (1973).
16. F. Coceani and L. S. Wolfe. On the action of prostaglandin
    E_1 and prostaglanidns from brain on the isolated rat stomach.
    Can. J. Physiol. Pharmac., 44: 933-950 (1966).
17. L. S. Wolfe, F. Coceani and C. Pace-Asciak. Brain prosta-
    glandins and studies on the action of prostaglandins on the
    isolated rat stomach. In: Nobel Symp. II, Prostaglandins,
    Stockholm. S. Bergstom and B. Samuelsson, eds., pp.265-276
    (1967).
18. R. J. Flower. Drugs which inhibit prostaglandin biosynthesis.
    Pharmacol. Rev., 26: 33-67 (1974).
19. H. O. J. Collier and W. J. F. Sweetman. Antagonism by fenamates
    of prostaglandin $F_{2\alpha}$ and of slow reacting substance on human
    bronchial muscle. Nature, 219: 864-865 (1978).
20. E. L. Tolman and R. Partridge. Multiple sites of interaction
    between prostaglandins and non-steroidal anti-inflammatory
    agents. Prostaglandins, 9: 349-359 (1975).

21. L. Sorrentino, F. Capasso and M. Di Rosa. Indomethacin and
     prostaglandins. Eur. J. Pharmac., 17: 306-308 (1972).
22. F. Lembeck and H. Juan. Interaction of prostaglandins and
     indomethacin with algesic substances. Naunyn-Schmiedeberg's
     Arch. Pharmacol., 285: 301-313 (1974).
23   J. P. Famaey, J. Fontaine and J. Reuse. Effect of high
     concentrations of non-steroidal anti-inflammatory drugs on
     prostaglandin-induced contraction of the guinea-pig isolated
     ileum. Prostaglandins, 13: 107-114 (1977).
24. H. Karpaanen and J. Puurunen. Antagonism of $PGF_{2\alpha}$-induced
     secretion of gastric acid by mefenamic acid and other fenamates.
     Naunyn-Schmiedeberg's Arch. Pharmacol., 294: (Suppl) R7 (1976).
25. A. Bennett, M. A. Carroll and G. J. Sanger. Sodium
     flufenamate antagonises the potentiation by prostaglandins
     of noradrenaline-induced vasoconstriction in rat mesentary.
     Br. J. Pharmac., 66: 449P (1979).
26. E. W. Horton and I. H. M. Main. A comparison of the biological
     activities of four prostaglandins. Br. J. Pharmac. Chemother.,
     21: 182-189 (1963).
27. E. W. Horton and I. H. M. Main. A comparison of the actions
     of $PGF_{2\alpha}$ and PGE_1 on smooth muscle. Br. J. Pharmac.
     Chemother., 24: 470-476 (1965).
28. M. Hamberg, P. Hedqvist, K. Strandberg, J. Svensson
     and B. Samuelsson. Prostaglandin endoperoxides IV. Effects
     on smooth muscle. Life Sci., 16: 451-462 (1975).
29. D. M. Engineer, U. Niederhauser, P. J. Piper and P.
     Sirois. Release of mediators of anaphylaxis: Inhibition of
     prostaglandin synthesis and the modification of release of
     slow reacting substance of anaphylaxis and histamine. Br. J.
     Pharmac., 62: 61-66 (1978).
30. A. Bennett, K. G. Eley and G. B. Scholes. Effect of prosta-
     glandins E_1 and E_2 on human, guinea-pig and rat isolated small
     intestine. Br. J. Pharmac., 34: 639-647 (1968).
31. A. Bennett, K. G. Eley and H. L. Stockley. The effects of
     prostaglandins on guinea-pig isolated intestine and their
     possible contribution to muscle activity and tone. Br. J.
     Pharmac., 54: 197-204 (1975).
32. B. Fleshler and A. Bennett. Responses of human, guinea-pig
     and rat colonic circular muscle to prostaglandins. J. Lab.
     Clin. Med., 74:872 (1969).
33. A. Bennett and A. Fleshler. Prostaglandins and the gastro-
     intestinal tract. Gastroenterology, 59: 790-800 (1970).
34. V. Petkov, R. Radomirov, O. Petkov and S. Todorov. The
     character of the antagonism by polyphloretin phosphate of
     contractions to prostaglandins E_1 and $F_{2\alpha}$ in guinea-pig ileum.
     J. Pharm. Pharmac., 30: 491-498 (1978).
35. A. Bennett, C. N. Hensby, G. J. Sanger and I. F. Stamford.
     Identification of arachidonic acid metabolites in the human
     gastrointestinal tract, and the ways in which some of these
     affect the longitudinal muscle. In: The Prostaglandin System:

Endoperoxides, Prostacyclin and Thromboxanes. F. Berti and G. P. Velo, eds., pp.356-366. Plenum Press, New York and London (1980).

36. S. M. M. Karim. The effect of polyphloretin phosphate and other compounds on prostaglandin-induced diarrhoea in man. Annals Acad. Med., 3: 201-206 (1974).

37. K. E. Eakins. Prostaglandin antagonism by polymeric phosphates of phloretin and related compounds. Ann. N.Y. Acad. Sci., 180: 386-395 (1971).

38. A. Bennett, D. Pratt and A. Schechter, Unpublished.

CYTOPROTECTION AND ENTEROPOOLING BY PROSTAGLANDINS

André Robert

Department of Experimental Biology
The Upjohn Company
Kalamazoo, Michigan 49001, U.S.A.

Prostaglandins (PG) influence a variety of gastrointestinal functions. One of the most prominent effects is the inhibition of gastric secretion by several PG of the E and A type (1,2,3). Presumably because of this anti-secretory effect, these PG were also shown to inhibit ulcer formation (4,5,6) and to accelerate the rate of ulcer healing (7,8). More recently, another property of several PG, called "cytoprotection", was reported. It is the ability to protect the mucosa of the stomach and the intestine against inflammation and necrosis when this mucosa is exposed to noxious agents. Such noxious agents include nonsteroidal anti-inflammatory compounds (NOSAC), (9,10,11) such as aspirin and indomethacin, necrotizing agents such as absolute ethanol, 0.6 N HCl, 0.2 NaOH, 80 mM taurocholate, and even boiling water (12,13,14,15,16,17). The severe gastric hemorrhagic lesions produced by any of these agents are completely prevented by a variety of PG. In this report, we will present evidence showing that cytoprotection is a property separate from the antisecretory effect of PG.

One of the side effects of PG, when administered at high doses, is the development of diarrhea. The diarrhea is of the secretory type, and originates in the small intestine. Soon after administration of a high dose of a PG, either orally or subcutaneously, fluid accumulates in the small intestine (18,19,20), a phenomenon called "enteropooling" (21). The enteropooling fluid is then carried to the large intestine. Because of its abundance, this fluid is not sufficiently reabsorbed and is expelled as diarrhea. Although most PG with biological activity can exert enteropooling, two of these do not show this property. They are PGI_2 (prostacyclin) and PGD_2. Not only are these PG not enteropooling,

393

but they exert an antienteropooling effect, that is, they block
enteropooling produced by other PG and even by cholera toxin
(22,23). We will present data on the process of enteropooling
caused by PG and cholera toxin.

Cytoprotection by Prostaglandins

Administration of aspirin and indomethacin, either orally or
subcutaneously, can damage the gastric mucosa in animals as well
as in humans. For such lesions to develop, however, a certain
amount of acid must be present in the stomach (24). Therefore, by
preventing acid secretion or by neutralizing acid already formed
in the lumen, one can inhibit aspirin-induced lesions. This is
why antacids, anticholinergics and histamine H_2 blockers have
been used to prevent such lesions. However, we have shown that
PG inhibit aspirin lesions by a mechanism other than reducing
gastric acid secretion (11). The following studies demonstrate this
point.

Female rats were fasted for 24 hrs. On the following day,
they were given 100 mg/kg of aspirin, orally, in 1 ml of hydrochloric acid at various concentrations from 0.005 N to 0.35 N.
The animals were killed 1 hr after the administration of aspirin.
Gastric lesions were found in the corpus, the portion of the
stomach secreting acid and pepsin. They consisted of mulitple
hemorrhagic ulcerations with necrotic foci. The number of lesions
increased with the concentration of acid. Thus, when aspirin was
suspended in water, only 1.5 lesions per stomach were found. When,
on the other hand, aspirin was suspended in 0.35 N HCl, as many
as 16.2 lesions per stomach, on the average, were counted.

In other groups of animals, various substances were administered
prior to the oral treatment with aspirin, in an attempt to prevent
aspirin-induced lesions. These substances were: 16,16-dimethyl
PGE_2, at doses of 0.05 to 1.5 µg/kg, subcutaneously, cimetidine,
150 mg/kg intraperitoneally, and probanthine, at a dose of 5 mg/kg,
subcutaneously. Table 1 shows the results. Cimetidine and
probanthine completely inhibited aspirin-induced lesions when
aspirin was suspended in water or in 0.005 N and 0.05 N HCl. When
the normality of HCl was 0.15, the inhibition produced by cimetidine
was only of the order of 57%, and that by probanthine of 68%.
When aspirin was suspended in 0.35 N HCl, neither cimetidine nor
probanthine inhibited gastric lesions produced by aspirin (p<0.05).
In contrast, 16,16-dimethyl PGE_2 given subcutaneously at a dose
of 1.5 µg/kg (a dose that is about 100th of the threshold anti-
secretory dose), prevented nearly completely aspirin-induced
gastric lesions, even when aspirin was suspended in 0.35 N.

This result shows that agents such as cimetidine and probanthine
can inhibit aspirin-induced gastric lesions only in the presence of

TABLE 1

Effect of a prostaglandin, imetidine and probanthine
on gastric lesions produced by acidified aspirin

| | Vehicle | 16,16-Dimethyl PGE$_2$: µg/kg | | | Cimetidine 150 mg/kg | Probanthine 5 mg/kg |
		0.05	0.5	1.5		
Aspirin in:						
Water	1.5	2.5	0	0	0	0
0.005 N HCl	8.2	3.7*	0*	0*	0*	0*
0.05 N HCl	8.5	7.8	0*	0*	0*	0*
0.15 N HCl	11.0	10.8	0*	0*	4.7*	3.5*
0.35 N HCl	16.2	14.2	7.2*	1.2*	14.2	9.9

16,16-Dimethyl PGE$_2$ orally, cimetidine intraperitoneally, probanthine
subcutaneously, 30 minutes before aspirin. Aspirin given orally in
1 ml. Animals killed 1 hour after aspirin (200 mg/kg).

Numerals represent average number of lesions per stomach in each group.

Six rats per group. *: P<0.01.

moderate gastric acidity, wheras the protection disappears by raising
the concentration of acid. On the contrary, 16,16-dimethyl PGE$_2$,
as a representative of cytoprotective PG, protects the stomach
regardless of the acid content of gastric juice. It is clear,
therefore, that cytoprotection by PG is a property independent of
any effect on acid secretion, and is not exhibited by cimetidine
and probanthine..

Enteropooling by Prostaglandins and Cholera Toxin

Several PG when given either orally or subcutaneously stimulate
fluid accumulation in the small intestine of several species
(18,19,20,21). This is illustrated in Figure 1. Cholera toxin
exerts a similar effect, although enteropooling is delayed by 30
to 60 minutes and reaches values much higher than those obtained
with PG.

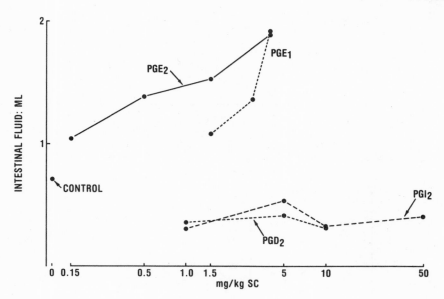

Fig. 1.   Enteropooling effect of prostaglandins.
          Intestinal fluid collected 30 minutes after treatment.
          PGE_1 and PGE_2 are enteropooling, PGI_2 and PGD_2 are not.
          Eight rate per point.

        Prostacyclin (PGI_2) and PGD_2, however, exert the opposite
effect.   They are not enteropooling and in fact inhibit the enteropooling effect of other PG, such as $PGF_{2\alpha}$ and 16,16-dimethyl
PGE_2, as well as enteropooling caused by cholera toxin (Figure 2).
Indomethacin has also been reported to inhibit cholera toxin-
induced enteropooling (25,26), and we have confirmed those results.

        More recently, in the course of studies with cholera toxin,
we found that the mere finger handling of the small intestine,
through laparotomy, exerted a marked pro-enteropooling effect.
The results of such a study are illustrated in Figure 3.   This
pro-enteropooling effect of gut handling was directly related to
the length of intestinal segment being handled.   At least 40 cm
of the small intestine, measured from the ileo-cecal junction,
had to be handled manually for this pro-enteropooling effect to
take place.   Maximum enteropooling is obtained when the whole length
of the small intestine (approximately 100 cm) was handled.
Similarly, handling of the small intestine enhanced the enteropooling
effect of PGE_2.

        The mechanism by which physical handling of the small intestine
favors enteropooling by either PG or cholera toxin is unknown.
Since indomethacin blocks this enhancement caused by handling, it

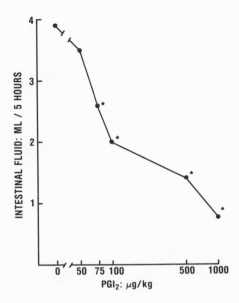

Fig. 2. PGI$_2$ inhibits enteropooling produced by cholera toxin.
PGI$_2$:subcutaneously every hour. All animals received
cholera toxin, 20 µg, intra-jejunally, and were killed
5 hours later. The anti-enteropooling effect of PGI$_2$
was dose dependent. Six rats per point. *: P<0.01.

may be that handling stimulates the local release of PG. More
studies are needed to explain the pro-enteropooling effect of
intestinal handling.

Clinical Applications

Gastric cytoprotection by PG suggests that these compounds
might be useful for the prevention and treatment of hemorrhagic
gastritis due to administration of nonsteroidal antiinflammatory
compounds. Two studies have already shown that occult bleeding,
produced in humans by either aspirin (26) or indomethacin (27),
is prevented by oral treatment with PGE$_2$. It is likely that the
gastritis itself caused by these anti inflammatory compounds
is also prevented by the PG treatment.

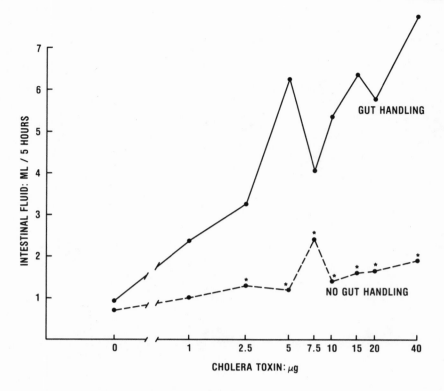

Fig. 3. Gut handling stimulates enteropooling produced by
cholera toxin. The small intestine was handled with
fingers immediately prior to intra-jejunal administration
of cholera toxin, 20 µg. Six rats per point. *: P<0.01.

REFERENCES

1. A. Robert, J. E. Nezamis and J. P. Phillips. Inhibition of
   gastric secretion by prostaglandins. Am. J. Dig. Dis.,12:
   1073-1076 (1967).
2. A. Robert, B. Nylander and S. Andersson. Marked inhibition of
   gastric secretion by two prostaglandin analogs given orally to
   man. Life Sci., 14: 533-538 (1974).
3. S.M.M. Karim, D. C. Carter, D. Bhana and P. A. Ganesan.
   Effect of orally and intravenously administered prostaglandin
   15(R)-15 methyl E_2 on gastric secretion in man. Adv. Biosci.,
   9: 255-264 (1973).
4. A. Robert, J. E. Nezamis and J. P. Phillips. Effect of
   prostaglandin E_1 on gastric secretion and ulcer formation in the
   rat. Gastroenterology, 55: 481-487 (1968).
5. A. Robert, D. F. Stowe and J. E. Nezamis. Prevention of duodenal
   ulcers by administration of prostaglandin E_2 (PGE_2). Scand. J.
   Gastroenterol, 6: 303-305 (1971).

6. A. Robert, J. R. Schultz, J. E. Nezamis and C. Lancaster.
    Gastric antisecretory and antiulcer properties of PGE_2 15-
    methyl PGE_2, and 16,16-dimethyl PGE_2. Intravenous, oral and
    intrajejunal administration. Gastroenterology, 70: 359 (1976).
7. W. P. Fung, S. M. M. Karim and C. Y. Tye. Effect of 15(R)-
    15-methyl prostaglandin E_2 methyl ester on healing of gastric
    ulcers. Controlled endoscopic study. Lancet,II: 10-12 (1974).
8. J. Rybicka and K. Gibinski. Methyl-prostaglandin E_2 analogues
    for healing of gastroduodenal ulcers. Scand. J. Gastroent.,
    13: 155-159 (1978).
9. A. Robert. Antisecretory, antiulcer, cytoprotective and
    diarrheogenic properties of prostaglandins. In: Advances in
    Prostaglandin and Thromboxane Research, Raven Press, New York,
    507 (1975).
10. B. J. R. Whittle. Mechanisms underlying gastric mucosal damage
    induced by indomethacin and bile-salts, and the actions of
    prostaglandins. Brit. J. Pharmacol., 60: 455-460 (1977).
11. A. Robert, A. J. Hanchar, J. E. Nezamis and C. Lancaster.
    Cytoprotection against acidified aspirin: comparison of prosta-
    glandin, cimetidine and probanthine. Gastroenterology, 76:
    1277 (1979).
12. A. Robert, J. E. Nezamis, C. Lancaster and A. J. Hanchar.
    Gastric cytoprotective property of prostaglandins. Gastro-
    enterology, 72:1121 (1977).
13. A. Robert, A. J. Hanchar and C. Lancaster. Antisecretory and
    cytoprotective effects of prostacyclin (PGI_2). Fed. Proc., 37:
    460 (1978).
14. A. Robert, J. E. Nezamis, C. Lancaster and A. J. Hanchar.
    Cytoprotection by prostaglandins in rats: prevention of gastric
    necrosis produced by alcohol, HCl, NaOH, hypertonic NaCl, and
    thermal injury. Gastroenterology, 77: 433-443 (1979).
15. A. Robert. Cytoprotection by prostaglandins. Gastroenterology,
    77: 761-767 (1979).
16. T. K. Chaudhury and A. Robert. Prevention by mild irritants of
    gastric necrosis produced in rats by Na-taurocholate. Fed. Proc.,
    37:303 (1978).
17. T. K. Chaudhury and A. Robert. Prevention by mild irritants
    of gastric necrosis produced in rats by sodium taurocholate.
    Dig. Dis. Sc., in press (1980).
18. N. F. Pierce, C. C. J. Carpenter, H. J. Elliott and W. B.
    Greenough. Effects of prostaglandins, theophylline, and
    cholera exotoxin upon transmucosal water and electrolyte movement
    in the canine jejunum. Gastroenterology, 60:22 (1971).
19. J. H. Cummings, A. Newman, J. J. Misiewicz, G. J. Milton-
    Thompson and J. A. Billings. Effect of intravenous prostaglandin
    $F_{2\alpha}$ on small intestinal function in man. Nature (Lond.),
    243:169 (1973).
20. C. Matuchansky and J. J. Bernier. Effect of prostaglandin E_1
    on glucose, water, and electrolyte absorption in the human
    jejunum. Gastroenterology, 64:1111 (1973).

21. A. Robert, J. E. Nezamis, C. Lancaster, A. J. Hanchar and
     M. S. Klepper. Enteropooling assay: a test for diarrhea
     produced by prostaglandins. Prostaglandins, 11:809:828 (1976).

22. A. Robert, A. J. Hanchar, C. Lancaster and J. E. Nezamis.
     Prostacyclin (PGI_2) and PGD_2 prevent enteropooling and diarrhea
     caused by prostaglandins and cholera toxin. Fed. Prod., 38:
     1239 (1979).

23. A. Robert, A. J. Hanchar, C. Lancaster and J. E. Nezamis.
     Prostacyclin inhibits enteropooling and diarrhea. In: J. R.
     Vane and S. Bergström, eds., Prostacyclin, Raven Press, 147-158
     (1979).

24. D. A. Brodie, B. J. Chase. Role of gastric acid in aspirin-
     induced gastric irritiation in the rat. Gastroenterology,
     53: 604-610 (1967).

25. H. I. Jacoby and C. H. Marshall. Antagonism of cholera
     enterotoxin by anti-inflammatory agents in the rat. Nature,
     235: 163-165 (1972).

26. R. E. Gots, S. B. Formal and R. A. Giannella. Indomethacin
     inhibition of Salmonella typhimurium, Shigella flexneri, and
     cholera-mediated rabbit ileal secretion. J. Infect. Dis.,
     130: 280-284 (1974).

27. M. M. Cohen. Mucosal cytoprotection by prostaglandin E_2.
     Lancet, Dec. 8: 1253-1254 (1978).

28. C. Johansson,B. Kollberg, R. Nordeman and S. Bergstrom.
     Mucosal protection by prostaglandin E_2. Lancet,I: 317 (1979).

INTERACTIONS BETWEEN ASPIRIN AND OTHER COMPOUNDS IN ANALGESIC
MEDICINES ON GASTRIC MUCOSAL DAMAGE IN RATS

Lowie P. Jager, Ad J. M. Seegers and J. van Noordwijk
Department of Pharmacology, State University Utrecht
The Netherlands
and
Laboratory of Pharmacology
National Institute of Public Health
3720 BA Bilthoven, The Netherlands

INTRODUCTION

The erosive activity of aspirin on the gastric mucosa is
amply documented (12-15) and with regard to the mechanisms underlying this gastrotoxicity the following picture appears to emerge
from the literature. By inhibiting the endogenous production of
prostaglandins in the gastric wall aspirin weakens the defensive
capacity of the mucosa indirectly (28). Several types of prostaglandins are reported to stimulate production of mucus (2) or to
inhibit acid secretion (20) and all prostanoids tested seem to
exert a cytoprotective action in the gastrointestinal tract (10,18,
21). Furthermore, back diffusion of hydrogen ions from the stomach
lumen into the gastric wall through the broken mucosal barrier
seems to be essential for the development of gastric damage (6,5).

In contrast with the vast knowledge about activities of aspirin
by itself very little is known about the activities of drug mixtures
containing aspirin. The purpose of the present paper is to discuss
some recent observations on interactions between aspirin and other
compounds in non-narcotic analgesic drug mixtures used by man,
emphasizing gastric mucosal damage, as observed in rats.

Interactions on Aspirin-Induced Gastric Erosions

The rat stomach differs in several aspects from that of man.
Only the glandular part of the rat stomach is more or less
comparable to the human stomach (11) and it is in this part that
aspirin induces mucosal damage. As an animal model to study the

gastric erosive activity of orally administered drugs the rat is used by preference, not only because it cannot regurgitate but also because of its relatively high level of basal acid secretion; a condition which seems to be prevalent in humans prone to irritation of the stomach (3).

The severity of gastric erosions observed 17 h after a single oral administration of aspirin was found to be closely correlated with the logarithm of the dosage administered (Fig. 1). This relationship between erosion score and aspirin dosage was not affected when phenacetin was added in equal amounts. Addition of caffeine to the aspirin (dose-ratio 1:5) increased the erosion scores. Paracetamol in admixture with equal amounts of aspirin seemed not to induce gastric damage at all (23). Furthermore, male and female rats were found to be equally susceptible to the erosive activity of aspirin given alone or in admixture with the drugs mentioned (Fig. 1). Further investigation of the interactions between aspirin and caffeine or paracetamol revealed that both drugs increased or decreased the erosions induced by aspirin, respectively, in a log-dose dependent way (Fig. 2).

Interactions on Development of Aspirin Induced Gastric Damage

Elucidation of the interactions between aspirin and caffeine and aspirin and paracetamol was sought by studying the development of gastric damage with time. Treatments were applied which were known to have pronounced effects seventeen hours later. Already half an hour after its administration the mixture of caffeine with aspirin caused significantly higher erosion scores compared to those of either drug alone (Fig. 3).. Throughout the observation-period caffeine seemed to potentiate the erosive activity of aspirin by increasing both the number and the severity of the erosions. Surprisingly, the gastric damage induced by the mixture of paracetamol and aspirin during the first two hours hardly differed from that induced by aspirin administered alone. A second experiment with a higher time-resolution confirmed this observation. Analysis of the erosion score date indicated that during the first four hours the number of erosion foculi induced by the mixture of paracetamol and aspirin was not significantly different from that induced by aspirin alone (Fig. 4). Thus, paracetamol did not inhibit the induction of erosion foculi by aspirin, but apparently prevented the growth of foculi into erosions. Moreover, after two hours the foculi started to disappear and eight hours after administration of the mixture the stomachs seemed not to be damaged at all.

Interactions on Gastric Acid Output

As already outlined in the introduction the presence of hydrogen ions in the gastric lumen is supposed to be an essential prerequisite for the development of gastric damage (5). Caffeine

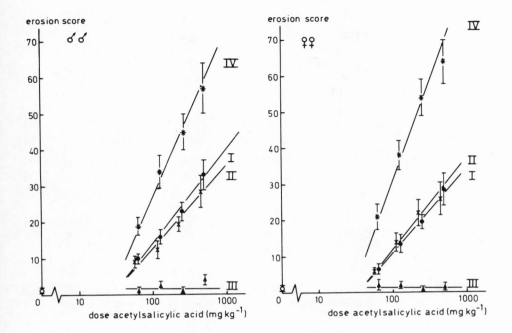

Fig. 1.   Relationships between the amount of aspirin administered
orally to starved male and female rats and the erosion
score (m ± SEM) observed 17 h later.
•, I : aspirin; x, II : aspirin and phenacetin (dose ratio,
1:1); ▲, III: aspirin and paracetamol (dose ratio, 1:1);*,
IV : aspirin and caffeine (dose ratio, 5:1);o : vehicle,
5 ml.kg^{-1} 4% Tween-80 solution; n = 10.

is reported to stimulate acid secretion in patients with a
clinical history of gastrointestinal ulceration (3).   In man and
dog paracetamol did not affect the acid output (1,8).   In our
experiments with rats the acid secretion was stimulated submaximally
with histamine and the acid output of the perfused stomach was
measured.   The acid output thus measured is the resultant of the
secretion of hydrochloric acid by parietal cells and its absorption
and/or neutralization.   It was found that perfusion with saline
containing aspirin induced a rapid decrease in acid output, which
is likely due to an increase in the back-diffusion of hydrogen ions
(24).   Addition of paracetamol or caffeine to the perfusion fluid

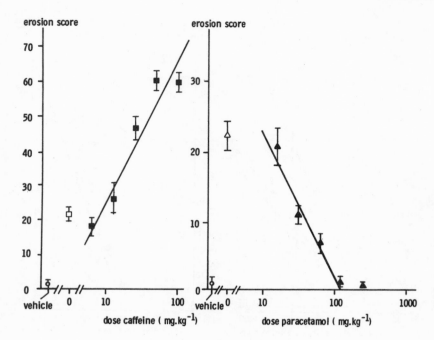

Fig. 2.   Interactions between aspirin and caffeine (left hand
          graph) or paracetamol (right hand graph) on gastric
          erosions observed 17 h after oral administration. □ ,
          Δ: aspirin 250 mg.kg⁻¹; ■ : aspirin (250 mg.kg⁻¹) and
          caffeine; ▲: aspirin (250 mg.kg⁻¹) and paracetamol; o:
          vehicle, 5 ml.kg⁻¹ 4% Tween-80 solution; n = 10.

containing aspirin did not affect this rapid reduction in acid
output. Paracetamol by itself did not alter the acid output. On
the other hand, perfusion with caffeine increased the acid output
in a log-dose dependent manner (Fig. 5). As caffeine does not
increase acid output until 80 min after the beginning of perfusion
and has no effect on the gastric mucosal barrier (4) it seems
likely that this delayed enhancement of acid output is a result of
an increase in acid secretion. Furthermore, it seems fair to
assume that this stimulatory effect is delayed mainly because
caffeine had to be absorbed by the stomach, and that an earlier
onset of stimulation of the acid secretion is to be expected when
intestinal absorption is involved. In corollary experiments
intravenous infusion of caffeine (4×10^{-6} mol.min⁻¹.kg⁻¹) increased
the acid output within 10 min.

        Thus, it seems reasonable to ascribe the potentiating effect
of caffeine in aspirin-induced erosions to the stimulation of acid

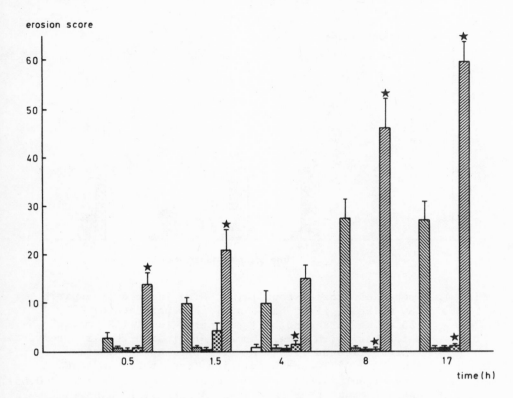

Fig. 3. Erosion development with time after oral administration of aspirin 250 mg.kg^{-1} (first bar); paracetamol 125 mg.kg^{-1} (second bar); caffeine 50 mg.kg^{-1} (third bar); aspirin + paracetamol 250 + 125 mg.kg^{-1} (fourth bar); aspirin + caffeine 250 + 50 mg.kg^{-1} (fifth bar). Erosion score of vehicle treated rats measured 4 h after oral administration of 5 ml.kg^{-1} 4% Tween 80 solution (open bar). m ± SEM, n = 10.*: Significant difference between erosion scores of aspirin alone and in admixture (P < 0.05).

secretion. Elevated levels of hydrogen ions facilitate both the induction of erosion foculi by aspirin and the development of foculi into erosions.

Localization of the Interaction between Aspirin and Paracetamol

In contrast with the caffeine-aspirin interaction, the observed interaction between paracetamol and aspirin cannot be explained easily within the current concepts of the pathogenesis of aspirin-induced erosions. Paracetamol does not affect the acid

number of erosions ⩽ 2 mm

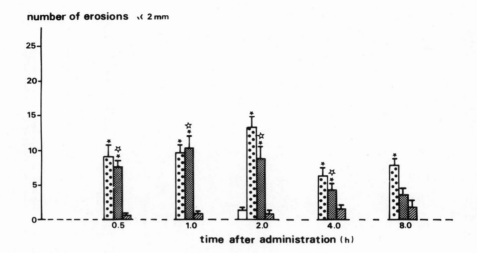

Fig. 4.   Number of erosion-foculi (m ± SEM) induced by aspirin
         (250 mg.kg⁻¹, first bar), aspirin + paracetamol (250 +
         125 mg.kg⁻¹, second bar) and paracetamol (125 mg.kg⁻¹,
         third bar) with time. Number of erosion-foculi observed in
         vehicle treated rats 2 h after oral administration of
         5 ml.kg⁻¹ 4% Tween-80 solution (open bar). n = 10.
        *:Significant different from vehicle treated rats (P < 0.05).
        ✰:Not different from rats treated with plain aspirin (P >
         0.05). (From Seegers et al., 1979b, with permission).

output, nor does it interact with aspirin on either the aspirin-
induced reduction of acid output or the induction of erosion
foculi by aspirin. The two latter observations seem to confirm
each other mutually. But how does paracetamol inhibit the
development of erosion foculi in the presence of comparable
levels of hydrogen ions? Furthermore, why does this favourable
effect of paracetamol become apparent only after two hours?
Moreover, why does phenacetin, known to be metabolized mainly and
rapidly into paracetamol (16,27) not produce similar effects?

An explanation might be a physico-chemical interaction
between aspirin and paracetamol in the acidic milieu of the stomach:
an ester of paracetamol and aspirin, benorylate, was found not to
damage the gastric mucosa (24). Semi-quantitative densitometric
analysis after TLC of the stomach contents 2, 10 and 60 min after
oral administration to rats of aspirin and paracetamol, alone and
in admixture gave comparable data, which were not different from
those obtained by analysis of the solutions before administration.

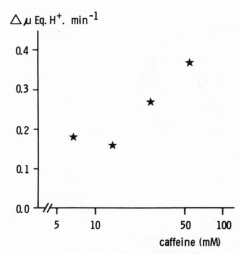

Fig. 5. Increase in acid output due to gastric perfusion with
caffeine. Anesthesized (Nembutal (R)) rats were perfused
with saline (1.1 ml.min^{-1} ; pH 7.0; 27° C); acid secretion
was stimulated submaximally with histamine (1.25 x 10^{-7}
mol.min^{-1}.kg^{-1}; iv);acid output before addition of
caffeine to the saline : 0.4 ± 0.06 µEq.H^{+}.min^{-1}.

In addition, the result of the analysis of the solution of the drug
mixture proved to be a summation of those of the single drug
solutions, thus, if there is a physico-chemical interaction in the
gastric lumen it is not detectable with the method used.

Another possibility might be that paracetamol only exerts its
erosion-decreasing activity after the drug has been absorbed and
reaches its site of action via the circulation. The results observed
with application of paracetamol at different times or via different
routes (Table 1) lead us to conclude that it can inhibit the
development of erosion foculi only when it is administered orally,
together with the aspirin. Furthermore, as the concentrations of
paracetamol in blood plasma one hour after oral administration of
phenacetin are comparable to the peak levels of paracetamol in
plasma after oral administration of equivalent amounts of
paracetamol the conclusion is warranted that neither uptake nor
target sites reached via the circulation are involved.

The lack of interaction between paracetamol and aspirin on
the induction of erosion foculi or on acid output makes it unlikely
that paracetamol affects absorption and accumulation of salicylate
in the gastric mucosa. To verify this suggestion the absorption of
paracetamol and aspirin administered orally, alone and in

TABLE 1

Effects of route and timing of the administration of paracetamol or phenacetin on their influence on aspirin-induced erosions in starved rats (n = 10).

Treatment Drugs	Dose mg.kg^{-1}	Route	Timing*	Erosion score after 17 h * (m ± SEM)
Aspirin	250	p o	-	26.6 ± 4.6[†]
Paracetamol	250	p o	-	0.5 ± 0.2
Phenacetin	250	p o	-	0.2 ± 0.2
Vehicle	-	p o	-	0.3 ± 0.1
Aspirin	250	p o		
+ paracetamol	125	p o	simult.	1.0 ± 0.5 [†]
+ phenacetin	125	p o	simult.	22.2 ± 3.9
+ vehicle	-	p o	simult.	22.2 ± 2.1
Aspirin	250	p o		
+ paracetamol	125	p o	1 h before	25.0 ± 2.7
+ phenacetin	147	p o	1 h before	22.0 ± 1.7
+ vehicle	-	p o	1 h before	27.3 ± 3.5
Aspirin	250	p o		
+ paracetamol	250	s c	simult.	15.5 ± 2.6
+ vehicle	-	s c	simult.	22.7 ± 1.6

Vehicle: 5 ml.kg^{-1} 4% Tween-80 solution
[†] : Different from the respective vehicle value (P < 0.05)
* : Time refers to the administration of aspirin.

admixture was studied (26). The results summarized in Fig. 6 confirmed the expectation that the accumulation of salicylate was
not affected by paracetamol. Surprisingly however, paracetamol
accumulated in the glandular part of the stomach, to an even
extent than salicylate. Moreover, aspirin stimulated this
accumulation and it increased the absorption of paracetamol in
the gastric mucosa, as shown for the glandular part of the
rat stomach in Fig. 7.

In summary the erosive activity of aspirin is not affected by paracetamol in experimental circumstances which supposingly lead to relatively
high levels of paracetamol in glandular mucosa before, during or
after oral administration of aspirin. Only when paracetamol is
administered orally an together with the aspirin 'healing' of
erosion foculi was observed and this coincided with the very high
levels of paracetamol in the glandular mucosa.

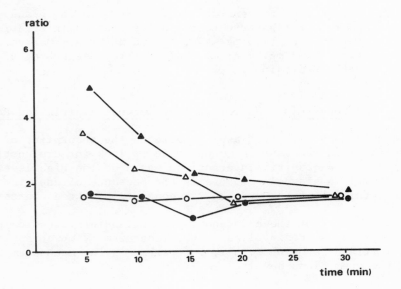

Fig. 6.   Mean ratios of glandular to ruminal tissue concentration
          of total salicylate (0,●) and paracetamol (Δ,▲) after oral
          administration to rats of aspirin (250 mg.kg^{-1}; 0),
          paracetamol (125 mg.kg^{-1}; Δ) and aspirin + paracetamol
          (250 + 125 mg.kg^{-1}; ●,▲). n = 8 (from Seegers et al.,
          1979b, with permission).

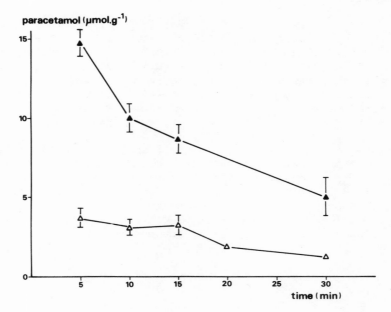

Fig. 7.   Paracetamol concentrations (m ± SEM) in the glandular
          part of rat gastric tissue after oral administration of
          paracetamol (125 mg.kg^{-1}; Δ) and aspirin + paracetamol
          (250 + 125 mg.kg^{-1}; ▲).   n = 8 (From Seegers et al. 1979b,
          with permission).

Hypothesis Concerning the Interaction between Aspirin and Paracetamol

        The observation that aspirin affects the absorption of
paracetamol in the gastric mucosa made us look for explanations of
the paracetamol-aspirin interactions based on the high levels of
paracetamol in glandular mucosa in the presence of aspirin.
The hypothesis put forward (24,25) consists of three contentions:

(i)   Inhibition of the endogenous prostaglandin production by
       aspirin is not involved in the mechanism by which aspirin
       initiates erosion foculi, but rather in the mechanism by which
       these erosions develop.

(ii)   Prostaglandins participate in the defensive responses of the
       stomach which are activated by the induction of erosion
       foculi.

(iii) An initial stimulation or a facilitation of the endogenous
       prostaglandin production by large amounts of paracetamol
       prevents the development of erosion foculi into erosions.

The first two contentions are largely based on the observations (7,9) that pretreatment with orally administrated small doses of irritants, including aspirin, which cause little gastric damage by themselves protected the gastric wall against larger doses of irritants. This protective effect of 'mild' irritants is mediated via endogenous prostaglandin production (Roberts, this conference). Thus, as the endogenous prostaglandin production in the presence of aspirin is activated by the erosion foculi, it seems unlikely that aspirin induces these foculi by inhibiting the prostaglandin production. Furthermore, parenteral administration of aspirin in general does not cause gastric damage., although it does decrease the endogenous prostaglandin production, as reflected in an enhanced sensitivity of the stomach to stress of oral administration of irritating agents. The protective activity of prostaglandins against gastric irritation is amply documented (18).

The third contention is based on the observation (17) that in vitro paracetamol stimulates the prostaglandin synthesis, presumable by acting as a cofactor. There are indications that paracetamol shares this property with other chemical related compounds, known for their reducing activity such as hydroquinone, glutathion and phenolic compounds (McDonald-Gibson, Collier, pers. comm.). In this context the observations of Kuehl et al. (9) are relevant. Phenolic compounds, similar to paracetamol, were found to facilitate the transformation of PGG_2 into PGH_2. As PGG_2 is supposingly a main mediator in the inflammatory response the anti-inflammatory effect of paracetamol could be due to a similar effect. Thus, inhibition of the PGG_2 formation by aspirin or stimulation of the transformation of PGG_2 by paracetamol could produce similar effects. This might apply for inflammation but it seems unlikely that PGG_2 is involved in the genesis of gastric damage by aspirin, because then also low levels of paracetamol (e.g. after pretreatment) should influence the erosive activity of aspirin. If, on the other hand PGG_2 and PGH_2 in the gastric wall are just 'normal' prostaglandins with cyto-protective properties not largely different from other prostanoids, then low levels of paracetamol should not influence the erosive activity of aspirin, as was observed. Moreover, the antagonistic interaction between aspirin and paracetamol on gastric damage might indicate that paracetamol influences the prostaglandin synthetase system in two ways: (i) A specific stimulation of the transformation of PGG_2 into PGH_2 and (ii) a 'non-specific' stimulation of the total enzym system. However, we are unaware of data which support or negate this.

In conclusion, it seems reasonable to assume that the high level of paracetamol in the glandular mucosa of the rat stomach after oral administration of paracetamol with aspirin at least protects the endogenous prostaglandin synthetase system against the

<u>TABLE 2</u>

Interaction between aspirin and paracetamol on inflammation* in rats

Treatment	Dose mg.kg^{-1}	Paw-diameter (m ± SEM) mm	Δ Paw-diameter (m ± SEM) mm
Aspirin	250	3.43 ± 0.06	+ 1.76 ± 0.16
Paracetamol	250	3.42 ± 0.04	+ 2.57 ± 0.29
Aspirin +paracetamol	250	3.40 ± 0.02	+ 0.92 ± 0.18
Vehicle	–	3.44 ± 0.02	+ 3.14 ± 0.18

*: Inflammation was induced by subplantar injection of 0.1 ml of a 1% carrageenan solution into the right hind-paw of each rat. Paw-diameter was measured immediately before and 4 h after this injection. Drugs were administered orally 1 h before the carrageenan injection.

Vehicle: 5 ml.kg^{-1} 4% Tween-80 solution. n = 8.

inhibition by aspirin and probably even stimulates this enzym system.

Other Interactions between Paracetamol and Aspirin

Having reached the conclusion that the interaction between aspirin and paracetamol on gastric mucosal damage is antagonistic, the question arises what kind of interaction between aspirin and paracetamol exists on 'therapeutic' effects. Therefore the anti-inflammatory, analgesic and anti-pyretic activity of aspirin and paracetamol alone and in combination were studied (22). The results, with regard to inflammation summarized in Table 2, suggest that the effects of the combination aspirin + paracetamol at least equal the sum of the effects of the drugs given alone. The additive interaction between aspirin and paracetamol seems to be in accord with the 'free-radical scavenger' theory as proposed by Kuehl et al. (9) and already mentioned in the previous paragraph. Furthermore, this observation and its interpretation stregthens the explanation proposed for the paracetamol-aspirin interaction in the stomach. Only when present in massive amounts stimulatory effects of paracetamol on the prostaglandin production _in vivo_ similar to those observed _in vitro_ are assumed.

ACKNOWLEDGEMENTS

The authors are indebted to Dr. A. A. van Kolfschoten for his kind permission to use the results obtained with subcutaneously injected paracetamol, presented in Table 1. We wish to thank Mrs. G. C. van den Bogaard and Mr. P. W. van Dorp van Vliet for their assistance in the presentation of this chapter.

This study forms part of project 101/76 of the National Institute of Public Health, the Board for the Evaluation of Medicines and the State University of Utrecht.

REFERENCES

1. A. Bennett and B. P. Curvain. Effects of aspirin-like drugs on canine gastric mucosal blood flow and acid secretion, _Br. J. Pharmacol._, 60: 499-504 (1977).
2. J. P. Bolton, D. Palmer and M. M. Cohen. Effect of the E_2 prostaglandins on gastric mucus production in rats, _Surg. Forum._, 27: 402-403 (1976).
3. R. Cano, J. J. Isenberg and M. J. Grossman. Cimet inhibits caffeine-stimulated gastric acid secretion in man, _Gastroenterology_, 70: 1055-1057 (1976).

4. T. E. Chvasta and A. R. Cooke. The effect of several ulcer-
    ogenic drugs on the canine gastric mucosal barrier, J. Lab.
    Clin. Med., 79: 302-315 (1972).
5. A. R. Cooke. The role of acid in the pathogenesis of aspirin-
    induced gastrointestinal erosions and hemorrhage, Am. J. Dig.,
    18: 225-237 (1973).
6. H. W. Davenport. Salicylate damage to the gastric mucosal
    barrier, N. Engl. J. Med., 276: 1307-1312 (1967).
7. L. J. Hayden, G. Thomas and G. B. West. Inhibitors of gastric
    lesions in the rat, J. Pharmacol., 30: 244-246 (1978).
8. K. I. Ivey and P. Settree. Effect of paracetamol (acetaminophen)
    on gastric ionic fluxes and potential difference in man, Gut,
    17: 916-919 (1976).
9. F. A. Kuehl, J. L. Humes, R. W. Egan, E. A. Ham, G. C.
    Beveridge and C. G. van Arman. Role of prostaglandin
    endoperoxide PG G_2 in inflammatory processes, Nature, 265: 170-
    172 (1977).
10. T. A. Miller and E. D. Jacobson. Gastrointestinal cytoproduction
    by prostaglandins, Gut, 20: 75-87 (1979).
11. E. Pernkopf. Beiträge zur vergleichenden Anatomie des Vertebra-
    tenmagens, Ztschr. Anat., 91: 329-390 (1930).
12. L. F. Prescott. Antipyretic analgesics, In: Meyler's Side
    Effects of Drugs, 8, M. N. G. Dukes, ed., Excerpta Medica,
    Amsterdam. pp.154-206 (1976).
13. L. F. Prescott. Ibid, Annual I, pp.64-85 (1977).
14. L. F. Prescott. Ibid, Annual II, pp.79-90 (1978).
15. L. F. Prescott. Ibid, Annual III, pp.78-89 (1979).
16. J. Raaflaub and U. C. Dubach. On the pharmacokinetics of
    phenatecin in man, Eur. J. Clin. Pharmacol., 8: 261-265 (1975).
17. J. Roback, A. Wieckowski and R. Gryglewski. The effect of 4-
    acetomidophenol (paracetamol) on prostaglandin synthetase
    activity in bovine and ram seminal vesicle microsomes,
    Biochem. Pharmacol., 27: 393-396 (1978).
18. A. Robert. Cytoprotection by prostaglandins, Gastroenterology,
    77 (1979).
19. A. Robert. Prostaglandins in gastrointestinal disease, In:
    Advances in Prostaglandin and Thromboxane Research, Vol. 6/7,
    Raven Press, New York, in press (1980).
20. A. Robert, J. E. Nezamis and J. P. Phillips. Inhibition of
    gastric secretion by prostaglandins, Am. J. Dig. Dis., 12:
    1073-1076 (1967).
21. A. Roberts, J. E. Nezamis, C. Lancaster and A. J. Hanchar.
    Cytoprotection by prostaglandins in rats, Gastroenterology,
    77: 433-443 (1979).
22. A. J. M. Seegers. Are non-narcotic analgesic drug mixtures
    rational? An evaluation of their pharmacological potency
    and gastric toxicity in rats. Thesis, State University
    Utrecht (1980).
23. A. J. M. Seegers, L. P. Jager and J. van Noordwijk. Gastric
    erosions induced by analgesic drug mixtures in the rat, J.
    Pharm. Pharmacol., 30: 84-87 (1978).

24. A. J. M. Seegers, L. P. Jager and J. van Noordwijk. Effects of phenatecin, paracetamol and caffeine on the erosive activity of acetyl-salicylic acid in the rat stomach: Dose-response relationships, time course of erosion development and effects on acid secretion, J. Pharm. Pharmacol., (in press) (1979a).

25. A. J. M. Seegers, L. P. Jager and J. van Noordwijk. An hypothesis concerning the protective action of paracetamol against erosions induced by acetylsalicylic acid in the rat stomach, In: Advances in Prostaglandin and Thromboxane Research, Vol. 6/7, Raven Press, New York, (in press) (1979b).

26. A. J. M. Seegers, M. Olling, L. P. Jager and J. van Noordwijk. Interactions of acetylsalicylic acid with acetaminophen and caffeine in the rat stomach: Pharmacokinetics of absorbtion and accumulation in gastric mucosa, (submitted) (1980).

27. G. E. Smith and L. A. Griffiths. Comparative metabolic studies of phenacetin and structurally-related compounds in the rat, Xenobiotica, 6: 217-236 (1976).

28. J. R. Vane. Inhibition of prostaglandin synthesis as a mechanism of aspirin-like drugs, Nature New Biol., 231: 232-235 (1971).

PROSTAGLANDINS IN RELATION TO CARCINOMAS IN MAN AND LABORATORY

ANIMALS

Alan Bennett

Department of Surgery
King's College Hospital Medical School
London, England

Various studies have shown that most tumours can produce
more prostaglandins (PGs) than the normal tissues in which they
arise (see Ref. 1). However, we still know little about which
types of PGs and related substances are formed,or about the effects
of many prostanoids and lipoxygenase products on tumour growth
and spread. Whereas the source of these substances is clear with
pure cell lines in culture, whole tumours contain numerous different
cell types which can form PGs. In the following account there are
brief discussions on PGs and cell growth, endocrine tumours,
breast cancer, malignant hypercalcaemia, unwanted effects of cancer
therapy, and beneficial effects of PG synthesis inhibitors in mice
with tumours.

PROSTAGLANDINS AND CELL GROWTH

Only a few prostaglandins have been studied on cell growth.
The effects of the different types vary, and whereas $PGF_{2\alpha}$ can
initiate cell proliferation in cultured mouse fibroblasts (2)
most studies with malignant or transformed cells in tissue culture
show an inhibition of proliferation by PGE_1 or PGE_2 (see Ref. 1).
Consistent with the PGE results is the finding that low concentrations of indomethacin (0.1-100nM) stimulated the growth of cultured
cells (3). However, a high concentration (0.1mM) inhibited cell
growth (4), so that the effect may depend on the extent to which
PG synthesis is reduced, or another action of the drug may be
involved. This is discussed more fully later.

In many types of cell, certain PGs can stimulate adenylate
cyclase, and the resulting cyclic AMP may influence proliferation.
This too is a confused area for many reasons, including the use of

high concentrations of agents, the indiscriminate use of cyclic
AMP analogues, the variation of adenylate cyclase activity and/or
the cyclic AMP content of tumours, and the importance of cell
calcium (5,6).

With adenocarcinomas removed from mice, the content of
arachidonic acid may be directly related to tumour growth (7).
Administration of PG synthesis inhibitors such as indomethacin or
flurbiprofen usually results in smaller tumours. However, this
reduction could be due to many factors apart from an effect on
tumour cell growth, such as a reduction in the numbers of inflammatory cells and exudate (8), and stimulation of the immune system
(9). Furthermore, the drugs inhibit the whole cascade of prostanoid
synthesis, and so increase the availability of precursors for
metabolism by lipoxygenase. It is therefore impossible to
attribute an effect to the reduced formation of any one prostanoid.
Nor can we exclude the possible importance of increased metabolism
of precursors by lipoxygenase, or actions of the drugs unrelated
to inhibition of PG synthesis.

Endocrine Tumours

Tumours of human endocrine glands are mentioned briefly
because they were the first to be examined with regard to PGs.
These tumours yield PG-like material (PG-lm) on extraction, but
whereas some authors reported that patients had raised blood
PG levels, other disagreed (see Ref. 1). A problem with the blood
measurements is that many PGs are substantially inactivated on
passage through the pulmonary circulation. Thus, it is probably
better to measure either the PG metabolites in peripheral blood
or the PGs in blood draining a tumour as an index of its ability
to release PGs.

Human Breast Cancer

Our interest in cancer arose from studies which indicate that
bone destruction by benign dental cysts may involve PGs (10).
We then wondered why certain cancers which spread to the skeleton
cause destruction of bone, and this started our investigation of
breast cancer.

We obtained samples of malignant and benign breast tumours
removed at surgery, and cut them into small pieces. After washing
with Krebs solution, one part was homogenized in acidified 50%
ethanol to indicate 'basal' amounts of PG-lm, and another part was
homogenized in Krebs solution to allow new synthesis of PGs from
endogenous precursors released during the tissue disruption (11).
The PG-lm was extracted (12) and then bioassayed using rat isolated
gastric fundus (11).

Extracts of homogenized human mammary carcinoma contained more

PG-1m than did those of benign tumours or normal breast tissue obtained from mastectomy specimens (13-15). Other workers later reported that incubated slices of breast carcinomas released substaintially more PGE- and PGF-like material than did normal tissue (16).

Our patients with malignant tumours were injected with ^{99}Tc-ethanehydroxydiphosphonate before or after surgery, and underwent skeletal scanning to assess the spread of tumour to bone. More patients whose tumours produced high amounts of PG-1m had bone metastases then did patients whose tumours produced low amounts (13-15). Since PGE and PGF compounds are substantially inactivated in the lungs and other tissues, we thought that the minute amounts of PGs remaining unmetabolised after release from the tumours would have little effect on the bone. It seemed more likely that malignant cells from the primary breast tumour which lodge in the bone might cause osteolysis by releasing PGs locally. This is consistent with studies in animals which demonstrate a relationship between PG synthesis and bone destruction by tumours (17-21).

Another factor aiding the growth of tumour in bone may be the calcium made available to the malignant cells by PG-induced osteoclast stimulation (6). Furthermore, certain PGs may act as calcium ionophores (22,23). It should be pointed out that in addition to PGs, human breast tumours can produce other bone-resorbing material which has not been identified but which may be osteoclast-activation factor (16).

Histological studies of tumours and resected lymph nodes indicated a tendency for the 'invasiveness' of the tumour to correlate with its PG-1m: malignant cells in the blood vessels, lymphatics or lymph nodes tended to occur more frequently in tumours which yielded most PG-1m on homogenisation (15). Perhaps PG-induced vasodilatation allows a greater escape of malignant cells from the tumour, so that more cells are available to form metastases.

It would be expected that the worse prognosis indicated by these PG findings would be reflected in a shorter survival time. This is indeed the case: death from cancer following breast surgery occurred most quickly in those patients whose tumours produced most PG-1m (24).

Hypercalcaemia

The relationship between PGs and hypercalcaemia is demonstrated by the findings that aspirin and indomethacin can prevent bone destruction by Walker tumour cells in rats (17), and that with tumours shown to produce PGE_2 indomethacin reduces their destruction of bone in vitro (19) and in vivo (18,20,21). Further-more, male hypercalcaemic patients with various solid tumours

excreted elevated amounts of PGE_2 metabolite in the urine, and in two
cases the raised excretion preceeded the appearance of hypercalcaemia
(25). Aspirin or indomethacin reduced both the excretion of
metabolite and the hypercalcaemia. In contrast, hypercalcaemia in
4 breast cancer patients did not respond to indomethacin (26). This
hypercalcaemia may have been due to other causes (e.g. bone
destruction by osteoclast activating factor, or direct bone
ressortion by tumour) or to other causes.

Unwanted Effects of Cancer Therapy

X-irradiation (27) or chemotherapeutic drugs (28) can increase
the amount of PGs extracted from tissues. Elevated PG synthesis
may therefore contribute to the side effects of treatment such as
the diarrhoea which can occur in patients receiving pelvic
irradiation for cervical cancer. This usually responds to aspirin,
and may therfore be due to PGs released in the incidentally-
irradiated intestine (29). In patients with head or neck cancer,
the severity of radiation-induced mucositis can delay treatment,
and it might be useful to give anti-inflammatory drugs prophy-
lactically. However, before this treatment is recommended, we
must await the results of our double-blind trial to assess the
effects of flurbiprofen on the inflammatory response and the
progression of malignant disease.

Beneficial Effects of Prostaglandin Synthesis Inhibitors in
Treating Animals with Tumours

The ability of indomethacin to inhibit destruction of bone
by tumours in rats and rabbits has already been discussed. Various
authors have shown that indomethacin reduces the growth of tumours
in mice (see Ref. 1). The meaning of this is not entirely clear
because the reduction in size might in some cases merely reflect a
smaller local inflammatory response (8). This cannot be the whole
explanation in the mouse experiments where indomethacin completely
suppressed tumour growth (8) or caused complete regression of
established tumours (30), or where hydrocortisone did not
significantly reduce tumour size (30). However, PGs can inhibit
the immune response (9) and indomethacin may act by restoring the
host's immune protection. Lynch et al (30), thought this
explanation unlikely with their murine tumours because they did
not detect tumour immunogenicity. In our experiments (31) the PG
synthesis inhibitor flurbiprofen reduced the growth of the murine
NC tumour which was thought (32) to be non-immunogenic. This may
no longer be entirely true, since lymphocytic infiltration of
tumours tended to increase when the mice were treated with
flurbiprofen (33).

We also showed that in mice with established tumours treated
with radiotherapy $\pm$ chemotherapy, administration of flurbiprofen
resulted in substantially smaller tumours (31). It seems likely

that flurbiprofen reduced the inflammation caused by the other
treatments, and the drug may have altered other factors such as an
immune response. Nevertheless, some of the effects of flurbiprofen
on tumour growth and the response to treatment may have been due to
an action on tumour cells. A high concentration (0.1mM) of
indomethacin, aspirin or sodium salicylate, which is nevertheless
within the range of blood concentrations obtained with therapeutic
doses of the salicylates, inhibited both the proliferation of rat
hepatoma and human fibroblasts in culture, and the synthesis of
protein and nucleic acid (4). Since the doses are higher than those
needed to inhibit PG synthesis in vivo, and salicylate has little
effect on PG synthesis in vitro, at least part of the reduction of
growth might not involve PGs. Non-steroidal anti-inflammatory
drugs also affect calcium transport (34) which may be important for
tumour growth (6). The ability of added PGE_2 to overcome the
effect of indomethacin (3,30) is not firm proof that indomethacin
acts by inhibiting PG synthesis: perhaps indomethacin inhibits
calcium transport and PGE_2 reverses this by acting as a calcium
ionophore.

The ability of non-steroidal anti-inflammatory drugs to
inhibit metastasis is potentially of great importance. In mice,
the development of soft tissue metastases can be reduced with
aspirin (35) and flurbiprofen reduced local recurrence after
tumour excision (36). The mechanism for this is not clear (1) but
one possibility not yet studied is that these drugs affect
vascularisation of the tumour. As in so many cases there are
species differences, and no significant effect was observed on
metastic spread in rats (17) or rabbits (20). The effect of such
drugs in man must await the clinical trials that are now in
progress. However, one piece of evidence consistent with their
safety is the use of corticosteroids in cancer therapy, and the
beneficial effect of tamoxifen; both these drugs inhibit PG
synthesis (37,38).

Perhaps our mouse experiments of greatest interest are
those designed to mimic the clinical situation by starting treatment with chemotherapy (methotrexate + melphalan) and flurbiprofen
just prior to tumour excision. The combined treatment increased
the survival time (36) and this did not seem to be due to an
increased bioavailability of the chemotherapeutic drugs. Thus
flurbiprofen neither displaced methotrexate from plasma binding
sites, nor increased the toxicity of large doses of chemotherapeutic
drugs given to mice without tumours (unpublished). Apart from the
various possible explanations discussed previously regarding
flurbiprofen and tumour growth, another idea for consideration is
'cytoprotection' by PGs. In the rat, PGs protect the stomach
from damage caused by various stimuli (39); perhaps flurbiprofen
removes a similar 'cytoprotective' effect of PGs on tumour cells,
and so increases their susceptibility to damage.

The possible contributions of PGs to the side effects of treatment, and the improved response when non-steroidal inhibitors of PG synthesis are used as adjunctive therapy in mice, suggests that similar drug combinations should be tried in cancer patients. However, non-steroidal anti-inflammatory drugs can cause gastric mucosal damage, and the question arises whether it is safe to give them with chemotherapeutic drugs. Chemotherapy is thought to cause most damage in rapidly dividing tissues, and gastrointestinal mucosa has a high turnover rate. Thus there is a theoretical possibility of increased damage when both types of drug are given together. Contrary to expectation, we found that treatment of rats with melphalan and methotrexate reduced the gastric mucosal damage caused by orally administered aspirin. The cytotoxic drugs appeared to increase mucus secretion and to stimulate gastric PG synthesis which may have exerted the 'cytoprotective' effect discussed previously (unpublished). It may follow that as far as human gastric mucosa is concerned, cytotoxic agents and inhibitors of PG synthesis are safe to give simultaneously by mouth. If the effects obtained in patients by combined treatments are similar to those obtained in mice, the adjunctive use of non-steroidal anti-inflammatory drugs could dramatically improve the therapy of malignant disease.

REFERENCES

1. A. Bennett. Prostaglandins and cancer. In: Practical Applications of Prostaglandins and Their Synthesis Inhibitors. S. M. M. Karim, ed., M.T.P. Press, Lancaster, pp. 149-188 (1979).
2. L. J. De Asua, D. Clingan and P. S. Rudland. Initiation of cell proliferation in cultured mouse fibroblasts by prostaglandin $F_{2\alpha}$. Proc. Nat. Acad. Sci., 72: 2724-2728 (1975).
3. D. R. Thomas, G. W. Philpott and B. M. Jaffe. Prostaglandin E control of cell replication in vitro. J. Surg. Res., 16: 463-465 (1974).
4. V. Hial, M. C. F. de Mello, Z. Horakova and M. A. Beavan. Antiproliferative activity of anti-inflammatory drugs in two mammalian cell culture lines. J. Pharm. Exp. Ther., 202: 446-454 (1977).
5. J. P. MacManus and J. F. Whitfield. Cyclic AMP, prostaglandins and the control of cell proliferation. Prostaglandins, 6: 475-487 (1974).
6. J. F. Whitfield, R. H. Rixon, J. P. MacManus and S. D. Balk. Calcium, cycli adenosine 3', 5'-monophosphate, and the control of cell proliferation: a review. In itro, 8: 257-278 (1973).
7. S. Abraham and G. A. Rao. Lipids and lipogenesis in a murine mammary neoplastic system. In: Control Mechanisms in Cancer. W. E.Criss, ed., Raven Press, New York, pp.363-378 (1976).

8. H. Strausser and J. Humes. Prostaglandin synthesis inhibition: effect on bone changes and sarcoma tumour induction in BALB/c mice. Int. J. Cancer, 15: 724-730 (1975).

9. O. J. Plescia, A. H. Smith and K. Grinwich. Subversion of immune system by tumour cells and role of prostaglandins. Proc. Nat. Acad. Sci., 72: 1848-1851 (1975).

10. M. Harris, M. V. Jenkins, A. Bennett and M. R. Wills. Prostaglandin production and bone resorption by dental cysts. Nature, 245: 213-215 (1973).

11. A. Bennett, I. F. Stamford and W. G. Unger. Prostaglandin E_2 and gastric acid secretion in man. J. Physiol., 229: 349-360 (1973).

12. W. G. Unger, I. F. Stamford and A. Bennett. Extraction of prostaglandins from human blood. Nature, 233: 336-337 (1971).

13. A. Bennett, A. M. McDonald, J. S. S mpson and I. F. Stamford. Breast cancer, prostaglandins and bone metastases. Lancet, 1: 1218-1220 (1975).

14. A. Bennett, E. M. Charlier,A. M. McDonald, J. S. Simpson and I. F. Stamford. Bone destruction by breast tumours. Prostaglandins, 11: 461-463 (1976).

15. A. Bennett, E. M. Charlier, A. M. McDonald, J. S. Simpson, I. F. Stamford and T. Zebro. Prostaglandins and breast cancer. Lancet, 2: 624-626 (1977).

16. M. Dowsett, G. C. Easty, T. J. Powles, D. M. Easty and A. M. Neville. $_n=49$ n breast tumour-induced osteolysis and prostaglandins. Prostaglandins, 11: 447-455 (1976).

17. T. J. Powles, S. A. Clark, D. M. Easty, G. C. Easty and A. M. Neville. The inhibition by aspirin and indomethacin of osteolytic tumour deposits and hypercalcaemia in rats with Walker tumour, and its possible application to breast cancer. Br. J. Cancer, 28: 316-321 (1973).

18. A. H. Tashjian, E. F. Voelkel, P. Goldhaber and L. Levine. Successful treatment of hypercalcemia by indomethacin in mice bearing a prostaglandin-producing tumour. Prostaglandins, 3: 515-524 (1973).

19. E. F. Voelkel, A. H. Tashjian, R. Franklin, E. Wasserman and L. Levine. Hypercalcemia and prostaglandins: The VX_2 carcinoma model in the rabbit. Metabolism, 24: 973-986 (1975).

20. C. S. B. Galasko and A. Bennett. Relationship of bone destruction in skeletal metastases to osteoclast activation and prostaglandins. Nature, 263: 508-510 (1976).

21. C. S. B. Galasko, R. Rawlins and A. Bennett. Timing of indomethacin in the control of prostaglandins, osteoclasts and bone destruction produced by VX_2 carcinoma in rabbits. Br. J. Cancer, 40: 360-364 (1979).

22. S. J. Kirtland and H. Baum. Prostaglandin E_1 may act as a calcium ionophore. Nature New Biol., 236: 47-49 (1972).

23. P. W. Reed. Calcium ionophore activity of prostaglandin endoperoxides and stabilized analogs of PGH_2. Fed. Proc., 36:673 (1977).

24. A. Bennett, D. A. Berstock, B. Raja and I. F. Stamford.
     Survival time after surgery is inversely related to the amounts
     of prostaglandins extracted from human breast cancers.
     Br. J. Pharmac., 66: 451P (1979).

25. H. W. Seyberth, G. V. Segre, J. L. Morgan, B. J. Sweetman,
     J. T. Potts and J. A. Oates. Prostaglandins as mediators of
     hypercalcemia associated with certain types of cancer.
     N. Engl. J. Med., 293: 1278-1283 (1975).

26. R. C. Coombes, A. M. Neville, P. K. Bondy and T. J. Powles.
     Failure of indomethacin to reduce hydroxyproline excretion or
     hypercalcemia in patients with breast cancer. Prostaglandins,
     12: 1027-1035 (1976).

27. V. Eisen and D. I. Walker. Effect of ionising radiation on
     prostaglandin-like activity in tissues. Br. J. Pharmac.,
     57: 527-532 (1976).

28. L. Levine. Chemical carcinogens stimulate canine kidney
     (MDCK) cells to produce prostaglandins. Nature, 268: 447-448
     (1977).

29. A. T. Mennie, V. Dalley, L. C. Dinneen and H. O. J. Collier.
     Treatment of radiation-induced gastrointestinal distress with
     acetylsalicylate. Lancet, 2: 942-943 (1975).

30. N. R. Lynch, M. Castes, M. Astoin and J. C. Salomon.
     Mechanism of inhibition of tumour growth by aspirin and
     indomethacin. Br. J. Cancer, 38: 503-512 (1978).

31. A. Bennett, J. Houghton, D. J. Leaper and I. F. Stamford.
     Cancer growth, response to treatment and survival time in mice:
     beneficial effect of the prostaglandin synthesis inhibitor
     flurbiprofen. Prostaglandins, 17: 179-191 (1979).

32. H. B. Hewitt, E. R. Blake and A. S. Walder. A critique of
     the evidence for active host defence against cancer, based on
     personal studies of 27 murine tumours of spontaneous origin.
     Br. J. Cancer, 33: 241-259 (1976).

33. D. J. Leaper, B. French and A. Bennett. Breast cancer and
     prostaglandins. A new approach to treatment. Br. J. Surg.,
     66: 683-686 (1979).

34. B. J. Northover. Effect of anti-inflammatory drugs on the
     binding of calcium to cellular membranes in various human
     and guinea-pig tissues. Br. J. Pharmac., 48: 496-504 (1973).

35. G. J. Gasic, T. B. Gasic, N. Galanti, T. Johnson and S.
     Murphy. Platelet-tumour-cell interactions in mice. The role
     of platelets in the spread of malignant disease. Int. J.
     Cancer, 11: 704-718 (1973).

36. D. A. Berstock, J. Houghton and A. Bennett. Improved anti-
     cancer effect by combining cytotoxic drugs with an inhibitor
     or prostaglandin synthesis. Cancer Treatment Reviews, 6:
     (Suppl), 69-71 (1979).

37. R. J. Gryglewski, B. Panczenko, R. Korbut, L. Grodzinska and
     A. Ocetkiewicz. Corticosteroids inhibit prostaglandin release
     from perfused mesenteric blood vessels of rabbit and from
     perfused lungs of sensitised guinea-pig. Prostaglandins, 10:
     343-355 (1975).

38. G. Ritchie. The direct inhibition of prostaglandin synthetase of human breast cancer tissue by 'Novaldex'. Reviews on Endocrine-Related Cancer (Suppl Oct. 1978), 35-39 (1978).

39. A. Robert. Effect of prostaglandins on gastro-intestinal functions. In: Prostaglandins and Thromboxanes. F. Berti, B. Samuelsson and G. P. Velo, eds., Plenum Press, New York, pp.287-313 (1977).

Index